"The biggest threat to _____ ____ _____ solvency, is the mismatch between the _____ etent science of medicine and the amaz_____ .ent pricing and allocation of it. Now come Silver and Hyman to frighten us with the facts, and to point to ways the biggest player in the health care game—the government—can stop making matters worse."

—George F. Will, Pulitzer Prize-winning columnist and author

"As CEO of Whole Foods, which spent more than $250 million on health care for our team members last year, I thought I knew how inefficient health care was. *Overcharged* opened my eyes to how truly dysfunctional America's health care system has become. This is not capitalism. Capitalism forces me to spend every day trying to provide greater value at a lower price. Silver and Hyman show that health care does not work that way—not because health care is special, but because Americans have let government and insurers control our health care dollars, and more of the same will only make things worse. Change will come, but only when consumers control their health care dollars and begin exerting massive pressure from below."

—John Mackey, CEO, Whole Foods Market

"This blood-boiling book will have you ready to root for serious change in our medical system where the patient—not third parties—is in charge."

—Steve Forbes, chairman and editor-in-chief, Forbes Media

"*Overcharged* is a compelling answer to the feeling of helplessness in health care. Charlie Silver and David Hyman take on medicine's problems and find a solution: the voice of consumers, empowered and in charge."

—David Cutler, Otto Eckstein Professor of Applied Economics, Department of Economics, Harvard University

"*Overcharged* uncovers all the flaws of the American health care system, from monopolistic drug-company pricing to the self-serving actions of physician specialty organizations to the pernicious impact of a broken fee-for-service system. Anyone who believes the medical care we provide in the United States is the best in the world will be shocked to learn the truth."

—Robert Pearl, MD, author of *Mistreated: Why We Think We're Getting Good Health Care and Why We're Usually Wrong*

"*Overcharged* presents a provocative point of view and thoughtful analysis on how to control surging U.S. health care costs without resorting to ideological clichés and simplistic thinking, all in a fun-to-read style."

—Michael L. Millenson, author of *Demanding Medical Excellence: Doctors and Accountability in the Information Age*

"Charles Silver and David Hyman's elegant book, *Overcharged*, reveals a stark truth that every informed citizen needs to know: our health system is broken. Their book is uniquely valuable, a tour de force of the root causes behind health system malfunction. *Overcharged* is powerful and beautifully written, filled with vivid examples of how, and why, Americans are short-changed. It will transform the way scholars and the public understand health insurance. Whatever your political persuasion, we need to all start with the core reality that Americans are ill-served by our health system."

—Lawrence O. Gostin, professor and founding O'Neill Chair in Global Health Law, Georgetown University Law Center

"Conventional wisdom says there are two things wrong with American health care: it is inefficient, ineffective, corrupt, often harmful, and overpriced—and not everyone has equal access to it. Obamacare targeted only the second criticism. *Overcharged* takes direct and accurate aim at the first. It shows [that] the cause of those failings is the insurance designs government creates or influences in both the public and private sectors— that the 'cost-unconsciousness' those designs promote also give[s] rise to 'quality neglect'—and that solving these problems requires putting individual patient-consumers back in the driver's seat with the incentives and information to make a difference, which requires reducing excessive government control. This point of view has never before been presented so persuasively and perceptively. *Overcharged* deserves serious attention."

—Mark V. Pauly, Bendheim Professor, Department of Health Care Management, Wharton School, University of Pennsylvania

"*Overcharged* shows [that] the outrageous prices and anti-competitive practices in U.S. health care are not the consequence of free markets, but of big government."

—Eamonn Butler, director, Adam Smith Institute

"The sheer complexity of health care can lead otherwise sensible people to abandon their confidence in basic economics. In this comprehensive yet impressively accessible book, Charles Silver and David Hyman call us back to basics and demonstrate that only genuine consumer pressure acting from below to demand value can fix American health care."

—Yuval Levin, editor of *National Affairs*

"Whether you are right, left, or center you'll find something in this book to make you happy, something to make you angry, and (because the writing is so good) something to make you laugh—ruefully. And whoever you are, there is a lot to learn from this book and its clear analysis of the mess that is our health care system. Different people will have different views of the authors' proposals, but no one will come away without new insight."

—Timothy M. Westmoreland, visiting professor of law, Georgetown University

"Americans lead the world in health care spending, and we are less healthy than others in comparably wealthy countries who spend much less. *Overcharged* shines light on every corner of the system, employing insights from the latest research to illuminate the numerous reasons behind our excessive spending. The book offers a number of proposals radically different from our latest attempts to bend the cost curve. Silver and Hyman provide a road map for the major overhaul our health care system desperately needs."

—Kathryn Zeiler, professor of law, Boston University

"Apologists dismiss each heartrending failure of the National Health Service as what you get from trying to do socialized medicine on the cheap. *Overcharged* reminds us that profligate socialism is no better."

—Daniel Hannan, member of the European Parliament

"Silver and Hyman powerfully demonstrate how the misguided incentives in our system—especially those generated by the party payment—push up the price of everything in health care and even distort the nature of care itself. Their examination of the unintended consequences of government efforts to control costs is a strong rejoinder to those hoping for the magic bullet solution of a single-payer system."

—David Goldhill, author of *Catastrophic Care*

"Read this insightful and witty book! If you're concerned about equitable access to medical care, you may be outraged—but you'll learn about profound failures of our health care system that you weren't aware of. And you'll be better prepared to offer compassionate solutions to our system's crises of cost and value."

—Gregg Bloche, professor of law, Georgetown University

"This fantastic book looks at the major faults of the supposedly free-market U.S. system. Clearly written and fun to read, it is essential reading for everybody in the business. There is no good universal solution, but

understanding the problems can help to make things better. This is a landmark publication of tremendous significance. What a great book!"
—Dr. Karol Sikora, dean,
University of Buckingham Medical School

"Wow! The stories in this book are so unbelievable, you will wish that they had been made up. Buy a copy and read it now—to find out all the ways in which things have gone wrong with the American health care system. It's just unreal."
—Luke M. Froeb, William C. Oehmig Chair of Free Enterprise and Entrepreneurship, Owen Graduate School of Management, Vanderbilt University

"In Europe and the United Kingdom, the U.S. health care system is often held out as an example of market mechanisms gone mad. We are asked to believe that insufficient state intervention is responsible for wealthy Americans receiving highly expensive, substandard treatment and for poorer Americans receiving no meaningful access to health care at all. *Overcharged* demolishes this myth. The unpalatable, social Darwinist tendencies of U.S. health care are frequently a direct consequence of government intervention, however well-intentioned. In contrast, where the market is able to thrive—for example, in competition in retail medicines—we see deprivation swiftly eliminated and universal access guaranteed. The case and analysis put forward in *Overcharged* have the power to change the health care debate on both sides of the Atlantic. It is a really important and illuminating contribution to the debate."
—Mark Littlewood, director general,
Institute of Economic Affairs

"A devastating description of the U.S. health care system and its pathologies. Anyone reading it would be stupid not to do their best to stay healthy."
—Ronen Avraham, professor of law,
Tel Aviv University

# OVERCHARGED

# OVERCHARGED

*Why Americans Pay Too Much for Health Care*

CHARLES SILVER

DAVID A. HYMAN

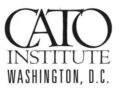

CATO INSTITUTE
WASHINGTON, D.C.

Paperback ISBN 978-1-944424-76-3
eISBN 978-1-944424-77-0

Library of Congress Cataloging-in-Publication Data available.

Jacket design: Jon Meyers.
Printed in the United States of America.

CATO INSTITUTE
1000 Massachusetts Ave., N.W.
Washington, D.C. 20001
www.cato.org

Library of Congress Cataloging-in-Publication Data

Silver, Charles, 1957-, Hyman, David A.
Overcharged : why Americans pay too much for health care / Charles
Silver, David A. Hyman.
page cm
Washington : Cato Institute, 2018.
Includes bibliographical references.
ISBN 9781944424770 (ebook) | ISBN 9781944424763 (pbk. : alk. paper)
1. Health Expenditures.        2. Health Care Costs.        3. Insurance,
4. Health—economics.      5. Health Care Reform—economics.      6. Economic Competition

HG9383
368.38/2          2018010551

*For Cindy, Katie, and Mabon, and Karen, Nathan, Benjamin, Rachel, and Eli*

# CONTENTS

Congress is just not capable of being the manager of a health care system and yet it's largely Congress today that has that responsibility. It hasn't worked for the last 50 years. It'll work even less in the next 50.

—Former U.S. Senator Thomas Daschle (D)[1]


We are putting people in a position where, when they are buying health care, it is like going to the grocery store and having a grocery insurance policy, where 95 percent of what you put in your grocery basket is going to be paid for by grocery insurance. Needless to say, if you had such a policy, you would eat differently, and so would your dog.

—Former U.S. Senator Phil Gramm (R)[2]


So you've got this crazy system where all of a sudden, 25 million more people have health care and then the people that are out there busting it, sometimes 60 hours a week, wind up with their premiums doubled and their coverage cut in half. It's the craziest thing in the world.

—Former President Bill Clinton (D) on Obamacare[3]

# PREFACE

The problems with America's health care system are many and varied. That's why there is no general guide to all of them. Instead, there are thousands of books and articles about specific difficulties, such as the mistreatment of prostate cancer in men, the politics of health care reform, outrageous hospital charges, or fraud in the prescription drug business.

Although many of these writings are excellent, they fail to convey a sense of the whole. An intelligent person wants to know, at the most general level, why our health care system is so dysfunctional. What are the root causes of spiraling costs, mediocre quality, and limited access? Why is more than $1 trillion—one out of every three dollars that passes through the system—lost to fraud, wasted on services that don't help patients, or otherwise misspent? Why do hospitalized patients receive bills that are laden with inflated charges, that come out of the blue from out-of-network providers, or that demand payment for services that weren't delivered? Why does the EpiPen, an old technology that contains $1 worth of medicine, cost $600? Do questions like these require separate answers? Or are the answers connected? Are there core drivers of the health care system's many pathologies?

We believe that an array of the American health care system's most important shortcomings stem from a few root causes. We also think that it is important to lay these fundamental drivers bare for everyone to see.

That is what we do in this book. We describe a range of different problems with the health care system, identify the structures that generate them and connect them, and show how they can all be addressed by means of reforms that reduce political control of the health care sector and that replace third-party payment for medical services with direct purchasing.

The need to think deeply and clearly about root causes could hardly be greater. As we write this, Republicans have been trying (so far with limited success) to repeal Obamacare. But they haven't figured out how to make the health care system better. Democrats are playing defense, but even they agree that Obamacare is in trouble and needs to be fixed.

Unfortunately, neither Republicans nor Democrats have the faintest intention of implementing policies with any real potential to make the health care system measurably better. Democrats see Obamacare as a solution, but all it really offered was more of everything that gave us the dysfunctional health care system we had before: more insurance, more Medicaid, more tax exemptions and subsidies, and more political control. Plowing tens of millions of new people and hundreds of billions of new dollars into a dysfunctional system was a recipe for disaster, as was giving even more control of that system to politicians. Republicans see Obamacare as the problem, but the health care system was riddled with pathologies long before Obamacare came along. Republicans haven't even focused on the problems that need fixing, much less offered serious proposals to address them.

To make health care better and cheaper for all Americans, we must change the way we pay for medical services. That is what this book explains. Our system costs too much and delivers too little because we pay for health care the wrong way. Instead of routing dollars through insurers, public payers like Medicare and Medicaid, and politicians, consumers must control the money. They must choose the health insurance plans and medical services they use and pay for them directly, the same way they choose and pay for goods and services of other types. If and when consumers take charge, the American health care system will quickly improve. Until then, it will not.

The prospect that Congress might reform the payment system will scare many people, as the possibility that it might repeal Obamacare already has. But if there is any lesson to be learned from the fight over

Obamacare, it is that Congress is unlikely to implement the changes we envision. Our proposals would subject medical providers to great pressure to deliver more while charging less. Health care providers want to operate without such pressure, so the lobbyists who represent them in Washington would do their best to kill our proposals long before they reached the floor of the House or the Senate.

Fortunately, even if our elected representatives leave private insurance, Medicare, and Medicaid as they are, pressure for improvement will build from below. It will come from people who are tired of being overcharged and underserved, and who decide to do something about it by taking their business to providers who are better and cheaper. In other words, pressure to improve will come from consumers who buy medical treatments directly.

There are millions of these people already, including those who bought high-deductible Obamacare policies, and those who obtained high-deductible policies through their employers. They are driving the expansion of the retail health care sector, which makes cheap and convenient services available to anyone who walks through the door. And, as time goes by, the uninsured population will grow because both private insurance and public programs are bound to shrink. Comprehensive insurance will become ever more expensive, so fewer healthy people will buy it, particularly now that the modest tax penalties Obamacare once imposed on the uninsured are gone. As the declining ratio of tax-paying workers to tax-consuming seniors wreaks havoc with Medicare's finances, Congress will have to cut back on benefits, increase seniors' deductibles and copayments, and raise the eligibility age, lest the deficit explode. Rising costs will pressure states to put clamps on Medicaid too, meaning that a greater traction of the rising cost of health care will be shouldered by the poor and near poor.

Like it or not, the country seems bound to have many more people who are financially responsible for their own health care. With a little luck, their purchasing decisions will force health care providers to improve without any help from Congress.

We wrote this book to communicate the underappreciated-but-hopeful message that health care will get better and cheaper as consumers exert pressure from below. Of course, there will be plenty of turmoil along the way. Health care providers will use every means at their disposal to ensure that tax money and insurance dollars continue to flow into their coffers. Medicare and Medicaid recipients will experience uncertainty and deprivation as their benefits are frozen or curtailed. Congress will feel great pressure to make insurance more affordable by dispensing subsidies and exempting all amounts spent on health care from taxation. But we are confident that pressure from an army of buyers who have to pay for medical treatments themselves will increasingly bring ordinary market forces to bear on American health care providers, to good effect.

It was a challenge to write this book. The enormity of the health care system made it a daunting project just to learn about the major pathologies. Every day brought new stories about health care fraud, surprise medical bills, prescription drug prices, doctors fighting turf wars against other medical professionals, and the politics of replacing Obamacare. Finishing the project meant making hard choices about what to put in and what to leave out. Every chapter is likely to cause some readers to wonder why we left out a favorite example or ignored a cherished topic. In the chapter on health care fraud, for example, we eventually decided to ignore anything new that didn't involve at least $500 million in ill-gotten gains. Even then, we had more material than we could use.

Academic research on health care, of which there is an enormous amount, presented other challenges. In a book of this type, which is intended to provide a coherent, high-level account of the entire health care system for a general audience of intelligent readers, we can discuss only general themes and the leading works that develop them. And we cannot go into even those works in much detail. We therefore strove to set out the basic insights and most important findings, and to do not much more than that. Readers who want to read the literature in greater depth are welcome to begin their journey by using the many citations we provide.

## ACKNOWLEDGMENTS

We received help with this book from many sources. First and foremost, we would like to thank Matthew Spitzer, of the Pritzker School of Law at Northwestern University and the Searle Center on Law, Regulation, and Economic Growth, for sponsoring a conference on our first draft of this manuscript. We are also grateful to Derek Gundersen for handling the conference arrangements, and to the individuals who participated in the program and provided helpful comments and advice: Bernie Black, Michael F. Cannon, John R. Graham, David Johnson, Ram Krishnamoorthi, David Meltzer, Michael Millenson, Jean Mitchell, Harold Pollack, Rita Redberg, Greg Ruhnke, and Kathy Zeiler.

Our editors at the Cato Institute—Robert Garber, Jason Kuznicki, Eleanor O'Connor, Peter Van Doren, and especially Michael Cannon—who reviewed the draft manuscript helped us enormously too. They provided extensive comments on every chapter that challenged us to deepen our analyses, sharpen our focus, clean up the language, and consider new ideas. We are grateful for their help, and we're happy to say that the book is much better because of them.

Michael Cannon also gave us the opportunity to present some of our ideas at a conference of state libertarian think tanks sponsored by the Texas Public Policy Foundation. We are grateful for the many helpful comments we received from the policy analysts who attended that program.

Brigitte Silver, then a young attorney fresh out of the University of Virginia Law School, was in on the ground floor of this book, which initially focused on health care fraud. Fortunately, the study of that dismal subject did not render her as cynical as it has us. We thank her for her efforts and hope she retains her optimism for many years to come.

Over several years, we have presented draft chapters of the book to students in seminars on health law and policy, some of whom went on to develop the ideas those drafts contained in greater detail than we had. We benefited from their thoughts and their work. We also published ideas from the book as short columns on The Health Care Blog. We wish to thank John Irvine and Jonathan Halvorson for giving us that opportunity. We placed op-eds in other publications as well and thank Chris Roberts, who handles public relations at the University of Texas School of Law, for editing them and finding homes for them.

We are, of course, also grateful to the Georgetown Law Center, the University of Illinois College of Law, and the School of Law at the University of Texas at Austin for supporting our research over many years. The University of Texas School of Law in particular helped us by supporting our research assistants—Tim Elliott, Kevin Stewart, and Bryan Zubay—all of whom did terrific work. We cannot thank them enough. The Cato Institute provided research assistance too. Tom Capone and Michael Schemenaur helped us get the citations right, caught several math mistakes, and suggested important textual improvements.

Last, our wives, children, relatives, friends, and colleagues helped us develop our thinking too. The health care system touches everyone, and everyone has thoughts on how well it works and how it might be improved. Because health care was an enormous issue in the 2016 election, we often seemed to be involved in conversations about the subject nonstop. Whenever we mentioned that we were writing a book on the health care payment system, people would ask about our views and want to know how we would fix things. They'd often disagree, but they also supported our efforts to think hard about problems, often by sending us media reports of new developments or studies of which we were unaware. We're grateful for their encouragement, assistance, and patience.

# FOREWORD

Good health ranks very high among the things that most people value. And yet in America, a wealthy country recognized for its capacity to innovate and to fulfill consumer demands with creativity and efficiency, health care has seriously lagged in achieving these important goals. The cardinal symptoms of this failure are rarely contested. Despite spending more on health care than any other country, problems of access, cost, and quality abound. These failings have dominated public attention for extended periods yet have defied recurrent efforts at reform. Understanding these failures should be a major goal of social scientists, economists, health care providers, and funders, as well as an increasingly concerned populace.

Remarkably, reformers seem to inhabit two independent analytical universes. The great majority, including analysts and activists from across the political spectrum, start their quests with current symptomatology. Symptoms in hand, they compete to design and promote political solutions that ignore or pay insufficient attention to root causes. They propose legislative remedies they claim will address one or more symptoms, with insufficient access to insurance being the most urgent. These efforts, backed by a supporting cast of pundits, academics, and especially special interests, manage to maintain key elements of the status quo and their root causes while ignoring or resisting paths to more fundamental reform. The Affordable Care Act, potential versions of "single payer" health care, and most Republican proposals are examples of this approach, each failing in different ways.

The book in your hands emerges from an alternative but far more rational universe. Inhabitants of this universe insist on identifying root causes, the two most central of which are the intrusion of the political process into health care spending decisions and the resulting overreliance on insurance and other forms of third-party payment. Ironically, these root causes are what mainstream health analysts propose as solutions. In Charlie Silver and David Hyman's view, the incentives that result from these fundamental errors render health care transactions financially opaque, often absurdly so. These incentives enable and encourage health care providers—for whom opacity is a boon—to mistreat patients and to overcharge consumers and taxpayers. Together, incumbent providers and their political allies promote an increasingly tenuous fantasy that the dysfunctional status quo is both sustainable and capable of meaningful repair with only minor tweaks. Silver and Hyman lay bare the serious flaws in such thinking.

Astute diagnoses in hand, Silver and Hyman sketch potential remedies with an approach distinct from those that emerge from the other health care universe. For one, they are far too honest to offer a comprehensive legislative proposal that claims to be both politically achievable and capable of producing the necessary disruptive innovations.

But that honesty doesn't imply that their analysis and proposals are for naught. Quite the contrary: their insights are critical for those seeking a path to true reform, whether one fully agrees with their approach or simply learns from it. For those interested in new paths government might take, as opposed to the current approaches of Medicare and Medicaid, Silver and Hyman identify Singapore as a model worthy of attention. That approach uses mandatory and tax-advantaged personal health savings accounts, to which the government could add funds when necessary. Patients have control over how these dollars are spent, and funds become part of a person's estate if unspent. Moving in this direction would transform the incentives that send health care prices and quality in the wrong directions, and limit the self-serving dance between health care providers and politicians.

Silver and Hyman also identify many promising innovations that markets have developed in spite of those perverse incentives. Rather than

emerging from the minds of centralized economic planners, these innovations arise from the bottom up as entrepreneurs rush to meet the needs
of patients. Among such developments are the growth of "retail clinics";
entry into health care by companies such as CVS and Walgreens and perhaps eventually Amazon, Costco, and other entrants; and increased use
of medical tourism, both domestic and international. These innovations
are under threat from incumbent providers, insurers, and regulators, who
deceptively package their regulatory assaults as a defense of quality and
safety.

Stimuli for such efforts include the fact that many people remain
uninsured today—a far more perilous state in a world lacking price transparency or effective competition—and even the insured are increasingly
paying for more of their health care out of pocket. The number of patients
facing this reality and the dollar amounts at stake will likely increase,
providing opportunities for innovation that, if successful, could promote
much broader change, including new approaches to competitive pricing,
package deals, and other features widespread in many markets apart from
health care.

Silver and Hyman address several other critical areas pertinent to
health care. One is fraud in health care billing, a problem of enormous
magnitude often linked to inappropriate care. Third-party payment
facilitates fraud by removing patients and their unique knowledge and
interests from the payment loop. So does poor oversight by Medicare
and Medicaid—which apologists for those programs laud as indicating
administrative efficiency. Other areas include complex legislative and regulatory schemes that drive pharmaceutical prices and spending to their
current high levels. The authors' creative solutions to rework flaws of the
patent system deserve broader discussion.

In a book whose primary focus is on excessive health care prices and
expenditures, it is laudable that the final chapter addresses the morality
of health care. It is all too easy for proponents of universal insurance,
single-payer, and direct government provision of health care to claim the
moral high ground—and to portray ideas that would actually make health
care more universal as heartless simply because they don't promise impossible outcomes. Silver and Hyman show it is those who defend the status

quo whose position is morally untenable, no matter how well the complex nature of medicine may obscure responsibility for the resulting harms. They explain that Medicare and Medicaid are paternalistic and dishonest, the former serving as an intergenerational Ponzi scheme. They illustrate how incentives for over-insurance produce numerous avoidable welfare losses. They endorse a role for government to assist those in need but suggest mechanisms more respectful of the autonomy of the recipients and less likely to suppress innovation and efficiency.

Health care is complicated, and its current dysfunction needs urgent understanding and attention. *Overcharged* is just what the doctor ordered. We will be better off if it is widely read and discussed.

Jeffrey S. Flier, M.D.
Former Dean, Harvard Medical School
January 28, 2018

# INTRODUCTION

## The Republicans' Dilemma

Is Obamacare doomed? Well before President Donald Trump took office, the House of Representatives and the Senate had already voted to repeal almost all of the statute. When Trump defeated Hillary Clinton in the 2016 election, it seemed that the last remaining obstacle had disappeared. As we write this Introduction, however, Obamacare is still the law of the land. The House of Representatives passed a bill—the American Health Care Act—that supposedly "repeals and replaces" Obamacare, but the Senate did not. There, several measures failed, including the "repeal and replace" bill that was favored by the Senate leadership, the repeal-only bill that was preferred by the hard right, a "skinny repeal" bill that would have eliminated some features of Obamacare while leaving most of the program in place, and a last-ditch effort that would have repealed some provisions while devolving the law's spending and control over other provisions to the states. The 2017 tax reform law eliminated the tax penalties for being uninsured, but left the rest of Obamacare intact. And in both the House and the Senate, Democrats have supported Obamacare steadfastly, even though they admit it is in need of repair and falls far short of the goal of providing universal health care that many of them hoped to reach.

Whatever Congress ultimately does (or does not do), the reality is that Obamacare has been experiencing serious difficulties for years. Health care insurers are dropping out of its exchanges, people in many areas of the country have access to only one insurer, premiums are high and rising fast, many states have refused to expand their Medicaid programs, and the cost of funding those that did is enormous and growing. Obamacare also disappointed on many of the promises its proponents made. President Obama predicted that it would save $2,500 per family per year, but health care spending per capita substantially increased. Americans were told that poor people would get medical services from doctors' offices instead of emergency rooms (ERs) once they were covered by insurance or Medicaid, but they actually went to doctors' offices *and* ERs more often. Health care quality and efficiency remained stagnant, even though Obamacare was supposed to pressure providers to improve both. One article published in 2017 asked, "Why Are Medical Errors Still a Leading Cause of Death?"[1] Another observed that "Needless Medical Tests Not Only Cost $200B— They Can Do Harm."[2] In the Bloomberg Health-Care Efficiency Index, the United States continues to rank near the bottom of the heap.[3]

Obamacare did dramatically increase the number of Americans with some form of coverage for health care costs, so that promise was kept. But even the Medicaid expansion turned out to be a disappointment when leading health economists found that many people who were brought under the program's umbrella didn't value the benefit all that highly—and certainly wouldn't have purchased it had they been spending their own money.

But they were not doing that. Instead, Obamacare was spending our money—and doing so at a ferocious clip. Overall health care spending reached $3.4 trillion in 2016, more than $10,000 for each person in the United States. In an official report, government actuaries dryly noted that "2015 expenditure growth was primarily the result of increased use and intensity of services as millions gained health coverage, as well as continued significant growth in spending for retail prescription drugs."[4] Obamacare proved two things: people use more medical services when they are insured, and the health care sector will absorb as much money as we are willing to throw at it.

Because Obamacare failed to address many of the problems of the American health care system, the obvious question is: What comes next? As we write this book, it is impossible to be certain; but, even if the Republicans in Congress can unite behind a new program, it seems increasingly clear that the replacement will be some version of "Obamacare-lite." All the proposals that Congress considered in 2017 stripped out certain features of Obamacare while retaining others. Evidently, Republicans no longer think it is politically feasible to rip out Obamacare root and branch, even though that is what their most ardent supporters want.

Why such timidity, after running on a platform of outright repeal? Because Trump and the rest of the GOP face a dilemma. Although Republican party loyalists hate Obamacare's individual mandate (which required people to buy insurance), other features of the program are popular— especially the guarantee of coverage for people with pre-existing medical conditions and the provision allowing parents to keep their kids on their policies until the age of 26. (In fairness, support exists mainly when pollsters ask people whether they like these provisions; it drops dramatically when respondents are told how much these provisions cost.[5]) By eliminating these benefits, Republicans would immediately cause millions of Americans to lose insurance—including many children of the white upper-middle class. Rolling back the Medicaid expansion would cause millions of poor Americans to lose coverage as well. Outright "repeal" without some form of "replace" seems likely to result in loud protests and civil unrest.

The health care industry also opposes outright repeal. Providers don't want to treat millions of patients for free. That's why hospitals and many physicians have been major supporters of Obamacare's Medicaid expansion. They know that demand for health care services will drop sharply if millions of people lose their insurance. The medical establishment has a long history of lobbying aggressively to reverse even the threat of a modest reduction in the *rate of increase* in health care spending. If threatened with an actual reduction in revenue, it will go ballistic.

Insurance companies also lobbied aggressively to keep Obamacare, which delivered millions of new customers to them and has the potential to deliver millions more. What industry wouldn't want the enormous weight and power of the federal government forcing every person in the United States to purchase its products? And, for those unable to pay full freight, the government helped cover the premiums and out-of-pocket expenses. If the government wants the Obamacare exchanges to succeed, it will have to contribute enough money for insurers to find it worthwhile to stick around.

But insurers may not stick around now that the GOP has neutered the individual mandate while leaving the guarantee of coverage intact. The coverage guarantee enabled millions of high-cost sick people to buy heavily subsidized insurance. The insurance mandate was supposed to provide much-needed financial balance by requiring millions of low-cost healthy people to buy coverage too. By zeroing-out the mandate penalty while leaving the coverage guarantee in place, the GOP has guaranteed that insurers will either jack up their prices even higher or withdraw from the market even faster. Health care coverage will then be completely unavailable or so expensive that only the richest people can afford it.

It's a safe bet that Congress will neither force providers to take a haircut, bankrupt the insurance industry, nor anger millions of voters by depriving them of insurance. How Congress will finesse this tricky situation is anybody's guess. The most plausible prediction seems to be that it will do nothing, as long as it possibly can.

Rather than focus on the specifics of legislation that may or may not pass Congress in the next year or so, we think it is more useful to step back and explain why our health care system is so dysfunctional. That is what Part 1 of this book is all about. For those who cannot wait, there are five big problems with the current system for financing and delivering health care.

## PROBLEM #1: POLITICAL CONTROL OF HEALTH CARE SPENDING

Political control is the biggest obstacle to making health care more affordable. Obamacare made it through Congress because providers knew that health care spending would increase. Wall Street understood that too. After Obamacare was signed into law, stock prices for health insurers, hospital chains, and drug manufacturers soared. Why? Because Obamacare forced millions of people to buy insurance and put millions more on Medicaid. Once these people had coverage, it was predictable that they would use more medical services and bring billions in new revenue to health care providers doors. Obamacare also helped the sector by significantly reducing the need for charity care. Health care businesses lose money on services they provide for free, so this aspect of Obamacare delighted them.

Obamacare was far from the first government-funded financial bonanza for the health care sector. Every time Congress wades into this swamp, it winds up sending health care providers more money. In 2016, the federal government included $6 billion in pork barrel spending in the 21st Century Cures Act. In 2015, Congress enacted the Medicare Access and CHIP (Children's Health Insurance Program) Reauthorization Act, which will inflate the deficit by an estimated $500 billion over the next 20 years, to ensure that the payments doctors receive from Medicare keep increasing. Obamacare, with its coverage mandate, premium subsidies, and enormous Medicaid expansion, became the law in 2010. In 2009, the federal government blew $30 billion on electronic health records in the Health Information Technology for Economic and Clinical Health Act. In 2003, it committed to spending trillions of dollars on prescription drugs for seniors by enacting Medicare Part D. So long as Congress controls the health care economy, spending will only go up and up and up.

President Trump's about-face on drug price regulation provides more evidence of how things work in Washington, D.C. Right after taking office, he held a press conference at which he accused pharmaceutical companies of "getting away with murder" and threatened to authorize Medicare to bargain down prices.[6] But, when a draft of his executive order was floated a few months later, the tough talk had disappeared. In its place were proposals written by the Pharmaceutical Research and Manufacturers Association (PhRMA), the drug industry's lobbying arm. Vinay Prasad, a professor of medicine at Oregon Health and Sciences University, remarked that "[the] six-page document contains the kind of solutions to the cost-of-drugs problem that you would get if you gathered together all the executives of pharma and asked them 'What sort of token gestures can we do?'"[7]

Why the reversal? The usual reasons. Former industry insiders appointed to powerful positions in government dominated the task force that produced the draft, and the industry spent $10 million more on lobbyists than it had the year before.[8] According to a report by Kaiser Health News, "PhRMA, the drug industry's largest trade group, spent $7.98 million during the quarter—more than in any single quarter in almost a decade . . . topping even its quarterly lobbying ahead of the Affordable Care Act's passage in 2010."[9] Individual drug makers reached into their pockets too.[10] The millions of dollars that Pfizer and other pharma-associated interests "donated" to Trump's inaugural festivities couldn't have hurt either.[11] Political control of health care financing is the most fundamental reason health care spending always rises.

## Problem #2: Third-Party Payment

Third-party payment for most health care expenses compounds the problems created by political control of health care spending. Consider what happened to a mutual friend of the authors, whose stitches gave out after he sustained a minor wound. He went to a hospital-owned urgent care center in a strip mall and spent 30 minutes having his injury treated. He subsequently received a bill for $3,000, which he thought was absurd on its face, and likely fraudulent. However, the center granted a $1,170 discount based on its relationship with his insurance company, which then unquestioningly paid the "allowed" amount—$1,770—leaving him with a nominal bill of $60. When he saw that he personally owed so little, he shrugged his shoulders and paid the balance. Does anyone believe his reaction would have been the same if he had been responsible for the full $1,830 the center received—let alone the $3,000 list price? Does anyone believe that health care providers would send out such inflated bills if third-party payment were not the rule?

Proponents hailed Obamacare as a revolutionary transformation, but it really just doubled down on the failed strategy of third-party payment. The payment system was already funneling unprecedented amounts of money into the health care sector—and Obamacare threw gasoline on the fire by offering subsidized insurance and vastly expanding Medicaid. If cost control was ever the object, Obamacare was designed to fail.

At this point, many readers will object: Don't we need insurance and government programs to pay for health care because it is too expensive for us to afford on our own? Sometimes. But historically, cause and effect have run in the opposite direction. Medical services became expensive *after and because* they were insured. Before the role of third-party payers expanded dramatically during and after World War II, health care was cheap and people paid for it directly.

Spending really took off in the 1960s, when Medicare and Medicaid came online. As Professors Ted Marmor and Jon Oberlander write:

> In the first year of Medicare's operation, the average daily service charge in American hospitals increased by an unprecedented 21.9%. The average compound rate of growth in this figure over the next five years was 13%. . . . In the eleven months between the time Medicare was enacted and the time it took effect, the rate of increase in physician fees more than doubled, from 3.8% in 1965 to 7.8% in 1966. The average compound rate of growth in physician fees remained a high 6.8% over the next five years. In the first five full years of Medicare's operation, total Medicare reimbursements rose 72%, from $4.6 billion in 1967 to $7.9 billion in 1971. Over the same period, the number of Medicare enrollees rose only 6%, from 19.5 million in 1967 to 20.7 million in 1971.[12]

The problem isn't trying to guess whether the chicken or the egg came first. Third-party payment drastically increases health care prices and spending.

It is worth reflecting on how enormous the spending increase has been. In 2016, Americans spent about $3.4 trillion on health care. In 1960, we spent only $27 billion. That's an average increase of 9 percent per year. Had health care spending grown at the same rate as the general economy, it would have been about $220 billion in 2016, just under 7 percent of the figure it actually was.

As health care spending was exploding, however, the percentage of dollars that came directly from consumers (rather than being routed through the hands of third-party payers) drastically declined. In the early 1960s, patients paid about $1.80 out-of-pocket for every $1 spent by third-party payers. After Medicare and Medicaid were created, that ratio declined so steeply that, by the end of the decade, it was approximately $1 to $1. Today, consumers directly contribute less than 20 cents for every dollar shelled out by a third-party payer. The less direct responsibility consumers bear for the costs of medical services, the more total spending increases.[13]

Christy Ford Chapin, a history professor who published a column in the *New York Times* in 2017, got the connection between third-party payment and health care spending right. "With Medicare, the demand for health services increased and medical costs became a national crisis."

"The challenge of real reform," she continued, is that, "to actually bring down costs, legislators must roll back regulations to allow market innovation outside the insurance company model."[14] To bend the cost curve downward, we need to rely less on third-party payers and more on ourselves.

The fundamental cause of spiraling health care costs isn't aging, technology, defensive medicine, or any of the other causes that are commonly cited. It is that we too often let others buy medical treatments for us instead of paying for them ourselves. Worse, excessive reliance on third-party payers has convinced Americans that they cannot and should not pay for medical services themselves. Tens of millions of people who would never think of using insurance to pay their mortgages or their rent reflexively use their health care coverage to pay for doctors' office visits and other medical services that cost far less. To dig ourselves out of this hole, we have to learn to treat health care like everything else. We should pay for most medical treatments directly, the same way we pay for housing, transportation, electricity, water, food, and clothes. Insurance should be reserved for calamities.

### PROBLEM #3: THE PRICES ARE TOO DAMN HIGH!

You could not design a more expensive health care system than the one we have if you tried. It's not just that the U.S. health care sector is expensive. The payment system behaves as though its *purpose* is to move as much money as possible into the pockets of health care providers, and to avoid doing anything that interferes with that goal.

That is not its acknowledged purpose, of course. If you ask politicians, providers, or health care policy experts, they will offer a variety of more palatable rationales. They will say that the payment system is supposed to motivate providers to deliver high-quality care at reasonable cost, to protect the elderly and the poor from going without, or to provide all Americans with the best health care money can buy.

We are certain that many people sincerely believe these high-minded pronouncements, and many changes to the payment system may have been made with lofty goals in mind. But we are just as sure that none of these accounts describes what, over time, the payment system has become.

The reality of paying out trillions of dollars a year has turned our payment system into a well-oiled money-moving machine. The most accurate account of the system today is that it exists to move the largest possible number of dollars from the sources that feed it into the hands of health care providers. That is why health care spending sets new records year after year.

All of the payment system's basic features can be explained by assuming that its function is to move the largest possible number of dollars into the medical sector. Start with Medicare. To get the program enacted, President Lyndon Johnson and Congress effectively gave doctors and hospitals the keys to the federal treasury. At the outset, there were no controls on the prices providers could charge, the services they could perform, or total funding for the program. Medicare even guaranteed that hospitals would be profitable, and that as their costs rose their profits would increase. No one should have been surprised that prices and spending quickly spiraled out of control.[15] Over time, controls were added on the prices that providers could charge—but there were still no restrictions on the volume of services that could be performed or total funding.

Medicare also has few quality controls. It pays doctors who deliver services that are unnecessary, unproven, and even negligent. It pays hospitals when their patients experience avoidable complications or die from medical mistakes. Until quite recently, it made no efforts even to track the quality of care. Of course, if the purpose of Medicare's payment system is just to move money from taxpayers to providers, these pathological practices are readily explained.

The goal of moving money also explains why Medicare and Medicaid are plagued by fraud, waste, and abuse. The fastest way to enrich health care providers is to pay claims without checking to see that services were even provided. That's why these programs pay first and ask questions later—if ever. This approach, commonly known as "pay and chase," makes it easy for career criminals and Main Street providers to steal billions of taxpayers' dollars. And, once the money is gone, there is no hope of getting it back. In 2014, the Department of Justice had one of its best years ever, making fraudsters cough up $3.3 billion.[16] But that very same year, wrongdoers drained almost $100 billion from the Treasury by filing false Medicare and

Medicaid claims.[17] The feds are not even fighting the criminals to a draw; they are getting creamed.

An even worse problem is that it is often hard to tell the career criminals from the legitimate health care providers who happen to bill the Treasury for all manner of unnecessary services. The cost of unnecessary treatments and other forms of waste far exceeds the cost of fraud. Reputable authorities believe that the annual combined cost of fraud, waste, and abuse is *$1 trillion or more.* That's one dollar out of every three spent on health care in the United States. If the purpose of the payment system is to move money, rampant waste is easy to explain.

The same assumption explains why we overpay for prescription drugs. As we discuss in Chapter 1, Martin Shkreli, the notorious "pharma-bro," briefly became the most hated person in America after he raised the price of Daraprim, a medicine used to treat patients with AIDS and other illnesses, from $13.50 a tablet to $750. But, by the time he came along, pharma execs had been jacking up drug prices for years. Shkreli was also small beer. With fewer than 9,000 prescriptions for Daraprim being written each year, Shkreli's ill-gotten gains did not even amount to a rounding error on the share of the national health care budget spent on pharmaceuticals. As we explain in Chapter 2, other pharma execs have exploited patient populations that run into the millions.[18]

Hospitals also gouge patients.[19] A recent example focused on a pregnant woman who timed her arrival at the Boca Raton Regional Hospital a bit too late: she delivered her baby in the hospital's parking lot.[20] Seven months later, the hospital billed her $7,000, its full price for maternity care. Another Florida hospital charged a patient with a broken pelvis $32,767, even though he was wheeled into its ER and quickly wheeled out again because the hospital didn't have the necessary specialist. The bill amounted to $800 per minute.[21] A cyclist with road rash was billed $12,500; an uninsured woman with superficial cuts incurred a fee of $33,000; and a 35-year-old woman with burned fingers who spent an hour at St. Mary's Medical Center was hit up for $13,626.[22] The parents of a one-year-old with a cut finger were charged $629 for a five-minute visit and a Band-Aid.[23]

Why is price gouging so common? The dominance of open-ended third-party payment allows providers to charge whatever they want because patients are so insulated from prices they don't care enough to resist. The same dynamic also explains why money spent on medical services receives preferential tax treatment. Deductions for insurance premiums and medical savings accounts make it cheaper for Americans to buy health care than goods and services of other types. There is no good reason for this favorable tax treatment. Health care isn't intrinsically more important than food, housing, water, electricity, sanitation, or transportation. Most of the time, most people need other things more urgently than health care. It makes little sense to put health care on a plateau above everything else. Yet that is what tax deductions do. Once again, the payment system acts as if its primary purpose is to enrich the medical sector at the expense of the rest of the economy.

Researchers who focus on health care quality like to say, "Every system is perfectly designed to get the results it gets."[24] Americans pay twice as much for drugs and medical services as people in other developed countries because our payment system is perfectly designed to move money from the rest of us into the health care sector.[25]

## PROBLEM #4: HEALTH CARE QUALITY IN LAKE WOBEGON

If you ask any questions at all when your doctor refers you to a particular specialist or hospital, you will probably hear that the new provider is top-notch or the best in town. Just like the children in Garrison Keillor's mythical Lake Wobegon, in America's health care sector, all doctors and hospitals are above average.

Except that they aren't. Some doctors and hospitals are worse than others. To a mathematical certainty, 50 percent of them are below the median. Ten percent are in the bottom decile. These differences affect outcomes. Choosing the wrong surgeon can double or triple a patient's odds of dying on the operating table.[26] Rates of hospital-acquired infections (HAIs)—which afflict 650,000 people a year and kill 75,000, more than twice the number of fatalities caused by car crashes[27]—vary greatly across hospitals. Some are very good. Others, including some prestigious teaching hospitals, have terrible infection rates.

Even when their lives hang in the balance, however, few patients have any clue how good or bad their surgeon or hospital actually is. If you had an operation recently, you probably had no idea where your hospital ranked. You probably knew nothing about your hospital's postsurgical mortality and morbidity rates, either.[28] Even if you tried, you probably wouldn't have been able to find out how your surgeon's performance compared to others. This information is crucially important for patients, but many hospitals do not even collect it. Others have the information but keep it to themselves.

What happens when someone finally ranks providers by their actual performance? Then, a sort of reverse Lake Wobegon effect kicks in. Low-scoring providers rationalize their poor showings by asserting that their patients are sicker than average. Rather than confront the reality that not all health care providers are terrific, the industry blames its failures on patients.

Again, if we assume that the payment system's primary purpose is to move money into the health care sector, persistent subpar performance is easy to explain. Quality is not Job #1 because providers are not paid to deliver outstanding care. They are paid to treat patients, period. As a result, they deliver enormous volumes of care, including an ocean of services that are dangerous and unnecessary. And, with few exceptions, they will not voluntarily generate information that would help patients shop, because intelligent shopping has no upside for them.

### PROBLEM #5: OPAQUE PRICES

No consumer would buy a car, a computer, or any other costly item without knowing the price in advance. But, when it comes to medical treatments that cost thousands (or tens of thousands) of dollars, it is all but impossible to get a single, all-inclusive price for most things that will be done even at the time a service is delivered. Instead, patients receive bills after the fact and piecemeal, from every provider that happened to be in the neighborhood, some of whose charges are covered by insurance while others are not.[29] And every bill is filled with meaningless acronyms and phony charges that seem to have been plucked out of thin air. Why do patients need a Rosetta stone to make sense of their bills? Because opacity makes it easier for the payment system to move money to health care providers. How better to disguise what's going on than with confusing bills?

★★★★★★★

Having identified the major shortcomings of the health care system, we now briefly describe the four lessons that should be drawn from our work.

## Lesson #1: The Health Care System Is Full of Good People— But Good People Can't Save a Bad System

If we are right about the perverse incentives that are baked into our health care payment system, how do we explain the existence of islands of clinical excellence where patients can go for topflight care at reasonable cost? These islands don't exist by accident. They are the result of careful planning and sustained efforts by conscientious frontline providers, backed up by outstanding business management.

The islands prove that good people sometimes prevail despite bad incentives. Unfortunately, good people cannot save a bad system, where the incentives encourage bad acts.

Consider the problem of central line–associated bloodstream infections (CLABSIs). CLABSIs are a particularly nasty form of HAI. Of the roughly 250,000 Americans who contract CLABSIs each year, almost one-quarter die, often after lengthy and expensive hospital stays. Although experience has proven that CLABSIs can be effectively eliminated with minimal inconvenience and at trivial expense, many hospitals' intensive care units (ICUs) still have high CLABSI rates.

It's easy to explain why CLABSIs are common. The problems we identify above have warped the payment system to the point where preventing CLABSIs is unprofitable. Thanks to political control, third-party payment, and the rest, hospitals literally make more money by treating patients for deadly infections than by preventing them. Patients spending their own money would never allow hospitals to profit by giving them infections. But because CLABSIs generate higher revenues, hospitals have no financial incentive to eliminate them.[30]

The same goes for other avoidable complications of surgery and medical errors. Hospitals can make more money by treating patients they have harmed than by preventing those harms in the first place.

Still, despite the extra money to be made by treating patients for avoidable infections, some ICUs have low CLABSI rates. Self-interest cannot explain the behavior of these high-performing units. What does?

The answer is wonderful and caring health care workers, administrators, and researchers who want to help patients. Hospitals and other health care providers employ hundreds of thousands of doctors, nurses, physician assistants, and other professionals who are committed to saving lives, regardless of the impact on their institutions' bottom lines. The successes that many ICUs have had in combating CLABSIs attest to the power of selflessness, as do millions of other miracles that health care workers have pulled off.

Good people have made the health care system better than it would otherwise be. But they have not made it better than it is—which is to say, expensive and mediocre. Why? Because incentives matter too. When quality is a losing proposition—as it is when hospitals make more money by harming patients than by treating them well—failures are easy to rationalize and the pressure to improve is reduced. When a hospital's mortality rate is unusually bad, it is not that the surgical practices used there are deficient; the problem is that the hospital's patients are unusually frail. When the information needed to benchmark a hospital's performance isn't readily available, the hospital's employees are not neglecting quality; they are too busy helping patients to waste time collecting data. The efforts of wonderful people cannot overcome a payment system that makes quality a money-losing proposition.

And let there be no mistake: under existing payment arrangements, quality improvement and cost reduction are often money-losing propositions. Doctors and hospitals have learned time and again that what is best for their patients is financially bad for them. In a market less distorted by political control and third-party payers, the interests of providers and patients would align more closely, and providers would be incentivized to serve patients better.

Popular rhetoric to the contrary, the problem is not that medical treatments are delivered by profit-seeking businesses. For-profit businesses add enormously to our quality of life. They bring us most of the goods and services we enjoy, including houses, cars, computers, cellphones, food, and millions of other things, all of which they deliver at prices we can afford. If consumers purchased medical treatments directly rather than via government bureaucracies and insurance companies, for-profit businesses would serve our health needs well too. The problem is our payment system, which breaks the link between profits and consumer satisfaction and makes it financially advantageous for providers to serve patients poorly.

### LESSON #2: IF THE BOTTOM LEADS, THE TOP WILL FOLLOW

Obamacare was doomed from the start. The core problems of health care are political control of spending and the overuse of insurance, and Obamacare offered more of both. The only reforms with real potential to transform our health system are those that give consumers control of health care dollars and require providers to compete for their business. We can rescue ourselves from the mess we have created by helping people buy medical goods and services and health insurance directly—the same way they buy other goods and services.

Politicians have little incentive to enact reforms that force providers to offer better treatments at less cost. For the better part of a century, industry groups have been paying politicians and lobbying them to do the exact opposite. Greater spending means more money for doctors, hospitals, drug companies, and insurers. That's why the health care sector always backs legislation that will increase spending and always opposes proposals that might reduce it. Mainstream health care providers will never support reforms that would subject them to market forces.

If change for the better is going to happen, consumers will have to exert pressure for it from below. Fortunately, CVS Health, Walgreens, Walmart, Costco, and many other retailers have opened new outlets for medical services that are inexpensive and as close as the nearest shopping mall. A growing number of treatments are sold directly to patients who pay for them with their own money. The list includes vision services like LASIK surgery, eyeglasses, and contact lenses; cosmetic procedures like Botox injections, breast augmentation, dental veneers, and tooth whitening; and medical treatments like in vitro fertilization, flu shots, tests for various illnesses, and vaccinations.

Services sold at retail have not been caught up in the same cost spiral that has affected the rest of health care. Their prices have held steady or declined. Why? Because patients who buy things with their own money comparison shop. They look for high-quality goods and services that are delivered conveniently and at a reasonable cost. They look for sales and discounts and will drive across town to save a few dollars. And, because they spend their own money, they buy only things that they value.

The retail sector responds by catering to consumers' desires. It offers convenient locations and times, transparent prices, and good quality. Many goods and services come with money-back guarantees. Retail medical outlets even have sales—something that your local hospital or doctor probably never does. That's what happens when providers compete for patients' dollars.

Retailers are good at figuring out how to sell things that people want at prices they can afford. Retailers also know how to make shopping easy and pleasant. That's why traditional health care providers are trying to prevent them from moving in. Like the old-line taxicab companies that want to stifle Uber and Lyft, they know that their business models can survive only as long as customers have no choice but to use them. Their best option is to thwart competition by excluding new entrants. These dinosaurs should be on the road to extinction, but they will use their political muscle to prolong their existence.

One of the medical establishment's most fundamental accomplishments has been to convince Americans that doctors alone should control the delivery of health care, even though few doctors know how to run a business. That is why many states have laws that require nurse practitioners and physician assistants to work under doctors' supervision, laws whose relaxation doctors continue to oppose even though patients' access to needed services would improve.[31] Many states also forbid the corporate practice of medicine, meaning that they won't let Costco or Walmart run hospitals or own other businesses that deliver health care to the public. There is no evidence—zero—that these laws improve the delivery of care. Their real purpose is to stifle competition, thereby enriching physicians and traditional hospitals.

In the crazy world of health care, doctors even set the prices Medicare pays for their services. Everyone else, from accountants to zookeepers, has to compete on price and gets what the market bears. But not physicians. The amounts they receive from Medicare are set, in large part, according to estimates of the time required to perform procedures. The estimates are prepared by a secretive American Medical Association (AMA) committee whose members know that higher estimates mean higher pay. As Tom Scully, a former head of Medicare once observed, "the concept of having the AMA run the process of fixing prices for Medicare was crazy from the beginning . . . . It was a fundamental mistake." [32] That should've been obvious to everyone, but what better way to send doctors lots of money than by letting them set their own rates? Worse, by jacking up the prices Medicare pays, doctors also rig the rest of the market. Private insurers follow Medicare in rough lockstep: a $1 increase in Medicare payments predicts a $1.30 increase in the price paid by private insurers. [33] The uninsured get the shaft because doctors and hospitals charge them inflated "rack rates," collect whatever they can, and ruin the credit ratings of patients who don't pay.

Only in the retail sector do health care providers face pressure to charge less. That's why prices there have held steady or declined, while in the rest of the health care sector they have soared. Americans could save huge amounts of money and receive better-quality treatments by letting retailers expand.

On rushing out of an interview abruptly, Mahatma Gandhi supposedly said, "There goes my people. I must follow them, for I am their leader." [34] Gandhi knew how mass movements work. America's politicians do too. When millions of us take our business to retail medical outlets and tell our elected representatives that we want more freedom to do so, they will be forced to stand up to the health care establishment. And once the norm of buying health care at retail outlets is established, there'll be no turning back.

### Lesson #3: To Beat 'Em, Leave 'Em

Providers may enjoy a local monopoly, but beleaguered patients can disrupt their cozy cartel by traveling elsewhere. The field of "medical tourism" is booming. By flying to other countries to get hip and knee replacements, cardiac surgeries, and other expensive procedures, Americans can save more than enough money to pay for the trip. By having heart surgery at a world-class hospital in India, an average American can save enough money to live on for a year.

For patients who don't want to leave the country, there's still some good news. They can break the stranglehold of local providers by traveling domestically to other cities and states. The average charge for a knee replacement in the United States is about $57,000.[35] But the Surgery Center of Oklahoma (SCO) will perform the operation for only $19,400.[36] Its posted price includes anesthesia, operating room charges, and surgical fees. The artificial joint will cost $4,000–$6,000 more, but the folks at SCO will tell you its price in advance and they will charge you only what it costs them. No absurd markups here. If you like, they will even show you the receipt. With the $31,000 or so that you'd save by having knee replacement surgery done at the SCO, you could fly to Oklahoma City, stay in its fanciest hotel, buy courtside tickets to a Thunder game, and have enough left over to install granite countertops in your house.

SCO's prices for many surgeries are low enough for middle-class people to afford. A mastectomy costs $5,000. A pacemaker implantation runs $11,400, hardware included. A patient with droopy eyelids will spend $4,150 for a blepharoplasty. Although it's never pleasant to write a big check for a medical service (or anything else), these amounts are comparable to the cost of many medium-ticket items that middle-class people save up for. A used car for a kid in high school or a family vacation might cost about as much as a mastectomy or blepharoplasty. To get these prices, though, patients have to schedule their procedures in advance and pay for them themselves. When patients ask SCO to deal with their insurers, it charges more.

And here's the really good news. If you don't want to travel at all, you can probably save a bunch of money right where you are. Just tell the folks at your local hospital that you'll have your knee replacement surgery done at the SCO unless they match its price. You may be pleasantly surprised by the response. When faced with the prospect of losing patients, many hospitals are willing to offer substantial discounts. Although some patients have adopted these strategies, they will remain at the margins until more consumers begin to control and spend their health care dollars themselves.

LESSON #4: BETTER HEALTH CARE (AND BETTER HEALTH)
THROUGH SELF-PAY

Saving money matters to patients who spend their own dollars. But when Medicare, Medicaid, or private insurers foot the bills, patients have little reason to care. That's a recipe for disaster. If the payment system were designed sensibly, self-pay would be the rule. Health care coverage would be reserved for disasters, just like other forms of insurance. Auto insurance covers major crashes, not small dings and certainly not oil changes. Life insurance kicks in when people die, not when they miss a day at work because of a sore throat. Homeowners' insurance covers damage inflicted by serious fires, water leaks, and windstorms—and it has sizable deductibles, to get homeowners to bear all of the costs of minor problems and to share the costs of major disasters.

Health care coverage should work similarly. Insurers should pay for highly complex and expensive procedures that relatively few people need in any given year. Patients should pay for routine stuff—like check-ups, diabetes monitoring, and allergy medications—just like they pay for gym memberships, running shoes, and other things that contribute to good health.

This will happen naturally if consumers purchase health insurance themselves. We expect the high price of first-dollar coverage will lead most consumers to purchase coverage only for remote health risks that involve expensive treatments. They will not buy comprehensive coverage for their bodies for the same reason they do not buy it for their homes or their cars: such coverage costs more than it is worth to the people who are making the decisions about how they wish to spend their own money. Only people who are unusually risk averse will find the price worth paying, and they will be free to do so if they want. Similarly, people who don't want to spend time shopping for providers may seek out "concierge practices" that offer most services under one roof and help with referrals when unusual needs arise. These plans resemble insurance but are better described as prepaid service arrangements. Some people will seek out these arrangements, but we expect most consumers spending their own money will want insurance that covers catastrophes and will self-pay for everything else.

One easy way to see the potential benefits of self-pay is to focus on governmental programs, like Medicare. When people think about Medicare, they naturally focus on what the program does. They talk about the millions of seniors it covers, the fact that it now pays for drugs as well as medical services, and so on. But just for a moment consider what Medicare doesn't cover—because the omissions shed light on the program's true purpose and on the advantages of self-pay arrangements. Suppose you are an elderly person with a condition that will probably kill you in a few months. If you want to pull out all the stops in the hope of staving off death for as long as possible, you are in luck. Medicare will pay for unlimited medical treatments during the last days of your life. It will pay an oncology clinic to pump you full of anticancer drugs. It will pay a hospital to prod you and poke you as often as you can stand. It will pay a surgeon to operate on you even though there is little or no chance that you will recover. The people who designed Medicare love to pay for intensive treatments, enabling the program to hand out buckets of money to health care providers.

But suppose that, instead of being injected, prodded, poked, operated upon, and generally made miserable, you would rather spend your final days at home and experience a dignified death surrounded by your family. To make that happen, you would like to make a few modifications to your home—so you can move around in a wheelchair more easily. You would also like to hire a personal assistant to help with bathing, changing clothes, eating, and pain management. Or maybe you would like to check an item off your bucket list by moving to a foreign country and spending your last days on the beach.

Now you are out of luck. Although Medicare has a limited hospice benefit, it will not pay for any of the other possibilities just listed—even though all of them combined would cost substantially less than dying in an intensive care unit after a lengthy hospital stay. To get what you want, you'll have to buy it yourself. Why does Medicare refuse to pay, even though these alternatives are a comparative bargain? Because the program will only buy something for seniors if the money goes into the pockets of health care providers. It is not set up to help beneficiaries die with dignity in the manner they prefer or to pay for services of any other kind. If you want expensive medical treatments, great. If not, you are on your own.

To really help seniors, Medicare should operate like Social Security. It should give beneficiaries money and let them decide how to spend it. That simple reform would put seniors in the driver's seat. It would also jump-start the bottom-up process of improving the health care system that we discussed above, by creating an army of direct-purchasing seniors who are bent on finding economical health care. What would work for seniors would work for everyone else too—particularly the poor, who are covered by Medicaid.

Government would still play a role by distributing money to persons in need. Recipients could use their stipends to purchase insurance against catastrophes or pay for ordinary care out of pocket. This approach isn't new. Food stamps enable poor people to buy groceries wherever they want, so they can look for the best deals. The Earned Income Tax Credit and the Child Tax Credit give poor people money they can use to pay bills of all types, including bills from health care providers and insurers. Social Security and veterans' disability payments do the same thing.

One source reports that, if all anti-poverty programs were replaced with simple cash transfers, at current spending levels, a poor family of four would receive an annual income near $70,000.[37] And those dollars would go a lot farther than they currently do. Instead of wasting money on a flawed system, people would maximize their bang for the buck by shopping for bargains and forcing health care providers (and other sellers) to compete for their dollars.

In sum, to a distressing degree, American health care looks and acts expensive by design. The payment system behaves as if its objective is to move the largest possible amount of money into the health care sector. It does that job extraordinarily well, and it will do it even better in the future because health care providers use every trick they can think of to make more money. But rising costs and high deductibles have already motivated many consumers to look for bargains in the retail sector. When it seems as natural to go to a local big box store like Target or Walmart for a medical treatment as it currently does to visit a doctor's office or an emergency room, people may finally see the rest of the medical sector for what it is: a fat and lazy industry that needs a swift kick in the pants.

We expect the health care sector to become more efficient and pro-consumer when and only when it is subjected to the same competitive forces that apply to the rest of the economy. If you want to see why we make such strong claims, read on.

## PART 1. MISDIAGNOSIS: THE PROBLEMS OBAMACARE SHOULD HAVE FIXED

The United States is "the most expensive place in the world to get sick."[1] Why? One big reason is that providers routinely game the payment system. Drug companies are experts at this. Chapter 1 describes how they first gain strangleholds on supply. Chapter 2 describes how they then charge whatever they want, knowing the payment system imposes no restraint on prices. Chapter 3 shows that shady conduct occurs at every point in the drug distribution chain and often involves the willing participation of pharmacists and physicians who profit by exploiting existing payment arrangements. It is easy to see why spending on prescription drugs, new and old, has gone through the roof.

Doctors game the payment system too. As Chapters 4 and 5 show, they deliver an ocean of services that patients don't need, such as excessive numbers of stents and cesarean deliveries. Chapter 6 describes how doctors regularly perform treatments that haven't been proven to work, many of which are found to be ineffective or harmful when they are finally studied with care.

Chapter 7 explains how public officials get in on the action. In return for sizable campaign contributions from health care providers and their lobbyists, they let the flow of cash into the health care sector continue and look for ways to increase it. When the campaign contributions are large enough, elected officials even go to bat for corrupt providers who face fraud investigations.

Some hospitals and doctors aren't satisfied with excess payments for garden-variety overuse and unnecessary care, and they turn to a life of crime—or at least abuse. Chapter 8 explains how hospitals "upcode" treatments, invent secondary conditions that patients don't have, and concoct phony bills. Chapter 9 shows how hospitals also conspire with doctors to maximize their revenues by capturing differences in payments based on the site of service, tacking on absurd charges, and gouging patients who are uninsured or treated by out-of-network physicians at their facilities. Chapter 10 describes how hospices, nursing homes, and home health care services play similar games and frequently charge for services that were never delivered.

Chapter 11 shows how some doctors operate pill mills that supply the street with dangerous drugs—likely contributing to the rising death toll from overuse of prescription narcotics. Ambulance companies and durable medical equipment suppliers cheat the system regularly too, as do domestic and international criminal gangs. As Chapter 12 explains, there are far too many malefactors for the police to catch. For every one police put away, two more pop up. That is why the same types of fraud succeed again and again and again.

Chapter 13 explains that the quality of health care is often dangerously low because the payment system pays providers regardless of how well or poorly their patients fare. In fact, it often doles out more money to providers when patients experience complications than when they get well. Chapter 14 explains how incumbent health care providers have stifled competition so successfully that the government has to pay them extra to improve. In other industries, competition forces existing business to bear the costs of improving their products.

Although there have been repeated attempts to address these problems, all have failed because they have not changed the core incentives driving the system. We address that problem in Part 2.

# CHAPTER 1: PATENT NONSENSE

## A New Scandal Every Day

The pharmaceutical industry is awash in pricing scandals. New reports of abuses appear so often that anything we write here is likely to seem like ancient history by the time the book appears. When we composed the first draft of this chapter, no one had heard of Martin Shkreli, the now-infamous "pharma-bro." Shkreli's company, Turing Pharmaceuticals, gouged AIDS patients by raising the price of a drug called Daraprim from $13.50 to $750 per pill. Shkreli, who briefly became the most hated man in America, reveled in the attention and enjoyed trolling his critics. When he held a charity raffle in which the holder of the winning ticket got to punch him in the face, he boasted of having received an offer of $78,000 for the privilege.[1] Shkreli reportedly paid $2 million for the only copy ever made of the Wu-Tang Clan's album *Once Upon a Time in Shaolin*.[2] Then he threatened to destroy it so that no one would ever be able to hear it but him.

The press couldn't get enough of Shkreli, but other drug company execs insisted on sharing the spotlight, so he was pushed to the back pages. One of his successors was Michael Pearson, the CEO of Valeant Pharmaceuticals. Pearson presided over annual double-digit price increases for all of Valeant's drugs. Heather Bresch, the CEO of Mylan, likewise demanded her 15 minutes of fame. Under her leadership, Mylan priced EpiPens, which are used for the treatment of anaphylactic shock and cost no more than $30 to manufacture, at $600 apiece.[3]

Other pharmaceutical executives wanted the public to believe that Shkreli, Pearson, and Bresch were deviants whose exceptional greed unfairly tarnished the reputation of the entire industry. This public relations strategy had an obvious shortcoming: there was nothing exceptional about Shkreli, Pearson, or Bresch. They used the same business strategy that all major drug companies have employed: gain control of the supply of a drug and then jack up the price. That is why, when other drug company CEOs pilloried Shkreli, he fired back in kind, asserting that they were as guilty as he was. And, as *Bloomberg* reported, "Shkreli Was Right: Everyone's Hiking Drug Prices."[4]

Many of the price increases have been spectacular. Over short periods of time, one diabetes drug quadrupled in price, while another rose by 160 percent. Bloomberg.com listed 73 branded drugs whose prices rose by 75 percent or more. Leading the pack was Xyrem, a narcolepsy treatment manufactured by Jazz Pharmaceuticals. Its price increased by a stunning 841 percent.[5] A 2014 article noted that drug prices seem to "defy gravity," with "prices doubling for dozens of established drugs that target everything from multiple sclerosis to cancer, blood pressure and even erections."[6] A 2017 article similarly noted that "prices for U.S.-made pharmaceuticals have climbed over the past decade six times as fast as the cost of goods and services overall."[7]

The effect of price increases has been to move enormous amounts of wealth from consumers to drug companies. Americans spent $457 billion on prescription drugs in 2015 and are on pace to increase that amount by 6.7 percent every year through 2025.[8] A recent RXPrice Watch report by AARP found that older Americans who take an average of 4.5 brand-name prescription drugs per month incurred retail costs of more than $26,000 in 2015—more than the median annual income for Medicare beneficiaries.[9] Younger people are also caught in pharma's net: "prescription drug costs for Americans under 65 years old are projected to jump 11.6 percent in 2017. By comparison, wages are expected to rise just 2.5 percent in 2017."[10] Drug companies' profits reflect these wealth transfers. "After paying all research costs and other costs of doing business, pharmaceutical manufacturers earn profits that average close to 20 percent of sales. The industry has consistently ranked as one of the most profitable industry sectors with returns that are more than double the median return for all industries."[11]

It is not surprising that drug makers use their control over the supply of medications to gouge consumers and payers. The companies are not charities, and the executives who run them are not philanthropists. Pharmaceutical companies are businesses, and like other businesses, they are run so as to maximize their profits.

That is why it is dangerous to give drug companies monopolies. Give a business—any business—a monopoly and it will extract wealth from consumers by charging the monopoly price. And that is what patents do: they give drug companies monopolies on the sales of new medications. No wonder an article recently published in the *Journal of the American Medical Association* concluded, "the primary reason for increasing drug spending is the high price of branded products protected by market exclusivity provisions granted by the U.S. Patent and Trademark Office and the Food and Drug Administration."[12]

Pharmaceutical companies spend lavishly to preserve their market advantages too. In California alone, the industry poured over $100 million into a campaign to defeat the Drug Price Relief Act, a ballot initiative that would have limited what the state paid for drugs.[13] At the federal level, drug companies are just as busy:

> Open Secrets data show that, between 1997–2015, Congress accepted $3.3 billion in campaign contributions from the pharmaceutical/health products sector, 43% more than they received from insurance, the second most politically influential industry. That averages out to about $181 million annually over that 18-year period.[14]

Although large in absolute terms, these dollars are chump change for Big Pharma. That is why reforms with real potential to bring down drug prices are never seriously proposed at the federal level, despite the number of scandals in which drug companies are involved. The industry and its army of lobbyists nip them in the bud.

Examples compiled by Alfred Engelberg, a former counsel to generic drug makers, show how large the stakes are relative to the amounts that pharma companies spend on lobbying. Consider Lipitor, a cholesterol-fighting statin, to pick just one. An extension of its patent term and a second extension for pediatric testing gave Pfizer, Lipitor's manufacturer, an additional 1,393 days of marketing exclusivity, during which it took in $24 billion extra in sales revenue. Across the industry, patent extensions for statins generated $60 billion in extra revenue, while extensions for pediatric testing generated $5 billion on top of that.[15]

## EPIC PRICES FOR EPIPENS

At root, the strategy that Mylan used to turn the humble EpiPen into a cash cow is the same as that used by the rest of the industry: gain a monopoly and exploit it. The EpiPen is a decades-old technology for injecting epinephrine, a medicine that helps people who suffer from dangerous allergic reactions to things like peanuts, insect bites, milk, or bee stings. When a person is experiencing anaphylaxis, an allergic reaction that can cause the throat to swell and the airway to close, an EpiPen can make the difference between life and death. Fortunately, epinephrine is cheap. The medicine inside an EpiPen costs about $1.

Mylan sells millions of EpiPens a year. Its customers include schools, emergency medical technicians, and parents whose kids have allergies. Amie Vialet DeMontbel was one such parent. Her son's milk allergy was so severe that he wore a mask to protect himself from accidental exposure. She needed two EpiPens for him—one to take to camp and one to keep at home. The price? More than $1,200 for the pair. Mylan asked her to shell out more than her monthly mortgage payment for injectors that contained $2 worth of epinephrine.[16]

EpiPens were not always so pricey. They used to sell for less than $100. But from 2004 to 2016, Mylan raised the price by more than 450 percent, after adjusting for inflation. Why? Not because the cost of epinephrine or the injectors had gone up. They had not. If anything, Mylan's product costs should have declined, owing to improvements in manufacturing processes and economies of scale.

The simple truth is that Mylan raised the price of EpiPens because it could. The market was not competitive because Mylan held a patent on the design of the injector. Injectors made by a competing manufacturer experienced dose-regulation problems. There was no generic substitute either, partly because Mylan had used a lawsuit and a "citizen petition" to delay generic entry.[17] Armed with a monopoly, Mylan could force buyers to fork over every last dollar—so it did. Then its managers and shareholders pocketed the extra cash. Bresch, Mylan's CEO, saw her total compensation rise from $2.4 million in 2007 to $18.9 million in 2015, a 671 percent increase that followed on the heels of Mylan's acquisition of the right to make EpiPens.[18] In 2016, Mylan's chairman, Robert J. Coury, received nearly $100 million in salary, plus another $59 million in retirement benefits and other payments.[19]

Although the real explanation for EpiPen price gouging was simple greed, Mylan ran a sophisticated public relations campaign to deflect attention from the truth. Its position was that the price hikes were justified because of "the value the product provides." This is an argumentative gambit that many drug companies use. Trouble is, it only works with people who don't understand basic economics. The "value a product provides" sets a ceiling on the amount that a consumer would rationally pay for it, but it does not dictate what the price should be and has little bearing on the price a product will command in a competitive market. The competitive price is the smallest amount that a manufacturer can accept while still making a profit. That is why competitive markets are good for consumers. They force prices down to the lowest levels that sellers will accept for the last unit produced, not up to the highest prices that consumers will pay.

Suppose that a diner who loves steak would willingly pay up to $100 for a steak dinner. Now suppose that any of a dozen local restaurants could charge $25 for the meal and still make a profit. When restaurants compete, which price will prevail: $100 or $25? The latter. Why? Because the restaurants will try to gain the diner's business by undercutting each other's prices, and this will continue until they all charge $25. That the meal produces $100 in value for the diner does not matter. And the price would remain the same if the diner actually valued the meal at $500 or even $5,000. Competitive markets favor buyers, not sellers, because they drive prices down to the lowest sustainable levels.

Mylan did not have to charge a competitive price, however, because it had no competition. Neither did Kaleo Pharma, the maker of Evzio, an injector for the opioid-overdose preventive naloxone. It had a monopoly, so it raised prices too. In January of 2016, the injector twin-pack sold for $937.50. Three months later, the price was $4,687.50.[20] The increase had nothing to do with research costs or any other costs. Generic injectable naloxone has been on the market since 1971.[21] Kaleo charged more for Evzio because it was the only injector supplier.

Other commentators agree that pharma companies raise prices because they can. Dr. David Belk, who blogs at True Cost of Healthcare, studied the average price that retail pharmacies paid for more than 100 branded medications from 2012 to 2015. Their prices rose an average of 56 percent, roughly 16 times the rate of inflation over the same period. "So, why are the prices of these drugs going up as quickly as they are?" Dr. Belk asked. "One reason is that there's nothing to stop the pharmaceutical companies from raising their prices."[22]

Findings like Dr. Belk's put the lie to the pharmaceutical sector's claim that executives like Shkreli, Pearson, and Bresch are outliers. In the first quarter of 2016, "more than two-thirds of the 20 largest pharmaceutical companies said [that] price increases boosted sales of some or most of their biggest products." The companies involved were industry leaders, including Pfizer, Biogen, Gilead Sciences, Amgen, and AbbVie.[23] Pfizer raised the prices on 133 brand-name drugs in 2015 alone, with more than three-quarters of the increases exceeding 10 percent. Merck & Co. raised the prices on 38 drugs.[24] Exploiting monopolies is the name-brand pharma sector's business model.

### CORNER THE MARKET, RAISE THE PRICE

Monopolies are not new. Aristotle's *Politics* explains how the Greek philosopher Thales cornered a market more than 2,000 years ago:

> Thales, so the story goes, because of his poverty was taunted with the uselessness of philosophy; but from his knowledge of astronomy

he had observed while it was still winter that there was going to be a large crop of olives, so he raised a small sum of money and paid round deposits for the whole of the olive-presses in Miletus and Chios, which he hired at a low rent as nobody was running him up; and when the season arrived, there was a sudden demand for a number of presses at the same time, and by letting them out on what terms he liked he realized a large sum of money, so proving that it is easy for philosophers to be rich if they choose, but this is not what they care about. Thales then is reported to have thus displayed his wisdom, but as a matter of fact this device of taking an opportunity to secure a monopoly is a universal principle of business. . . .[25]

Few pharmaceutical execs have heard of Thales, but they all know how to corner markets. They often use patents to do this, but they find other ways too.[26] A 2016 Senate report describes one time-tested strategy:[27]

1. Identify a "sole-source" drug—a drug that has only one manufacturer.
2. Verify that the drug is the "gold standard" for treating an illness. This ensures that doctors will keep prescribing it if the price rises.
3. Determine that the market for the drug is small. Competitors are unlikely to enter small markets even when prices are high. Plus, small patient populations lack political power and can't protect themselves from price gouging.
4. Acquire the right to produce the drug and close the distribution network. This prevents patients from acquiring the medicine other than via approved outlets. It also makes it hard for potential competitors to acquire the samples they need in order to gain U.S. Food and Drug Administration (FDA) approval for generic equivalents, in the event the market is large enough to justify entry.
5. Maximize profits by raising prices, and keep prices high as long as possible. When challenged, deflect criticism by emphasizing the value the drug has for patients and cite the high cost of research and development (R&D).

The Senate report describes how four pharmaceutical companies used this strategy to gouge consumers for drugs that had been off-patent for decades. None of the companies spent any money on R&D or did anything to make the drugs better. They simply gamed the system, which paid whatever price the pharmaceutical companies set.

Martin Shkreli used this strategy repeatedly. He first employed it at a company called Retrophin, which raised the price of Thiola, a drug used to treat kidney stones, from $1.50 per pill to $30. Then he acquired Turing Pharmaceuticals and increased the price of Daraprim from $13.50 per tablet to $750. In Great Britain, Daraprim sold for less than $1.[28] When asked why he set the price so high, Shkreli said, "the ugly, dirty truth" was that Turing's "shareholders expect me to make the most profit."[29] Shkreli owned the lion's share of Turing's stock, of course, so the expectations he reported were mostly his own.

The owners of Novum Pharma expected to make money too. They raised the prices for three skin treatments—Aloquin, Alcortin A, and Novacort—after acquiring the rights to make them. In 2015, Aloquin cost $241. By late 2016, the price was $9,561, an almost 40-fold increase. The price hikes for Alcortin A and Novacort were similarly spectacular.[30]

There are variations on the basic five-step approach. Questcor, a subsidiary of Mallinckrodt, used one to raise the price of Acthar Gel, a life-saving treatment for infantile spasms of multiple sclerosis, by 85,000 percent. Questcor acquired the rights to make Achtar, a drug that was off-patent, in 2001 and began increasing the price. Then, in 2013, it outbid its competitors for the right to make Synacthem, a competing medication. Since in controlled the entire market, Questcor was free to charge whatever it wanted. And what it wanted was $34,000 per vial for a medicine that previously cost $40. The Federal Trade Commission got wind of the problem and intervened. It fined Mallinckrodt $100 million and required it to allow a competitor to make Synacthem.[31]

## WHY ISN'T COMPETITION KEEPING PRICES LOW?

Economic theory says that, for old drugs, the strategy of cornering the market shouldn't work. Producers can't overcharge consumers if competitors can enter the market and make money by undercutting those excessive prices.

Yet this strategy has worked over and over again. Prices for many old drugs have risen spectacularly. The cost of tetracycline, an antibiotic that's been around for decades, went from 3.4 cents per tablet to $2.36—a 67-fold increase in just one year. Erythromycin, another antibiotic, "had three separate price increases of at least 100 percent, with the price of the drug increasing from $0.24 per tablet in the first quarter of 2010 to $8.96 per tablet in the first quarter of 2015."[32] These aren't isolated examples. According to one report, 222 old drug groups saw prices at least double from November 2013 to November 2014. For 17 groups, prices rose by a factor of 10 or more.[33]

An economist might explain the increases just reported by suggesting that barriers to entry prevented potential competitors from offering these products, so that existing manufacturers had de facto monopolies even though the drugs were old. That may sometimes be true, but it cannot be the whole story. Spectacular price increases occurred for old generic drugs that were made by several companies. Eight of the 10 drugs with "the biggest percentage price hikes in 2014 were generic medicines made by multiple manufacturers."[34]

The story of ursodiol, a generic treatment for gallstones, is particularly vexing. It is a decades-old drug that is made by eight companies and that used to be cheap—45 cents per capsule. Then, in 2014, Lannett Co. raised its price to $5.10 "and one by one its competitors followed suit—with most charging nearly the same price." One of those competitors was Mylan—the maker of the EpiPen is also one of the largest producers of generic drugs in the world. It had stopped manufacturing ursodiol in 2012 but got back into the market after the price spiked. And when it did, it didn't undercut other sellers. Instead it charged $4.95 per capsule, about the same price.[35]

## ERECTILE PRICING

Why does competition exert less influence in drug markets than it does elsewhere? One likely explanation is "parallel pricing," which occurs when supposed competitors maintain or raise prices in lockstep. We call it "erectile pricing," rather than parallel pricing, because we observed it when studying Viagra and other erectile dysfunction (ED) drugs.

In the late 1990s, Pfizer's "blue diamonds" sold for $7 apiece. But they didn't stay that cheap for long. Over the ensuing decade, Pfizer raised the price repeatedly. For a few years, it did so every January. Then, after encountering little resistance, it did so twice a year and made the increments larger. By 2009, the price had doubled. By 2011, it had tripled. By 2012, Viagra went for $24 per pill.[36]

Most of these steep price increases for Viagra occurred after Eli Lilly brought Cialis to the market in 2003. The arrival of a competing ED drug should have exerted downward pressure on prices. Viagra and Cialis work by a similar mechanism, so men who responded well to one drug should have been happy to buy the other.[37] Many should have bought whichever drug was cheaper, and their willingness to change drugs should have encouraged Pfizer and Lilly to compete on the basis of price. It didn't. Pfizer and Lilly short-circuited comparison-shopping by charging similar amounts and raising prices in tandem:

> Cialis . . . was introduced in November of 2003 at a wholesale base cost of $8.10— the exact price of Viagra at that time. Since then, Pfizer and Lilly have raised the cost of Viagra and Cialis at about the same rate. Since 2005, however, Cialis has been slightly more expensive than Viagra, with a maximum difference of $1.50 per pill. Currently [in 2009], the wholesale base cost for Cialis is $16.67, or about 47 cents more per pill than Viagra. Since its introduction, the cost of Cialis has risen 105%.[38]

Erectile pricing even survived the arrival of a third big ED drug: Levitra. This is truly perplexing. With Pfizer and Lilly marching in lockstep, Bayer AG, Levitra's manufacturer, could have stolen the market by selling Levitra for less. It didn't. Instead, it matched Pfizer and Eli Lilly move for move. "When Levitra was introduced in 2003, it cost pharmacies $8.49 per pill," almost exactly the same as Viagra and Cialis.[39] In 2012, Levitra's price was over 300 percent higher, just like the other two. Bayer AG understood how the game was being played, so it marched in lockstep with the others.

Can this behavior be explained on any basis other than that the manufacturers coordinated their prices? AccessRX, an online pharmacy that is the source of some of our pricing information, offered two hypotheses. One was that charges went up because "consumers [were] willing to pay high prices. None of the top ED drugs ha[d] yet reached a price ceiling above which consumers won't go."[40] This explanation is unpersuasive, for a reason already explained. Competition is supposed to drive prices down to the lowest levels that sellers will accept. Consumers might be willing to spend more, but that is irrelevant to the price at which a drug should change hands in a competitive market.

AccessRX's second hypothesis centered on patents. Because only Pfizer could sell Viagra, only Eli Lilly could sell Cialis, and only Bayer AG could sell Levitra, each manufacturer could gouge its customers. This explanation for erectile pricing is no better than the first one. Its glaring flaw is that patents create exploitable monopolies only when there are no adequate substitutes for a drug. Viagra, Cialis, and Levitra *are* substitutes for one another. Consequently, men should have shifted to whichever drug was cheaper, exerting pressure on Pfizer, Lilly, and Bayer to compete for business by charging less. That each company had a patent on its particular ED drug should not have prevented competition from working.

To see the point, suppose you had a patent on Gala apples. Could you charge $100 a bag for them? Not when Fuji, Red Delicious, Ambrosia, Envy, and a host of other varieties sell for a whole lot less. If a bag of tasty Ambrosia apples costs $8, you might be able to charge a bit more for Galas—say $9—if consumers like them more. But if you tried to charge $100, you would get no buyers at all. Consumers would purchase other varieties, and your apples would rot on the shelves.

The same goes for Viagra, Cialis, and Levitra. Because the drugs are close substitutes, each manufacturer would have risked losing customers by charging more than the others. The only way they could all raise prices and hold onto market share was by acting in concert. And that is what they did. The fact that the drugs were patented doesn't explain how they were able to march in lockstep for so many years.

Erectile pricing occurs with other medicines too. Insulin is a drug used by millions of Americans afflicted with diabetes. It is off-patent and made by three companies, so it should be reasonably priced. It is not.

The past two decades have seen stunning price increases. Short-acting insulin, which cost about $21 in 1996, went for about $275 in 2017.[41] And, just as with ED drugs, the prices went up in lockstep, even though there were two companies making short-acting insulin. Prices for long-acting insulins, which also had two makers, rose in tandem too.[42]

## TIT FOR TAT AS A PRICING GAME

Why does erectile pricing happen in drug markets? Many medicines are made by only a few companies, all of which are repeat players in pricing games and have learned to employ a strategy known as "tit for tat." Whatever one company does, the others do in turn. When one raises prices, the others follow suit, knowing that if they play follow the leader, they will all get rich. The incentive to steal the market by charging less disappears because every manufacturer knows that other makers will cut their prices too, if it does. An outbreak of price competition would leave all manufacturers poorer—so they all raise prices instead of reducing them.

Ideally, tit-for-tat pricing would be unsustainable, and efforts to keep prices high would collapse, because individual producers could increase their profits by reducing their prices and stealing market share from their competitors. That appears to happen in the pharmaceutical market sector less often than it should.

Third-party payment contributes to this failure of competition. Heavily insured patients who fork over the same copays regardless of which drugs they use will not respond to rising prices by switching to lower-cost alternatives. They will buy what their doctors recommend, and their doctors will not care much about price, knowing that their patients are insured. Third-party payment may weaken drug makers' incentive to compete for market share.

Competition among pharma companies may also be less robust than it should be because they have learned not to invade each other's turf or, perhaps, because they face costs that discourage them from doing so. When Turing bought the rights to Daraprim, Shkreli bet millions of dollars that his company would make enough money by raising the drug's price to justify the investment. He would not have taken that

gamble had he thought that another company would rush in and undercut Turing's price.

Why was Shkreli so confident that no other company would compete? One reason was that the market for Daraprim was small. Only
about 9,000 prescriptions for it are written each year. That is probably
the main reason why, even before Shkreli showed up, only one company
was making the drug. Plus, any company that wanted to enter the market with a generic version of Daraprim would have had to spend time
and money obtaining FDA approval. These factors probably led Shkreli
to conclude that potential competitors would take a pass.

Shkreli's confidence may also have reflected the fact that extraordinary
price increases had become old hat for generic drug companies. A 2016
federal government report found that 315 of 1,441 established generics
had "at least one extraordinary price increase of 100 percent or more
between first quarter 2010 and first quarter 2015."[43] (Because manufacturers had hiked the prices for some of these drugs more than once, the
total number of extraordinary increases was actually 351.) Many of these
increases were truly enormous. "Out of the 351 extraordinary price
increases, 48 were 500 percent or higher and 15 were 1,000 percent or
higher."[44] Shkreli may have figured that competitors wouldn't undercut
Turing's price on Daraprim because they hadn't started price wars when
other generic companies engaged in price gouging.

Mylan, of EpiPen infamy, provides a nice case study of the power
drug manufacturers have to raise prices on generic drugs. In the first
half of 2016, Mylan raised prices for two dozen drugs by more than
20 percent and boosted prices for seven others by more than 100 percent.
It raised the price of ursodiol, used to treat gallstones, by 542 percent; the
price of metoclopramide, a treatment for gastroesophageal reflux disease,
by 444 percent; and the price of dicyclomine, which combats irrita-
ble bowel syndrome, by 400 percent.[45] Other generics that experienced
price hikes were captopril, a blood pressure treatment, which jumped
more than 2,700 percent; the asthma drug albuterol sulfate, whose price
rose more than 3,400 percent; and the antibiotic doxycycline, which
increased by a whopping 6,300 percent. All three increases occurred
over a period of just one year.[46]

For present purposes, the important point is not just that these extraordinary price spikes occurred; it is that prices stayed high long after they were raised because other makers did not compete. The simple story of competition driving down prices did not play out the way it usually does. As the Government Accountability Office (GAO) observed in the report on generics quoted above, "the extraordinary price increases generally persisted for at least 1 year and most had no downward movement after the extraordinary price increase." "Most" is an understatement. Of the 248 extraordinary price hikes that occurred between 2010 and 2014, 242 (98 percent) persisted for at least a year. Thus, after manufacturers raised the prices for these generic drugs by a factor of two or more, the prices stayed high, apparently because potential competitors refrained from starting price wars.

The frequency of extraordinary price increases is rising too. In the 2010–2011 period, 45 generic drugs had extraordinary price increases. From 2014 to 2015, 103 did—more than twice as many. Evidently, generic makers are learning that they can raise prices with impunity.

Is any of this illegal? Not necessarily. Antitrust law prohibits manufacturers from entering into anti-competitive agreements, such as fixing prices and dividing markets. But producers can legally play follow the leader when setting prices, and they can also voluntarily decline to compete with other manufacturers on any given product.

Whether illegal collusion occurred is currently under investigation.[47] Near the end of 2016, two former executives of Heritage Pharmaceuticals, Inc., pled guilty to price-fixing charges,[48] and 20 states filed a civil suit against Heritage, Mylan, Teva, and three other generic-drug makers, alleging that the defendants engaged in price fixing in the markets for antibiotics and diabetes treatments.[49]

Before closing this section, it is worth noting that Shkreli's gamble didn't pay off. He was indicted on securities fraud charges for unrelated wrongdoing, resigned his position at Turing, and was fired from the CEO position he held at another company, KaloBios. Also, soon after he raised Daraprim's price, Express Scripts, the country's largest pharmacy benefits manager, convinced a compounding pharmacy to sell a substitute product for $1 per pill.

Tim Worshall, an economist, offered the last development as evidence that drug markets continue to work, and competition certainly seems to have brought down the cost of Daraprim.[50] But the evidence shows that, when pharmaceutical companies raise prices for generic drugs, the increases usually stick. The puzzle is why, in the case of Daraprim, Express Scripts bothered to sponsor a competitor. Cost does not seem to be the answer. Express Scripts is an enormous company—number 22 on the Forbes 500 list in 2017. Turing's price for Daraprim would not have registered in Express Scripts' bottom line, even had it been much higher than it was.

So why did Express Scripts stick a finger in Shkreli's eye? Paraphrasing an old MasterCard ad:

The cost of Daraprim? $750.

The publicity to be gained by beating up the poster boy for pharma's pricing abuses? Priceless.

## If Patenting a Drug Once Is Good, Patenting It Repeatedly Is Terrific

Companies that make branded drugs like having monopolies and will do almost anything to protect them. A common strategy in the pharmaceutical game—known as "evergreening"—is to obtain a second patent before the first one expires.[51] Drug companies can obtain these secondary patents by tweaking their drugs in various ways. For example, the original patent on Prilosec, a remedy for heartburn, expired in 2001, but the manufacturer effectively extended its monopoly by getting a second patent on the pill's coating. The second patent lasted until 2007.[52] Another common tactic is to develop and patent a timed-release formulation. In each case, the drug manufacturer aggressively markets the new drug to physicians, switching as many patients as possible to the new pill. Once patients have been switched, generic entry (which is, by law, limited to the previous version of the drug) has a far smaller impact on the drug manufacturer's profits.

Some drug manufacturers take this strategy one step further. They withdraw the original drug to "encourage" physicians to put all of their

patients on the new one. This "hard switch" version of "product hopping" effectively eliminates the impact of generic competition, because
the old drug is no longer available. Although generic drug manufacturers and antitrust enforcers can go to court to challenge evergreening and
product hopping, doing so is costly and time-consuming. In the interim,
brand-name drugs will continue to fetch high prices, at the expense of
taxpayers and ordinary consumers.

Evergreening is widespread. According to the National Institute
for Health Care Management, roughly two-thirds of the 1,035 drugs
approved by the FDA from 1989 through 2000 were modified versions
of existing drugs. Looking at the period running from 2005 to 2015,
researchers Robin Feldman and Connie Wang found

> a startling departure from the classic conceptualization of intellectual
> property protection for pharmaceuticals. . . . Rather than creating
> new medicines, pharmaceutical companies are recycling and repur-
> posing old ones. Every year, at least 74% of the drugs associated with
> new patents in the FDA's records were not new drugs coming on
> the market, but existing drugs. . . . Of the roughly 100 best-selling
> drugs, almost 80% extended their protection at least once, with almost
> 50% extending the protection cliff more than once. . . . The problem
> is growing across time.[53]

Patents are supposed to encourage drug makers to take big risks by
investing in the original research that is needed to discover new drugs.
Far more often, though, they enable manufacturers to forestall generic competition by tweaking branded drugs that already exist. In other
words, drug makers are gaming the patent system to generate additional
profits on drugs that are already known to work. The deadweight social
losses caused by the high prices that these evergreening strategies help
maintain offset whatever benefits the tweaks may confer on patients.

The study by Feldman and Wang "definitively shows that stifling competition is not limited to a few pharma bad apples. Rather, it is a common
and pervasive problem endemic to the pharmaceutical industry."[54] A business practice this common must be profitable, and this one certainly is.
A study of popular brand-name drugs found that prices remained high

and even increased when manufacturers obtained line extensions after the original patents expired.[55] The gains were large. To pick but one example, during a 12-month period, Cardizem CD, a calcium-channel blocker used for the treatment of hypertension, generated more than $735 million in retail sales, the majority of which "could have been avoided if generic versions were used in lieu of expensive new extensions."[56]

## PAY-FOR-DELAY SETTLEMENTS

Evergreening isn't the only way that branded companies keep out generic competition. They can use "pay-for-delay" settlements to accomplish the same end. A recent Supreme Court case shows how the strategy works. In 2003, Solvay Pharmaceuticals obtained a patent on a testosterone drug called AndroGel. Later that year, two other drug companies, Actavis, Inc., and Paddock Laboratories, applied to the FDA for approval to sell a generic equivalent. Paddock later sold a part interest in its application to Par Pharmaceutical, another generic drug manufacturer.

Congress wanted to encourage generic drug manufacturers to challenge patents that might be invalid, so it gave the first generic manufacturer that files a certificate with the FDA 180 days of marketing exclusivity if it proves in court that a patent is invalid. For example, if Actavis had successfully challenged Solvay's patent on AndroGel, it would have received the exclusive right to sell a generic equivalent for six months.

But Actavis didn't do that. Instead, after locking horns with Solvay in patent litigation, Actavis and Solvay voluntarily settled the litigation on the following terms in 2006:

> Actavis agreed that it would not bring its generic [version of AndroGel] to market until August 31, 2015, 65 months before Solvay's patent expired. . . . Actavis also agreed to promote AndroGel to urologists. The other generic manufacturers [i.e., Paddock and Par] made roughly similar promises. And Solvay agreed to pay millions of dollars to each generic [maker]—$12 million in total to Paddock; $60 million in total to Par; and an estimated $19–$30 million annually, for nine years, to Actavis.[57]

Got that? Solvay promised to pay Actavis, Paddock, and Par hundreds of millions of dollars to stay out of the market for nine years, during which time they would encourage urologists to prescribe Solvay's AndroGel. Drug monopolies are so valuable that brand–name manufacturers are willing to pay enormous bribes to keep potential competitors from invading their turf. The money for these bribes came from taxpayers and everyone else who paid artificially high prices for AndroGel.

But why couldn't another generic drug company just start making testosterone and steal the market from Solvay? That would be illegal. As noted above, Congress gave the first company that files a certificate and challenges a patent (here, Actavis) the exclusive right to market generic testosterone for 180 days—and the 180-day period begins to run only when *that company* enters the market. Because Actavis agreed to postpone its entry for nine years when settling with Solvay, other generic drug companies would have to wait nine and a half years to start selling their versions. By bribing Actavis, Solvay blocked *all* competitors, and preserved its lock on the market.

Working together, Solvay and Actavis were more powerful than either was alone. Solvay's patent gave it control of the market for testosterone gel. Actavis' FDA filing gave it the power to prevent other companies from competing with Solvay, even if Solvay's patent was invalid. Solvay's lawsuit against Actavis was really a means of creating a contract—the settlement agreement—that ensured lasting cooperation between the two. Solvay showered Actavis with riches because Actavis helped it preserve a monopoly on testosterone gel that was worth far more.

If you think Solvay's pay-to-delay settlement smells fishy, you're in good company. The U.S. Federal Trade Commission (FTC) sued all of the companies involved in the deal, accusing them of engaging in an illegal restraint of trade. The federal district court dismissed the FTC's complaint, but the Supreme Court reinstated it in 2013. A trial will eventually decide whether the FTC prevails. The central factual question is whether the companies sought to impede competition or attempted in good faith to resolve a lawsuit over patent validity.

Many settlements raise this question. From 2005 to 2009, there were 66 such deals, according to a 2010 FTC report entitled "Pay-for-Delay:

How Drug Company Pay-Offs Cost Consumers Billions."[58] Back then, the FTC estimated that these competition-stifling agreements cost consumers $3.5 billion a year in higher prices for prescriptions drugs. In more recent years, the number of settlements has risen—there were 40 pay-to-delay settlements in 2012 alone—and the burden on consumers has multiplied. In 2013, two consumer advocacy groups estimated that pay-to-delay settlements involving 20 popular name-brand drugs cost consumers $98 billion by delaying sales of generic versions.[59]

Unfortunately, the Supreme Court used the wrong standard when assessing the Solvay litigation. The Court asked whether the brand-name manufacturers that paid generic drug companies to stay out of their markets were trying to limit competition or settle lawsuits in good faith. The brand-name drug companies that are involved in these lawsuits are seeking to maximize their profits, first by patenting the products and then by keeping the patents alive as long as possible, using pay-for-delay settlements (and other means). Any settlement that keeps a patent in place necessarily prevents generic competition. It follows that all these companies are, in fact, trying to limit competition. But, when an original patent, which also prevents generic competition, is obtained in good faith, how can an attempt to preserve the monopoly in the face of a legal challenge differ qualitatively from the earlier attempt to get the patent itself? Finally, even if the FTC prevails in this case, its victory will come more than a decade after the settlement between Solvay and Actavis.

### PITY THE GOUT SUFFERERS

It should be clear by now that pharmaceutical companies will use all available tools to gain pricing power. And there are more tools than just patents and cornering markets for generics. Another option involves proving that existing drugs work. We are serious. A drug maker can gain a monopoly on the supply of an existing drug just by showing that it helps patients.

A famous example of the use of this strategy involves colchicine, a medicine widely used to treat gout, rheumatism, and other inflammatory illnesses. Colchicine was first described as a medical treatment around 1500 BCE. Benjamin Franklin, himself a gout sufferer, is said to have brought *Colchicum* plants back to the United States after serving as envoy to France. The medicine has been widely available in pill form here since the 1800s.

Colchicine used to be cheap. For years, a pill cost about a dime. Then, in January 2011, the price suddenly increased to $5.[60] At the same time, generic manufacturers exited the market. The only version available in the United States was a branded drug named Colcrys, manufactured by Mutual Pharmaceutical, Inc. (MP). Overnight, colchicine was transformed from an inexpensive medicine with many producers into an expensive drug with only a single source.

How did a drug company gain a stranglehold on the market for this ancient medication? By proving that it worked. You might think there was never any doubt about this, and many gout sufferers would agree. Because colchicine was so old, no company could patent it, so no company had ever tested its efficacy in the sort of clinical trials the FDA requires for new drugs. Although the FDA requires proof of effectiveness for drugs brought to market after 1961, drugs already being sold to the public at that time were grandfathered. Consequently, many old drugs had no formal FDA approval. Colchicine was one of them.

The FDA wanted to do something about these unapproved drugs, so in 2006, it launched its Unapproved Drugs Initiative. It warned manufacturers that, because colchicine and other old drugs were technically unapproved, their grandfathered status could be revoked at any time. It then offered the companies a bribe in the form of a three-year exclusive on the right to sell any old drug they proved to be effective.

MP took the bait. It conducted a small study of the effect of colchicine involving 185 patients who were followed for one week, and then it applied for approval with the FDA.[61] In late 2010, the FDA granted MP's application and warned all other manufacturers to stop shipping colchicine.[62] Having become the sole supplier, MP raised the price from 10 cents to $5.[63] MP incurred little cost and effectively no risk in obtaining its monopoly position. As Dr. Edward Fudman, a rheumatologist, observed, "There [were] over 16,000 articles on Pub Med for colchicine, with 254 indexed as clinical trials. . . . Doing one trial in patients and a few drug interaction studies [did not] justify marketing exclusivity and a 50-fold increase in price."[64]

When it comes to marketing exclusivity, colchicine is actually a twofer. It is both an old drug and an "orphan" drug. Orphan drugs are medicines that treat rare diseases. They are called orphans because when an illness affects few people, the market is too small for most drug companies to take on the expense of developing and obtaining approval for new treatments. To encourage the development of drugs to treat these orphaned populations, Congress enacted the Orphan Drug Act (ODA), which gives manufacturers seven years of marketing exclusivity plus other incentives, including federal grants, tax credits for clinical trial costs, and a waiver of application fees.[65]

In the case of colchicine, the rare disease is Familial Mediterranean Fever (FMF), a painful and potentially lethal autoimmune illness that afflicts about 100,000 people worldwide. By holding clinical trials, MP gained a lock on sales of colchicine to FMF victims as well. Again, MP did not invent colchicine; it just tested its efficacy and safety. This modest expense justified a modest reward. But, instead, the FDA provided three years of marketing exclusivity for all purposes other than the treatment of FMF and a seven-year monopoly for FMF.

Not surprisingly, MP's gambit harmed both patient populations. Researchers at the Harvard Medical School studied about 217,000 enrollees in an insurance database who were diagnosed with gout or FMF from 2009 to 2012. They found that, owing to the price increase, the likelihood of receiving a prescription for colchicine dropped by 0.5 percent per month for gout suffers and by 7.6 percent per month for sufferers of FMF. At the same time, medical spending for the two groups rose by 55 percent and 38 percent, respectively. In other words, "the FDA action resulted in a reduction in colchicine initiation and an increase in cost."[66] Giving MP a monopoly caused a huge social loss.

A more recent orphan drug example involved deflazacort, a treatment for muscular dystrophy that has long been available in other countries for about $1,000 a year. After Marathon Pharmaceuticals gained FDA approval for deflazacort as an orphan drug in 2017, Jeffrey Aronin, the company's CEO, announced that the drug would henceforth cost $89,000 a year in the United States.[67]

No one should have been surprised. "In 2014, the average annual price tag for orphan drugs was $111,820."[68] When Express Scripts, the pharmacy benefits manager, analyzed the orphan drugs in its formulary, it found four that cost $840,000 a year and another 29 that cost more than $336,000 a year. That is why applications to have the FDA designate medicines as orphan drugs have gone through the roof. In 2015, the agency received a record 472 such requests and awarded 354 designations, 22 percent more than in the previous year.[69]

Researchers contend that drug makers are gaming the ODA by using it to obtain monopolies on drugs they expect to be prescribed widely. As evidence, they offer the fact that 7 of the 10 drugs that achieved blockbuster status in 2014—meaning that their sales exceeded $1 billion—were approved as orphans but were then prescribed by physicians for off-label uses.[70] For example,

> rituximab, which was initially FDA approved for use in the treatment of follicular non-Hodgkin's lymphoma, is the number 1 selling medication approved as an orphan drug. It is currently used to treat a wide variety of conditions, ranks as the 12th all-time bestselling medication in the United States, and generated over $3.7 billion in US sales in 2014.[71]

In the words of Martin Makary, a professor of health policy at Johns Hopkins School of Medicine,

> What's happening is that a drug company develops a medication to treat a specific cancer [that afflicts a small population], and will submit [it] to the FDA as intended for a very targeted subset of the cancer population. . . . Once a drug is approved, companies can seek additional indications for populations [that are far larger]. And this is a pattern with most of the orphan drugs approved by the FDA.[72]

In short, drug makers are gaming the orphan drug approval process. They are using it to gain monopolies over drugs that are used to treat much larger patient populations than the ODA was intended to help.

## THE PERFECT STORM

Colchicine is hardly the only old medication whose price skyrocketed after FDA approval. The price of potassium chloride, used to treat low potassium levels in the blood, nearly doubled after Endo obtained the exclusive right to market the liquid version. When Flamel Technologies secured FDA approval for neostigmine methylsulfate, a medicine that reverses the effects of anesthesia, it raised the price from $17 a vial to nearly $100. The price of vasopressin, a medication used in cases of cardiac arrest, increased 10-fold after Pan Sterile obtained FDA approval for it in 2013.[73]

An especially interesting story centers on 17OHP, a drug that helps prevent premature births. It was available from compounding pharmacies and was exceedingly cheap.[74] Until 2011, that is. That's when the FDA approved K-V Pharmaceutical Company's (K-V) application to manufacture 17OHP as an orphan drug.[75] Obstetricians and patient advocacy groups like the March of Dimes (MOD) welcomed the approval because they expected K-V to standardize the manufacturing process and broaden access. They weren't aware of K-V's plan to maximize its profits, which it acted upon the moment the FDA's approval gave it the exclusive right to market the drug. Overnight, K-V raised the price of 17OHP from $300 for a 20-week course to $29,000. This took the annual cost of treating the 130,000 or so women who need 17OHP from $41.7 million to $4 billion. The vast majority of the extra money was pure profit for K-V, a fact that its stock price reflected. It went from $1.50 a share to nearly $13.[76]

But K-V didn't collect the money. In fact, the company went bankrupt in 2012.[77] In a stunning turn of events, the FDA reversed course and allowed compounding pharmacies to sell 17OHP too. Two days after the FDA announced that decision, K-V cut the price of 17OHP in half.[78]

Why did the FDA act? Much of the credit belongs to senators Sherrod Brown (D-OH) and Amy Klobuchar (D-MN), who called for a price gouging investigation after patients and physicians complained that K-V was ripping them off. At a hearing before the Senate Appropriations Committee, they raked FDA Commissioner Margaret Hamburg over the coals.[79] Presumably, Hamburg then told her subordinates to make the problem disappear.

K-V's checkered history didn't help either. The federal government had previously investigated K-V for making and distributing adulterated and unapproved drugs, leading to a consent decree that bound the company, two of its subsidiaries, and its principal officers.[80] Then, in March of 2011, as the FDA's 17OHP ruling was causing a ruckus, K-V's former chairman pled guilty to violations of the Food, Drug and Cosmetic Act for manufacturing oversized morphine pills.[81] His punishments included $1.9 million in fines and forfeitures and a 30-day jail term. As if this wasn't enough, the Justice Department was concurrently investigating K-V's Ethex subsidiary for defrauding Medicare and Medicaid by misrepresenting that two of its drugs were FDA approved when, in fact, they weren't.[82] We're guessing the FDA preferred opening the market for 17OHP to explaining why it put preterm babies at risk by helping a sketchy drug company with a criminal past fleece pregnant women.

K-V's use and abuse of the MOD added fuel to the flames.[83] K-V was a large contributor to the MOD. So, when it sought FDA approval for its brand of 17OHP, the MOD supported its application. Then, after the stunning price increase was announced, the MOD found that it had helped a greedy corporation put premature infants at risk. To salvage its reputation, the MOD's president demanded prompt action by K-V and threatened to "pursue alternative strategies" to ensure ready availability of 17OHP.[84] This appears to have been code for urging the FDA to allow other companies to enter the market.

Pregnant women. Premature infants. An angry March of Dimes. A dodgy and scandal-plagued drug company. A criminal guilty plea. Morphine. Absurd corporate greed. Politicians sensing blood in the water. This was a perfect storm—and nothing less could have prevented K-V's owners from becoming rich.

We know that it took extreme circumstances to stop K-V because other drug companies with similar exclusive rights over old drugs have fleeced consumers with impunity. Adams Respiratory Therapeutics reportedly raised the price of guaifenesin (i.e., Mucinex) 700 percent after gaining its stranglehold.[85] ACTH, a treatment for infantile spasms used since the 1950s, rose in price from $1,650 to $23,000 for a single vial "in what the company described as an 'orphan-style pricing model.'"[86] The best gauge for the impact of market exclusivity? Forty-three orphan drugs achieved blockbuster status—with sales exceeding $1 billion— after being approved by the FDA.[87] With revenues like these to be had, no wonder so many orphans were being adopted.

Marketing exclusivity hit asthma sufferers especially hard: "Pulmicort, a steroid inhaler, generally retails for over $175 in the United States, while pharmacists in Britain buy the identical product for about $20."[88] A month's worth of Rhinocort Aqua cost more than $250 here when it sold for less than $7 in Europe.[89]

Again, none of this should surprise anyone. When a private drug company has a monopoly on a product, it will charge monopoly prices. That's how it maximizes profits, and maximizing profits is what companies do. That's an observation, not a judgment. Businesses that produce pharmaceuticals are neither better nor worse than businesses of other sorts. Give a business a monopoly on air travel, electricity, cable TV, or groceries and it will behave like a monopolist. (If you noticed that every time you asked for a higher salary your employer promptly obliged, what would *you* do?) Drug companies are no different. The mystery is why anyone expects them to behave differently.

NICE PLANET YOU'VE GOT HERE—SHAME IF ANYTHING HAPPENED TO IT

Consider a famous example involving albuterol, another widely used treatment for asthma, which afflicts about 40 million Americans. Albuterol is dispensed by means of inhalers—hand-held pumps that deliver measured doses of mist for people to breathe in. Prior to the mid-2000s, all inhalers were powered by chlorofluorocarbons (CFCs). These inhalers worked just fine, but CFCs were found to be depleting the ozone layer, and there was strong international support for banning their production and use. Of course, inhalers accounted for a tiny fraction of the CFCs that were being released into the atmosphere—less than 0.01 percent.[90]

Manufacturers typically hate environmental regulations that require them to redesign their products, and many of them did oppose restrictions on CFCs. But not the pharmaceutical industry. It *supported* the CFC ban. Eight pharmaceutical firms even formed an organization called the International Pharmaceutical Aerosol Consortium (IPAC) to come up with a new ozone-friendly propellant.[91] Why was the industry so gung-ho? Because the need to develop new inhalers that operated without CFCs meant that pharmaceutical companies could get new patents on inhaler-delivered drugs that were about to go generic. The CFC ban thus gave drug companies a perfectly legal and practically mandatory way to evergreen their patents.

Perversely, the new inhalers they came up with were powered by hydrofluorocarbons (HFCs). HFCs don't break down the ozone layer, but they do contribute to climate change. Seeing this, several scientists and one generic drug company proposed that the old CFC-based inhalers be exempted from the international ban. Given the tiny quantity of CFCs that inhalers released into the air, an exemption would have made perfect sense. But it would also have spoiled the drug companies' plan to evergreen their patents, *so the drug companies lobbied against it*.[92] Got that? Drug companies spent money to ensure that the government would force them to redesign their products. It worked, too. In 2005, the FDA approved an outright ban on CFC-based inhalers.

The result? Generic drug companies were kept out of the market for inhaler-delivered medications, and the prices for those medications went through the roof. "Albuterol, one of the oldest asthma medicines, typically costs $50 to $100 per inhaler in the United States, but it was less than $15 a decade ago, before it was re-patented."[93] Nationwide, the FDA estimated that the switch to new inhalers increased health care spending by $8 billion over a ten-year period, while conferring a trivial benefit on the environment. And whatever minimal good may have been done for the ozone layer was offset by the aggravation of climate change stemming from the use of HFCs. Everyone lost. Except Big Pharma.

### DEATH WITH INDIGNITY

Six states allow people with terminal illnesses to end their lives on their own terms, using drugs prescribed by physicians.[94] Secobarbital, a generic drug that has been on the market for decades, is commonly used for this purpose. It should therefore be cheap, and it once was. "In 2009, a lethal dose of secobarbital (100 capsules) cost less than $200 (less than $2 per capsule)."[95] Today, however, the same amount of the drug costs $3,000. Why? At first, the price crept up slowly, rising to $1,500. Then Valeant Pharmaceuticals acquired the rights to make secobarbital and doubled the price. The timing coincided with the introduction of California's End of Life Option Act. From Valeant's perspective, people in straits so desperate that they want to end their lives are just one more group of buyers waiting to be gouged.

Rising prices for drugs (both branded and generic) are impoverishing Americans. Although there are many reasons why "drug prices keep defying the law of gravity," monopolies obtained by patents and other means are a primary cost driver.[96] We let drug companies acquire monopolies in a system that is designed to pay whatever they ask, then we are surprised that they act like monopolists and take us for every thing they can. We suggest some fixes for these problems in later chapters. For now, the main lesson is that health care providers do and always will seek to maximize their profits, just like businesses of other kinds. Any suggestion to the contrary is patent nonsense.

## CHAPTER 2: NO LIMITS

### PRICE IS NO OBJECT

Chapter 1 focused on strategies that makers of branded and generic drugs use to raise prices, with special focus on patents and other monopolies. But what about a drug's initial launch price? We now turn to this issue.

Pharmaceutical manufacturers, like all profit-seeking businesses, charge as much as they can for their products. But, unlike other businesses, pharmaceutical companies sell their wares into markets where there are no meaningful limits on the prices they can charge. This is why one often hears that drug companies raise prices simply because they can.

The absence of a price constraint explains why new drugs are often introduced at prices that will impoverish consumers—while making the companies that sell them rich. Consider the recent batch of drugs that treat hepatitis C, a disease that afflicts more than 3 million Americans. For years, it was treated with interferon, with unimpressive results (and significant side effects). Then, in 2014, Gilead Sciences introduced Sovaldi, the first real cure. Gilead marketed it at the astronomical price of $1,000 per pill, which meant that a full course of treatment cost $84,000.[1]

"Never before has a drug been priced this high to treat a patient population this large," observed Steve Miller, the chief medical officer at Express

Scripts, the country's largest pharmacy benefits manager.[2] It would have cost $268 billion to buy Sovaldi for all Americans infected with hepatitis C. To put that number in perspective, in 2012—just two years earlier—Americans spent $261 billion on all prescription drugs *combined*.[3]

Sovaldi helped Gilead rack up about $18 billion in profits in 2015.[4] And it wasn't the only super-priced drug that Gilead was selling. A year after introducing Sovaldi, Gilead began marketing Harvoni, a two-drug combo that paired Sovaldi with another agent. Harvoni cost $94,500, "a jaw-dropping price that raised howls of anger from insurers and spurred calls for drug price controls."[5] But Gilead had payers over a barrel. Sovaldi and Harvoni were the only effective hepatitis C treatments available. Consequently, they set the standard of care, and doctors immediately began prescribing them. Payers that denied access to these medications would be forcing hepatitis C victims to suffer physically and emotionally, and they would have sentenced some of them to death.

But at $1,000 or more per pill, access to Sovaldi and Harvoni would bust the budgets of most countries. In England, the National Health Service (NHS) "caused delays in providing treatment to many of the estimated 160,000 hepatitis C patients, while others were unable to obtain the medications due to rationing."[6] High-risk patients were treated first while nonurgent patients were made to wait. This triaging occurred because the NHS didn't have enough money to treat everyone. An NHS spokesman candidly observed,

> It is utterly naive to pretend that the NHS could instead somehow have "magicked up" several billion pounds in one year, for this one condition, without that meaning damaging cuts in other critical services such as mental health, cancer or primary care. That's not a failure of planning; that's just the reality of the financial circumstances facing us.

In the United States, state Medicaid programs shelled out $1.3 billion for Sovaldi in 2014.[7] But they too rationed access to these medicines. Given the potential financial exposure, rationing was inevitable. By some estimates, half of those with hepatitis C were on Medicaid or other taxpayer-funded insurance.[8]

Hepatitis C sufferers naturally wanted these medicines immediately. They filed class action lawsuits in which they accused Medicaid programs and other payers of violating the law by refusing to cover medicines that were approved by the U.S. Food and Drug Administration (FDA).[9]

Veterans were also left out in the cold. About 190,000 vets have hepatitis C. Covering them all would have required a massive increase in funding for the U.S. Department of Veterans Affairs (VA)—which wasn't going to happen. To give but one example, the VA's Greater Los Angeles Healthcare System treats 4,000 vets with hepatitis C. At $84,000 apiece, the cost of giving Sovaldi to all of them would have exceeded the facility's total budget. Many infected veterans were therefore denied a curative treatment.

Prisoners were excluded too. The Centers for Disease Control and Prevention estimates that "one-third of the 2.2 million people in jails and prisons in the United States have hepatitis C."[10] But prison facilities could not handle the financial shock of paying for Sovaldi or Harvoni, so less than 1 percent of infected state prisoners were given the drugs.[11]

Medicare was in a different situation. It could not ration access, because it is set up to pay—and pay, and pay. The result was that Medicare spending on "catastrophic" prescription drug coverage (where Medicare foots the bill for drug costs above a high threshold) skyrocketed. From 2013 to 2015, spending on catastrophic prescription drug coverage went from $27.7 billion to $51.3 billion, an 85 percent increase.[12] Sovaldi and Harvoni were major cost drivers, accounting for $0 in spending in 2013, $3.5 billion in 2014, and $7.5 billion in 2015.[13]

> "The incentive is to price it as high as they can," said Jim Yocum, senior vice president of Connecture, Inc., a company that tracks drug prices. Medicare is barred from negotiating prices, "so you max out your pricing and most of that risk is covered by the federal government."[14]

Of course, with all pharmaceutical companies jacking up their rates, the impact on total spending is enormous. Medicare pays for almost one-third of all retail drugs, and spending through Part D is rising at 7 percent per year.[15] Sen. Chuck Grassley dryly observed, "it may be that some drug companies are taking advantage of government programs to maximize their market share."[16]

What about the costs incurred by private insurers, which are ultimately reflected in subscribers' premiums? Sovaldi, Harvoni, and the other super-expensive drugs we discuss below didn't affect their costs immediately, partly because many insurers refused to pay for them or limited access to the sickest patients at the highest risk of dying. Express Scripts flatly refused to cover Harvoni. It steered patients to AbbVie's Viekira Pak, a competitor that reached that market later and costs thousands of dollars less.[17] But the costs are likely to mount with time, as insurers come under political pressure to pay for super-expensive drugs. Given time, Big Pharma will bankrupt us all.

Why were Sovaldi and Harvoni so expensive? Everyone wants to know. The pills are cheap to produce. They cost about $1 each to make, according to a 2015 Senate report that was based on the records of Pharmasset, the company that Gilead purchased to acquire the rights to Sovaldi.[18] The same report put total research costs associated with Sovaldi—including those incurred by both Pharmasset and Gilead—at less than $1 billion. Gilead's revenues on sales of Sovaldi returned that amount in just a few months. Even factoring in the cost of Gilead's unsuccessful research, Sovaldi is priced far higher than Gilead's research and development (R&D) costs could ever justify.

Gilead argues that at $84,000 Sovaldi is still a good deal because, by curing hepatitis C, it reduces the number of liver transplants and other expensive medical treatments infected people will need. In other words, Solvadi confers value that exceeds its cost. We addressed this argument in Chapter 1. When new and innovative products are sold in competitive markets, their prices are forced down to the lowest levels their makers can accept while still earning a profit. The benefits the products generate for consumers set a ceiling on the amounts that consumers will pay, but real sales prices normally fall well below the ceiling, as a result of competition. By saying that Sovaldi saves money, Gilead is simply deflecting attention from the fact that it is profiting wildly from sales of the drug.

An employee of Express Scripts made the same point in a column entitled "The Sovaldi Tax: Gilead Can't Justify The Price It's Asking

For Hepatitis C Therapy."[19] As he noted, if Solvadi is worth $84,000 because of downstream health savings, then "all antibiotics have been vastly underpriced since the introduction of penicillin some 60 years ago." See the point? Every medical treatment (indeed, every good or service of any kind) that is worth buying generates benefits that consumers value above its price. That is why consumers buy them.

Antibiotics are a great example. They've generated trillions of dollars' worth of benefits by preventing and curing infections and by saving countless lives. But in competitive markets, antibiotics are priced on the basis of what it costs to make them, not in light of the benefits they yield. Competition pushes prices down to producers' costs, and consumers enjoy the "surplus"—that is, the difference between the actual price and the highest price they would willingly pay. That's why competitive markets are famously pro-consumer. They *minimize* sellers' profits.

Sen. Bernie Sanders, the former Democratic presidential candidate, once published a missive stating that Gilead's $1,000 per pill price for Sovaldi was, "pure and simple, an abuse of monopoly power." He urged the VA to "break the patent" on the drug by invoking a federal law that would have permitted other companies to manufacture the drug for use by the VA.[20] The VA did not act on the suggestion; but, when Gilead went about trying to justify Sovaldi's price in the way it did, it as much as admitted that Sanders was right. The company sought to maximize its profits by charging as much as it thought it could get away with, and then used a phony argument to hide what it was doing.

## This Is Not Capitalism

When denouncing the price of Sovaldi, Senator Sanders also took aim at John Martin, Gilead's CEO. He claimed that Gilead put Martin's $190 million compensation package ahead of the welfare of America's veterans. Now Sanders was engaging in bad economic analysis, coupled with political grandstanding. The directors and officers of Gilead are supposed to run the company for the benefit of its shareholders. The responsibility of caring for America's veterans rests with the U.S. government, not Gilead.

And the shareholders are doing very well. After Gilead spent $11 billion to acquire Pharmasset, the company that invented Sovaldi, its stock went through the roof. Future sales of hepatitis C drugs have been said to account for at least half of Gilead's $127 billion market capitalization.[21]

John Martin's net worth has skyrocketed too. Sovaldi launched him onto Bloomberg's Billionaires Index.[22] That may irk Bernie Sanders, a committed socialist, but great wealth does not bother committed capitalists like us. We believe that enormous risks justify enormous rewards when ambitious undertakings succeed. *If* Pharmasset/Gilead took big risks by inventing and testing Sovaldi, then big rewards are warranted, just as they are when companies invent and bring to market other new products, like electric cars, smartphones, or flat screen TVs. Maybe Senator Sanders doesn't understand that, but anyone with a basic knowledge of economics will get the point.

How big a risk Pharmasset/Gilead took is, however, an open question. Public funds helped pay for the research that led to the invention of Sovaldi. Much of the original work on hepatitis C was done in universities by academics who received grant funding from the National Institutes of Health (NIH). Raymond Schinazi, one of the scientists whose work the NIH supported, founded Pharmasset in the late 1990s after leaving his position at the Emory School of Medicine. Over 20 years, his lab received at least $7.7 million from the NIH.[23] After acquiring Pharmasset, Gilead spent tens of millions of dollars to complete Sovaldi's clinical trials, but scientists from the NIH were involved in those trials too.[24] These facts complicate any judgment of how much risk Pharmasset/Gilead actually incurred.

What is true of Gilead and Sovaldi is also true of other pharma companies and other drugs. About half of the most transformative drugs invented during the past 25 years had their origins in research that was supported with public funds.[25] When a group of prominent doctors accused Vertex Pharmaceuticals of overcharging for Orkambi, a two-drug combination of cystic fibrosis medications that costs $259,000 per patient per year, Stuart Arbuckle, Vertex's chief commercial officer, fired back by arguing that the research needed to produce new drugs "is highly expensive and risky."[26] As a generalization, that is surely correct. But, as the doctors noted in response, Vertex didn't develop its

cystic fibrosis treatments alone. They argued that the company was prof-
iting from support provided by others, including the NIH and the Cystic
Fibrosis Foundation, both of which helped underwrite basic research.[27]
Vertex certainly incurred costs and bore risks, but whether they justify
Orkambi's price is hard to determine.

The list of drugs that were developed in part with public funds
is lengthy and includes several that generated enormous revenues for
pharma companies. Pfizer reportedly earned $77 billon on sales of Xala-
tan, Lyrica, and Enbrel, all of which "were discovered as a result of federally funded academic research."[28] Gilead Sciences made billions on HIV
drugs that "include emtricitabine, a drug discovered at Emory University under a federally funded research grant."[29] Johnson & Johnson is said
to have made "one third of its pharmaceutical revenue between 2011 and
2015 (about $30 billion) from sales of Remicade—a federally funded dis-
covery made at New York University."[30] Many examples could be added
to these. Because pharma companies draw heavily upon public-funded
research, it is difficult to quantify the risks they incur.

Government domination of the demand side of the market further
complicates the picture. Only in the health care sector can a company
charge whatever it wants for an FDA-approved product and be confident
that public payers will fork over the money. In other markets, demand
curves slope downward—meaning that, as the price gets higher, fewer
customers want the product. Gilead ran no such risk. A similar dynamic
also explains why Pharmasset was worth $11 billion. Had substantial
sales of Sovaldi not been guaranteed at whatever price Gilead decided to
charge, Pharmasset would have been worth far less.

Finally, looking at the big picture, one might well conclude that
pharma companies are not high-risk operations at all. That is the conclusion that Stan Finkelstein and Peter Temin reach in *Reasonable R X:
Solving the Drug Price Crisis*. They point out that, although research is
risky at the level of individual drugs, no similar risk exists at the company level for large firms. To the contrary, the stocks of big drug companies have performed better than those of comparable companies in other
industries and have grown consistently, across both companies and years.
Investors in large drug makers haven't taken big risks.[31] Finkelstein and

Temin offer several explanations for this finding, including the pricing strategies that drug companies employ and the law of large numbers, which ensures a predictable flow of discoveries when companies test hundreds of thousands of molecules.

The idea that large risks merit large rewards is certainly true, but it doesn't apply to drug companies in quite the same way that it applies to others. Public support for research and the dominance of public payers reduce drug companies' risks enormously, making it difficult to assess whether the returns on brand-name drugs bear any reasonable relationship to the risks and costs actually incurred. That said, the fact that many pharmaceuticals had some amount of public support during their development does not justify breaking patents at the whim of public officials either. That would undermine the incentive to innovate by making patent rights unreliable. It would also expose the United States to lawsuits under the Takings Clause of the Constitution. We discuss an alternative way of incentivizing drug makers in Chapter 19.

### THE COMING PRICE CRAZINESS

Sovaldi is neither the only specialty drug on the market nor the most expensive. In 2014, columnist Joe Nocera wrote about Kalydeco, a treatment for cystic fibrosis that works wonderfully for the 2,000 or so suffers who have a specific genetic mutation. Kalydeco costs $300,000 a year—more than five times the median household income—and people have to take it for their entire lives. It would cost $600 million a year just to treat this small population. Nocera asked the relevant question: "How are we, as a society, going to pay for it?"[32] Regrettably, he gave no answer.

The number of expensive specialty drugs being brought to market makes the need for an answer especially urgent.

- Blincyto, a chemotherapy agent for acute lymphoblastic leukemia, fetches $178,000 for a standard course, making it the most expensive cancer treatment in the world.[33]
- A year's supply of Gleevec, another leukemia agent, costs $106,000.[34]

- Keytruda, made by Merck, costs $150,000 per year.[35]
- Opdivo and Yervoy, both made by Bristol-Myers Squibb, run $143,000 and $120,000, respectively.[36]
- Perjeta, made by Roche, works in tandem with Herceptin, and the combination costs $188,000 for a typical 18-month treatment. Pairing Perjecta with Kadcyla, another new drug, will cost even more.[37]
- Spinraza, a new treatment for spinal muscular atrophy, is projected to cost $750,000 for the first year of treatment and $375,000 a year after that.[38]
- Ravicti and Carbaglu, both of which are used to treat metabolic disorders, cost $794,000 and $585,000 per patient per year, respectively.[39]
- Lumizyme, which treats a condition that causes progressive muscle weakness, runs $626,000 per patient per year.[40]
- Actimmune costs $572,000 per patient per year. It treats conditions that can disrupt normal immune system functioning and normal bone formation.[41]
- Soliris, which prevents the destruction of red blood cells, costs $543,000 per patient per year.[42]

All these medications target orphan populations. For example, about 1,000 people a year are diagnosed with the kind of leukemia for which Blincyto is appropriate. Consequently, unless prescribed in large volumes for off-label uses, none of these drugs are individually likely to break the bank.

Even so, their cost is concerning. One reason is that many of these drugs confer few benefits on patients. "The 72 cancer therapies approved from 2002 through 2014 gave patients only 2.1 more months of life than older drugs," but 11 of the 12 approved in 2012 were priced above $100,000 per course of treatment.[43] The tally was even higher in 2016, when the approved drugs cost an average of $171,000 a year. "Although the high prices can lead patients to think they're getting the Mercedes of cancer drugs, research shows that a medication's price has no relationship to how well it works."[44] The situation is so bad that "[a] group of academic researchers has demanded an end to cancer medicines costing more than $100,000 a year."[45]

Drug makers don't seem to care what academics think about pricing. Consider the new CAR (chimeric antigen receptor) T-cell cancer treatments that are coming on line. Kymriah, a therapy for leukemia, provides an obvious example. After obtaining FDA approval, Novartis set Kymriah's price at $475,000, a level that, in the words of Dr. Leonard Saltz, chief of gastrointestinal oncology at Memorial Sloan Kettering Cancer Center in New York, "shattered oncology drug pricing norms."[46] And that's just the price of the drug. Kymriah requires lengthy hospital stays and can have serious side effects, incuding immune system reactions, stroke-like symptoms, and coma. Some patients who receive it need bone marrow transplants and other expensive procedures. The total cost per patient could reach $1.5 million. The only good news is that Novartis will charge for the drug only if patients go into remission within one month of treatment—but it is not clear whether hospitals will pass those savings on to patients and their insurers. Kymriah is also only the first of many other CAR T-cell treatments that are currently being developed—21 according to the most recent report.[47]

The number of pricey specialty drugs is truly alarming and makes their aggregate cost enormous. According to a 2016 report by the Center for Policy and Research at America's Health Insurance Plans, the health insurance industry's main lobbying shop, "specialty drugs account for less than 2 percent of all prescriptions, [but] they make up roughly 30 percent of spending on all prescription drugs."[48] "That is projected to grow to 50% in 2017, according to Express Scripts, the pharmacy benefits manager."[49] The growing number of high-priced specialty drugs is a primary reason that total spending on prescription drugs is expected to exceed $590 billion by 2020, up from $337 billion in 2015.[50]

An even bigger problem is the precedent these drugs set. If an anti-cancer drug can sell for $150,000, why shouldn't a new medicine that treats a more common illness or condition command the same price? If society is willing to spend $150,000 to cure one person's medical problem, how can it refuse to spend the same amount on someone else? Given that the average annual price of a specialty drug—$53,384—now rivals the median household income in the United States, the prospect of a flood of high-priced drugs is deeply troubling.[51]

Sovaldi brought this problem home to roost. Prescription drugs are not subject to normal market forces. Once drugs are proven effective and approved by the FDA, government payers and private insurers will fall into line and pay whatever amount drug manufacturers ask for. Upon its introduction, Sovaldi became the treatment of choice for hepatitis C because it works better and has fewer side effects than the medicines it replaced. Cost doesn't figure in the equation. But, thanks to political control of health care and the dominance of third-party payment, new drugs are not sold into markets where consumers' willingness to pay limits the prices that manufacturers can charge. Congress has not been willing or able to limit prices either. And calls for Medicare and other public payers to negotiate prices are an empty threat unless they are prepared not to cover a drug at all. The result is that drug companies can write their own tickets by developing new drugs and getting doctors to prescribe them.

The problem is real and about to explode, as the race to develop drugs that treat large populations is on. In 2014, the FDA approved Saxenda, a new weight-loss medication requiring daily injections. Its price? One thousand dollars a month, and the minimum recommended course is four months. Upward of 100 million American adults could benefit from Saxenda, meaning that the cost of giving everyone the minimum course would be $400 billion. Novo Norodisk, Saxenda's manufacturer, may not rake in that much money because other companies have new weight-loss drugs on the market too. But Big Pharma, one of the most profitable business sectors for many years, will keep looking for big hits.

Two other drugs that may help break the bank are Praluent and Repatha. Both are cholesterol-lowering injectable medications that were recently approved by the FDA and are alternatives to statins. They cost $14,600 and $14,100 a year, respectively. Because they are maintenance drugs, patients must take them their entire lives. Currently, between 4 million and 5 million Americans are thought to be candidates for using these drugs. The cost of treating just this population would exceed $70 billion a year. But the bad news doesn't end there. Cardiologists are currently debating the desirability of using these new drugs on the entire population of adults with a history of cardiovascular disease. That's 15 million people. At \$14,000 per person per year, the annual price tag would come to more than \$200 billion.[52]

Of course, cardiologists won't be left out of the party. They will receive procedure fees for injecting the drugs and monitoring their patients—and the larger the patient population that receives the drug, the greater the fees. Judging from their expressed eagerness, cardiologists will soon be giving these drugs to millions of people. At a cardiology meeting that took place just two days after the FDA approved Repatha, a reporter for *MedPage Today* discovered that many doctors had already written prescriptions.[53] The initial group of recipients were patients for whom other treatments were not working as well as their doctors wanted. But several cardiologists also said that they expected use to expand beyond this group quickly, a phenomenon they described as "script creep." "[A]lmost all of the cardiologists . . . estimated that 10% to 15% of their patients would be on [Praluent or Repatha] by this time next year."[54]

Not surprisingly, pharmacy benefits managers are "strictly controlling who can use [these drugs], demanding proof from doctors that patients have high cholesterol and have already tried statins. . . . Express Scripts had rejected half the prescriptions" it received.[55] But the constraint may only be temporary. A reporter who interviewed Dr. Steven Miller, Express Scripts' chief medical officer, wrote that the doctor believes that use of these medications could "explode if new information shows that the drugs can prevent heart attacks, strokes and death."[56] Dr. Miller himself offered the opinion that they could "grow to the largest class of drugs in history."[57]

Are the prices for all of these drugs justified? And how would we know? In ordinary markets, we depend on people spending their own money to sort these things out. Lots of people thought the iPhone was worth \$700. Very few people thought Google Glass was worth \$1,500. But in pharmaceutical markets, the dominance of third-party coverage and public payers means that this approach will not work. So how should we analyze the issue of whether these costs are worth incurring?

One approach is to study the cost-effectiveness of the drug, and then back into the price that would be justified by the drug's efficacy.

The Institute for Clinical and Economic Review (ICER), a nonprofit organization that studies just these issues, analyzed the cost-effectiveness of Praluent and Repatha. It concluded that "the price that best represents the overall benefits these drugs may bring to patients would be between $3,615 and $4,811 [per year], representing a 67% discount off the list price."[58] And, if we want to keep overall health care spending within reasonable bounds, ICER concluded that the price would have to fall to $2,177. But, as we have explained already, neither market forces nor regulations pressure drug manufacturers to take account of these factors when setting prices. Simply stated, there are no constraints on what they can charge.

### Will Sex Pills Break the Bank?

Sex sells. Erectile dysfunction (ED) drugs show that, so it should come as no surprise that pharmaceutical companies have women's sexual performance in their sights too. In 2015, the FDA approved Addyi, a treatment for premenopausal women who suffer from "hypoactive sexual desire disorder" (HSDD).[59] In hope of influencing the FDA's decision, Sprout Pharmaceuticals, Addyi's creator, helped finance a lobbying campaign called "Even the Score," which brought together several women's groups. "Even the Score" argued that men have drugs that enhance their sex lives, so women should too. Never mind that Addyi is "at best minimally effective and c[an] cause side effects like low blood pressure, fainting, nausea, dizziness and sleepiness," shortcomings that led the FDA to deny approval in 2010 and again in 2013.[60] Never mind that birth control pills intensify these side effects. And never mind that Addyi is especially dangerous when combined with alcohol, a substance that has accompanied sex on occasion. Men are free to take drugs that may cause heart palpitations and four-hour erections, so equity demands that women wanting to improve their sex lives should be allowed to take risks too.

"About 16 million U.S. women are estimated to have some degree of low sexual desire,"[61] and Sprout had plans to make sure all of them heard about Addyi. It committed to hiring 200 sales reps to tout Addyi's virtues to 30,000 doctors with large numbers of female patients, especially OB/GYNs and psychiatrists. Sprout never put this plan in motion, however.

Shortly after the FDA approved Addyi, Valeant acquired Sprout for $1 billion.[62]

Sprout intended to peg Addyi's price to the cost of men's ED drugs, which were running $400–$430 for a one-month supply at the time. That linkage had no economic basis. HSDD and ED are completely different problems, which Addyi and men's ED drugs treat by completely different means. The R&D costs and the failure risks associated with the two types of medication surely differ too. The only reason given for connecting the prices was that if insurers were willing to pay a certain amount to improve men's sex lives, it would be fair to charge them the same amount to help women.

Valeant wasn't bound by Sprout's intentions, and it priced Addyi considerably higher. As of mid-2017, GoodRx showed an average cash price of $961 for a one-month supply.[63] By using a coupon and shopping around, a woman could knock $150 off the cost.

Price may be one of the reasons that Addyi hasn't become the blockbuster drug that Valeant and Sprout thought it would be. In hope of improving sales, Valeant relaunched the drug in 2017. Of course, the real problems could be the dangers that Addyi poses and its marginal effectiveness. Whatever the truth may be, one thing is certain. Pharma companies will keep on looking for new ways to make sex better, and when they find them, the "cures" won't come cheap.

## CHARITIES AND COUPONS

We close by noting that, even when pharmaceutical companies appear to be acting altruistically, there is usually a darker side to the story. For example, many drug manufacturers support charities that help cover needy patients' out-of-pocket costs. Celgene Corp., which makes pricey cancer treatments like Thalomid and Revlimid, does this. It donates upward of $100 million a year to the Patient Access Network Foundation (the PAN Foundation) and other charities that run patient assistance programs (PAPs). These programs provide financial assistance to patients who have difficulty bearing the deductibles, copays, and coinsurance costs associated with Celgene's drugs.

Questcor, another pharma company, supports a PAP too. After it acquired the rights to make H.P. Acthar Gel, a medicine invented in 1952, Questcor raised the price repeatedly and steeply. Acthar's price went from $40 a vial in 2001 to $38,000 in 2016. In 2014, Acthar "was the single most expensive drug, per patient, that the government paid for. . . . Of the 3,100 beneficiaries using Acthar, Medicare spent an average of $162,371. Total Medicare spending on Acthar was $504 million [in 2014], a 29 percent increase from the year before."[64] These staggering price increases required many patients to shoulder large payments associated with deductibles and coinsurance requirements. Ostensibly out of concern for them, Questcor "funded a charity"—the Chronic Disease Fund—"to help cover patient copays, taking the sting out of the drug's out-of-pocket cost to consumers."[65]

Kaleo, the maker of the Evzio naloxone injector, also donated to a PAP. When accused of gouging consumers by quintupling the price, it claimed to have done so "to cover the cost of a new patient-assistance program that lowers the out-of-pocket costs for people who cannot afford the product"—of which, at the new higher price, there must have been many.[66] Apparently, Kaleo's decisions to charge thousands of dollars more for Evzio was an act of charity.

On the surface, drug makers' relationships with the PAN Foundation, the Chronic Disease Fund, and other PAPs may seem fine, even noble. But when one considers the underlying economics, the motives of both the manufacturers and the charities seem more sinister. A *New York Times* reporter explained the economics simply. "[I]f a patient cannot afford out-of-pocket costs of $5,000 for a $100,000-a-year drug, the drug company gets nothing. But if the manufacturer or the charity pays the $5,000, the patient gets the drug and the company receives $95,000 from the patient's insurance company or Medicare."[67] If it costs less than $90,000 to make the drug—and additional units of most drugs are cheap to produce—the company still profits, despite making the contribution. Then, the company can enrich itself further by taking a charitable deduction for the $5,000 against its taxes. The PAP wins too, of course. In return for channeling funds from a manufacturer to patients who need the maker's drugs, a PAP can extract fees that cover its operating costs and pay its managers hefty salaries.

For drug companies, donations to PAPs are business investments. They give money expecting the charities to use most of it to help patients who, by using their products, will generate lucrative payments from government payers and private insurers. "A million-dollar contribution from a pharmaceutical company to a copay charity can keep hundreds of patients from abandoning a newly pricey drug, enabling the donor to collect many millions from Medicare."[68] No wonder the PAP business is booming. In 2014, pharma companies donated $1.1 billion to the seven largest charities that sponsor PAPs, more than twice the amount they gave in 2010. As Professor Joel Hay, the founding chair in the department of pharmaceutical economics and policy at the University of Southern California, observed, the charities "don't ever have to scrounge for money. It falls right to them."[69]

The troubling nature of the relationship between drug makers and PAPs comes into sharp focus if you ask why pharma companies use the charities as middlemen instead of reimbursing patients' out-of-pocket costs directly. The answer is that, when patients are on Medicare or Medicaid, the federal anti-kickback statute imposes criminal penalties on drug manufacturers who do that. The reason for prohibiting such payments is simple: deductibles, copays, and coinsurance requirements regulate drug consumption in desirable ways. They discourage overuse, and they motivate patients to use cheaper drugs instead of pricier ones that require government agencies and private insurers to pay more.

By sponsoring PAPs, then, Celgene, Questcor, Kaleo, and other pharma companies do something indirectly that they cannot legally do directly. This is the reddest of red flags. Civil and criminal prohibitions would mean nothing if people could freely circumvent them by acting through agents. For this reason, the federal government forbids charities from helping pharma companies funnel dollars to patients. In the words of an Advisory Bulletin issued by the U.S. Department of Health and Human Services Office of the Inspector General, "an Independent Charity PAP must not function as a conduit for payments or other benefits from the pharmaceutical manufacturer to patients."[70] In reality, of course, this is exactly what PAPs do. Although they are nominally separate organizations that decide how the donations they receive will be spent, their managers know that they must dole out funds to patients who use their sponsors' drugs. Otherwise, the corporate dollars will stop flowing. Pharma companies are in business to make money, not to support charities.

Professor Hay, who is quoted above, serves as an expert witness in a whistleblower lawsuit involving Beverly Brown, a former Celgene sales representative. Brown contends that the company's relationship with the PAN Foundation was corrupt. In Hay's opinion, Celgene's donations to the PAN Foundation were "a ruse to cover the fact that these payments were actually illegal kickbacks designed to hide the fact that Celgene was contributing these payments to the foundations to get Medicare patients to use more Thalomid and Revlimid."[71] In other words, Celgene's working arrangements with the charity "were designed to pay patient copays in violation of Anti-Kickback laws."[72] Dan Klein, the president and CEO of the PAN Foundation, rejects the accusation. He says that the PAN Foundation is just a charity that "helps people with life-threatening, chronic and rare diseases access critical medications by supporting their out-of-pocket costs."[73]

Klein is right that PAN "helps people," but it does so by helping drug companies skirt the law while also obtaining good public relations. The PAN Foundation took money from Valeant Pharmaceuticals International after that company raised the prices on two old treatments for Wilson's Disease by 2,600 percent. And shortly after Turing Pharmaceuticals—the company run by pharma bro Martin Shkreli—increased Daraprim's price by 5,000 percent, it created a PAP for toxoplasmosis sufferers with help from Patient Services Inc., another charity. Is it any wonder that, to an outsider, the entire PAP industry seems morally suspect?

Coupons serve the same purpose as PAPs. By freeing patients from out-of-pocket costs, they encourage consumption and insulate manufacturers from market forces that might otherwise limit what they can charge. But they really help drug companies maintain high prices only when patients are insured, because the money they receive then comes solely from insurers. For this reason, self-pay patients often find that coupons aren't available for them.

John R. Graham, a well-known health care policy expert and acting assistant secretary for planning and evaluation at the Department of
Health and Human Services, used Mylan's offer for an EpiPen Savings
Card to show how the scam works. The ad that touted the card promised that users would have to pay nothing out-of-pocket. When Graham applied for the card, he was asked whether he had private insurance.
When he answered "no," the offer of the card was rescinded. When he
reapplied and said "yes," his eligibility was confirmed. As Graham wrote:

> This is an extreme example of a coupon strategy used by some drug
> makers: Immunize the patient from the direct cost of the medicine so
> the health insurer has to pay a price much higher than the market can
> bear. Of course, the insurer might get a discount from the list price,
> but the uninsured patient will never benefit from that. Further, the
> above-market price is paid by patients through high insurance premi-
> ums, so nobody is really saving money. In Canada, where EpiPen is
> sold over-the-counter in drugstores to cash-paying customers, it sells
> for about $80, instead of over $600 in the [United States]. Much of that
> price differential is due to our overreliance on health insurance to pay
> for medical goods.[74]

Graham's closing observation—that high prices are "due to our overreliance on health insurance" is one of the themes of this book. Chapter 15
provides more detail on why health care is expensive *because* it is insured.

When consumers buy things with their own money, their willingness to part with cash places a natural ceiling on what they will pay, and
competition usually drives prices well below that ceiling. In the pharma sector, where insurance carriers and public payers foot the bills, this
ceiling has been eliminated. Consequently, the sky is the limit on what
drug makers can charge. Seeing this, drug makers have set absurdly high
prices for new drugs and have used a variety of strategies to hide what
they are up to. They have emphasized the value their products confer,
exaggerated their research and development costs, and supported charities purportedly to ease the burdens on patients. But the truth is that
they are gaming the payment system to siphon as much money as they
can from insurers, consumers, and taxpayers—ending up with far more
than they could in a free market.

## CHAPTER 3: VIAL MISDEEDS

### THE MONSTER

Fraud and abuse occur at every point in the drug distribution chain. Although most of the people who help bring drugs to market are honest, many are not. Consequently, the variety of schemes and scams is enormous. This chapter begins with a case involving a medical professional whom no one would ever suspect: an admired and successful local pharmacist.

In 2001, Kansas pharmacist Robert Courtney was worth over $18 million and enjoyed many of the trappings of wealth.[1] He owned a mansion, collected luxury cars, and took frequent ski trips to Colorado. He held an esteemed position in his church, to which he had pledged $1 million to the building fund.

No one knew that Courtney amassed his fortune by diluting prescription drugs. Make two doses out of one and you double your money. Altogether, Courtney diluted 98,000 prescriptions for 72 different drugs taken by 4,200 patients. He diluted all types of drugs, including chemotherapy medications and antibiotics. How many of his patients died who might have been saved? No one can say for certain. In 2002, Courtney pled guilty to a host of crimes and was sentenced to 30 years in jail.

When federal agents were first alerted to Courtney's misdeeds, they refused to believe his actions were intentional. According to FBI Agent

Judy Lewis, "everybody who sat around that table that day had the same feeling, which was: 'There's got to be another explanation. I don't care how it looks. No one could do this.'"[2]

Why did hardened FBI agents, who spend all their time dealing with criminals, react with disbelief? Pharmacists enjoy a wonderful reputation, and we trust them to do the right thing. Most of the time, we are right to do so. But our politically controlled, third-party payment system creates endless opportunities for pharmacists and other health care providers to enrich themselves by cheating. Persistent exposure to bad incentives is inherently corrupting. Although most providers draw the line at hurting people, when serious money is on the line, some do not. And because policing is so spotty, the immoral ones rarely have to worry about being caught.

Courtney's wrongdoing occurred over several years. Why did no one notice? One obvious reason: medical treatments fail all the time. Many cancer patients die even when they receive full doses of chemotherapy drugs. Some infections are antibiotic resistant. Until Courtney's scheme was discovered, the patients who died after receiving diluted drugs were thought to have lost nature's lottery. Neither they nor their loved ones had any reason to suspect a monster was at work. Courtney also flew below the radar of those whose job was to look for fraudsters.

Courtney's downfall was precipitated by, of all people, a sales rep for a drug company who received commissions when Courtney purchased drugs through him. Somehow he learned that Courtney was dispensing far more of his company's chemotherapy product than he was buying. He figured Courtney was giving him the end run by purchasing drugs on the black market, and he expressed this concern to a nurse who happened to work for an oncologist. The nurse passed the story on to her employer, who had been ordering chemotherapy meds from Courtney for years. The doctor sent one of Courtney's prescriptions to a lab. When the results showed that the drug was diluted, the oncologist contacted the feds.

Courtney is an outlier. Most pharmacists are honest. But with almost 300,000 of them dispensing medicines in the United States, if even 1 percent are not, that is a lot of pharmacists gaming the way we pay for drugs.

## Compounding the Problem

In 2012, an epidemic of fungal meningitis infected more than 700 people and killed 64 of them. It was the deadliest outbreak of the disease ever in the United States. The infections and deaths occurred because a compounding pharmacy, the New England Compounding Center (NECC), used unsafe procedures and expired ingredients when producing vials of a steroidal medication.

Barry Cadden, the owner of NECC, was not convicted of homicide, however. Instead, in 2017, a jury found him guilty on more than 50 counts of racketeering and mail fraud for having put misbranded drugs into interstate commerce with the intent to deceive. A judge sentenced him to nine years in prison. In October 2017, Glenn Chin, a second NECC pharmacist charged in connection with the outbreak, was convicted of racketeering, conspiracy, false labeling, and mail fraud, but acquitted of murder.[3]

As frauds go, the NECC case is fairly simple. NECC was a badly run outfit that made unsafe drugs and sold them to the public. Other schemes involving compounding pharmacies are more involved.

At Fort Hood, Texas, for example, 10 people allegedly bilked TRICARE, the health insurance program for soldiers and their families, out of more than $102 million by paying people $250 a month to use compounded creams for pain, scars, and migraine headaches, and for taking vitamins. The ringleaders, Richard Cesario and John Cooper, disguised the scam by characterizing the payments as compensation for participating in a medical study, and then billing TRICARE for the compounded creams and vitamins. They even created a charity, the Freedom From Pain Foundation, to make the payments seem legitimate. The study was a hoax. Cesario and Cooper also allegedly used the charity's funds to bribe doctors to prescribe their medications.[4] Cesario and Cooper had no education or licensing in the medical, nursing, or pharmaceutical fields.[5] Yet they took TRICARE for more than $100 million, and they lived lavishly. Their wealth included four houses in Texas, a fifth in Florida, more than a dozen bank accounts, and 21 motor vehicles, including "a Jaguar, a Maserati, a Ferrari, a Porsche, an Aston Martin and three Mercedes-Benz; two motor coaches; and one boat."[6]

Two other scams involving compounded creams occurred in
Florida, where separate groups of fraudsters milked private insurers and
TRICARE for $157 million and $175 million over two to three years.[7]
The smaller scam, which ran from October 2012 to December 2015,
involved A to Z Pharmacy in New Port Richey and several other
pharmacies located in Miami. Collectively, the conspirators submitted
$633 million in false claims to Medicare, TRICARE, and private insur-
ers, and received $157 million in payments. The leader of this scheme,
Nicholas A. Borgesano Jr., pled guilty in late 2017, bringing the total
number of guilty pleas to eight.[8] In his plea agreement, Borgesano admitted that he and his fellow conspirators "manipulated billing codes in the
reimbursement claims and submitted reimbursement claims for pharmaceutical ingredients they did not have."[9] They also "paid kickbacks and
bribes in exchange for prescriptions and patient-identifying information
used to further the scheme, including to a physician in exchange for the
physician signing prescriptions for patients he never saw."[10]

The larger scheme, which lasted two years and led to 16 indict-
ments, was run out of Boca Raton, Florida. Its mastermind was Clifford
Carroll, who joined several co-conspirators by confessing his guilt in
2017. Carroll and others also paid kickbacks to corrupt doctors and other
medical professionals for prescribing compounded pain medications. "In
some cases, the co-conspirators received as much as $31,000 for a single
tube of compounded cream medication from private insurance companies."[11] They bribed patients too, offering them payments disguised
as reimbursements for data collection. In an interesting twist, the conspirators purchased failing pharmacies and used them as fronts for their
operations, and they created call centers to encourage military veterans
and other patients who had previously been prescribed medications to
refill their prescriptions or obtain new ones.

According to a federal complaint filed in 2017, however, the mother
of all schemes involving compounding pharmacies—which is said to
have taken TRICARE, Medicare, other public and private payers, and
pharmacy benefit managers for more than $400 million in four years—
was centered in Hattiesburg, Mississippi. Advantage Pharmacy allegedly
pulled in at least $155 million. Two other outfits involved in the scheme,

World Health Industries and Medworx, are said to have collected about $120 million and $130 million, respectively. [12]

The complaint alleges that the pharmacies "maximize[d] profits from the fraud scheme" by "creat[ing] their own demand for compounded medications."[13] They did this by "engag[ing] a series of marketers to provide incentives to doctors to write prescriptions for compounded medications and divert patients to the pharmacies."[14] The marketers also identified "complicit doctors willing to write prescriptions for compounded medications for patients whom they never saw and where there was no determination of medical need."[15] The marketers recruited willing patients too, and compensated them by paying kickbacks. Can you imagine this happening if the patients were spending their own money? Neither can we. The dominance of open-ended third-party payment makes massive fraud possible—and easy to commit.

With such astonishing sums taken in, it is no wonder the people alleged to have run these scams became fabulously rich. Before setting up Medworx, Thomas E. Spell Jr., whom the feds identified as a principal architect, made less than $200,000 a year. "After managing Medworx for only 18 months, he was able to amass assets estimated to be worth more than $12 million."[16] As a group, the participants did extremely well. The assets seized by the government included 8 Florida homes that were collectively worth over $5 million, another 43 properties in other states, 24 vehicles, 5 planes, 2 boats, and 80 bank accounts containing a total of $15 million.[17] The principals seem to have been printing money.

To date, two people have been criminally charged in this scam, but the four "key" names referenced in a civil forfeiture filing have not yet been charged.[18] More details will presumably emerge as the drama plays out in court.

### THE OLD SWITCHEROO

When you go to the drugstore to buy aspirin, ibuprofen, or some other pain reliever, you know that capsules and tablets are interchangeable. An aspirin pill and an aspirin capsule contain the same ingredient: acetylsalicylic acid. You may prefer one to the other. You may find capsules easier to swallow or dislike the aftertaste of pills. Or you may not care and buy whatever's on sale.

Because capsules and tablets are so similar, people won't pay $25 for a bottle of aspirin capsules when a bottle of aspirin tablets can be had for $5. They will buy the tablets and save $20. This explains why retail outlets sell capsules and tablets for about the same price. Consumers care about the price, and their ability to switch deters overcharging.

Where third-party payment predominates, different ways of delivering the same amount of the same drug can fetch wildly different prices. Consider ranitidine, the generic form of a popular heartburn medication (Zantac), typically dispensed in tablet form. When the patent on Zantac expired, ranitidine tablets became the approved generic replacements for the original medication. Knowing that ranitidine tablets were cheap and would be in high demand, Medicaid set a low standardized reimbursement level. This payment was known as either a Federal Upper Limit or a state Maximum Allowable Cost (MAC). But no similar limit was placed on the capsule form of ranitidine—presumably because it was rarely used and there was no reason to expect it to be dispensed in large numbers.

This quirk in Medicaid's payment system made it much more profitable for pharmacies to dispense ranitidine capsules than ranitidine tablets. Illinois' Medicaid program paid only 34 cents per ranitidine tablet, compared to $1.36 per ranitidine capsule.[19] Tennessee's Medicaid program paid 32 cents per tablet and 87 cents per capsule.[20] Florida's Medicaid program paid 28 cents per tablet and 91 cents per capsule.[21]

The reverse was true for fluoxetine, the generic version of Prozac, the popular anti-anxiety drug. There, Medicaid set a MAC for capsules but paid higher prices for tablets. In Florida, a pharmacist who filled a Prozac prescription with fluoxetine capsules received 57 cents per capsule from the state, whereas a pharmacist who delivered fluoxetine tablets received $1.77 per tablet—three times as much.[22] Indiana's Medicaid program paid 69 cents per fluoxetine capsule and $1.91 per tablet.[23]

Medicaid even paid different prices when pharmacists delivered the same amount of the same medicine in the form of two tablets rather than one. Buspirone, the generic form of Buspar, another anti-anxiety drug, was normally prescribed in single 15 mg tablets, so Medicaid set a low MAC on that tablet dosage. But Medicaid's payment system set no MAC for 7.5 milligram (mg) buspirone tablets. The result was that a pharmacy that dispensed two 7.5 mg tablets would be paid more than a pharmacy that dispensed one 15 mg tablet, even though both pharmacies dispensed the same amount of buspirone. Michigan's Medicaid program paid more than five times as much for the two-pill combination as for the single buspirone pill—$1.70 vs. 28 cents.[24] In Tennessee, the single 15 mg tablet fetched 49 cents while the price for the pair of 7.5 mg pills was $1.93.[25] Florida, Indiana, Louisiana, and Virginia all paid at least three times as much for the two-pill combination as for the single pill.[26]

On a per-tablet or per-pill basis, these differences seem modest, but they can add up to big money for pharmacies that fill lots of prescriptions. Walgreens, CVS, and Omnicare, a large pharmacy specializing in long-term care facilities, collected hundreds of millions of dollars from Medicaid by swapping dosage forms.[27] Start with Walgreens. In July 2001, it decided to automatically switch all prescriptions for ranitidine tablets to capsules.[28] Walgreens' supplier for ranitidine capsules estimated that Walgreens would increase its annual profits by $75 million by making this one simple change.[29] Put differently, the company would force taxpayers to pay $75 million more than necessary to provide ranitidine to Medicaid enrollees. Fluoxetine tablets would become "the #1 Rx profit item in the company."[30]

Omnicare pulled a similar trick with fluoxetine and buspirone and reaped similar rewards. In a December 2001 email, Dan Maloney, the company's head of generic drug purchasing, reminded employees that "on average every Buspirone switch is worth about 38 dollars and [every] Fluoxetine 18 dollars."[31] In another email, he wrote of having "shared" with other managers a "financial analysis on the two drugs [fluoxetine and buspirone]" showing that the switches for both drugs "combined were worth well over half a million per month in profits."[32]

This wasn't even Omnicare's first pharmacy scam. It had previously been caught stealing from Medicaid by failing to reverse the charges for medications that were returned unopened after being prescribed for patients who had died. Omnicare was effectively on probation for that earlier offense, since it was subject to a Corporate Integrity Agreement with the feds.[33] But it still entered into the drug-switching scheme.

The drug-switching scam lasted only three years—but not because Walgreens or any other participant suddenly grew a conscience. Walgreens was caught by a whistleblower who filed a lawsuit accusing the company of filing false claims. When the federal government and several states' attorneys general joined the lawsuit, the heat became too much for Walgreens to bear. Separate lawsuits were filed against CVS and Omnicare. All three companies settled these cases. Omnicare paid almost $50 million, and Walgreens and CVS paid roughly $35 million each. All three companies denied wrongdoing, and none of their employees went to jail.

A closer look at the drug-switching scandal reveals a hidden player and an additional wrinkle common to all three lawsuits. Sources report that Par Pharmaceuticals, a manufacturer of generic drugs, figured out how to game Medicaid's pricing system and explained the scam to the pharmacies. Not coincidentally, Par also manufactured ranitidine capsules, fluoxetine tablets, and buspirone tablets in the 7.5 mg size. Par made money by selling these products—and to help increase its sales, it gave significant discounts to pharmacies that achieved target levels of drug conversions. Because Par was the only supplier of ranitidine capsules, fluoxetine tablets, and 7.5 mg buspirone tablets, it could charge monopoly prices and make much more money.

Par and the pharmacies needed one another to pull off the scheme. Par needed pharmacies to switch patients from the prescribed medications over to Par's products, and the pharmacies needed Par to supply medications in forms that were not subject to Medicaid's price caps. Thus, Par made money by selling drugs to Walgreens, CVS, and Omnicare, which made even more money by bilking Medicaid.

A whistleblower filed suit against Par in 2006. The federal government and numerous states joined the suit in 2011. However, in August 2017, these cases were dismissed on several technical grounds.[34] It remains to be seen whether the plaintiffs will appeal.

### Selling Salt and Sugar for $1,000 a Pound

Saline and dextrose intravenous (IV) bags are about as low-tech as it gets in health care. A saline IV bag contains salt and water. A dextrose IV bag contains sugar and water. Both cost less than 50 cents to manufacture and both sell for about $2, give or take a few cents. Would it surprise you to discover that Louisiana's Medicaid program paid $928 per bag for both? Eventually, Louisiana Medicaid wised up and sued Baxter International for fraud.

Louisiana wasn't the only state taken to the cleaners, and saline and dextrose IV bags weren't the only products whose prices were rigged. The story of how Louisiana, other states, and the federal government came to pay through the nose for saline solution, dextrose, and many other pharmaceuticals is one of the greatest scams in the history of health care. It centers on something called the average wholesale price (AWP).

For many years, Medicaid paid for drugs using a formula based on AWPs. But AWPs come in two varieties. There's the real AWP—that is, the amount pharmacies *actually* pay wholesalers for their products. And there is the phony AWP—that is, a higher number listed in a book that determines what Medicare and Medicaid pay. The real AWP for saline solution was a couple of bucks. But Medicare and Medicaid paid absurdly large amounts because drug companies listed phony AWPs that were far higher. The problem was not limited to saline; phony AWPs were pervasive.

Phony AWPs appeared in several pricing guides, the most prominent of which is called the *Redbook,* but the same analysis applies to them all. Pharmaceutical manufacturers and wholesalers would send numbers to the *Redbook* that were supposed to reflect the prices that wholesalers were actually charging pharmacies, but often did not.[35] For branded drugs, drug companies inflated the listed prices by roughly 20–25 percent. For generic drugs and other products, the sky was the limit. Because Medicaid and Medicare based their payments for drugs on the prices shown in the *Redbook*, both agencies greatly overpaid. Patients overpaid too, because their copayments were also based on phony AWPs.

Here's an example of how the scam worked. In April 2000, vancomycin, an antibiotic made by Abbott Laboratories, had a published

AWP of $68.77. Medicare paid 80 percent of the AWP less 5 percent, or $52.26. The patient contributed another 20 percent of the AWP: $13.75. But the vancomycin actually cost the pharmacy only $8.17.[36] That was the *real* AWP. The pharmacy thus made $57.84 in profit on an $8.17 drug, a risk-free return of about 700 percent.

The spread on vancomycin was exceedingly healthy, but the spread on some other drugs was far larger. A class action complaint filed by patient advocacy groups against more than a dozen drug companies contains the following allegation: "In the 2000 edition of the Redbook, Defendant BMS [Bristol-Myers Squibb Company] listed the AWP for a 20 mg vial of injectable Vepesid (Etoposide) as $1,296.65. BMS sold the exact same drug to a group purchasing organization for $70 per 20 mg vial."[37] When "reimbursed" at Medicare's rate, a $70 vial of Vepesid generated a profit of $1,161.82, a risk-free return of more than 1,600 percent.[38]

The spreads between real and phony AWPs grew so large in part because many drugs had several manufacturers who competed for pharmacies' business. To win, manufacturers had to offer larger spreads between their actual charges and the phony numbers they published in the *Redbook*. The race was actually a contest to see who could squeeze the most money out of the dumbest buyers around: Medicare and Medicaid. Pharmacies kept the competition going by switching to whichever manufacturer offered the largest spread.[39] The profits were enormous. According to the director of health care issues for the General Accounting Office, Medicare alone paid pharmacists almost half a billion dollars more than it should have in just one year.[40]

One can get a sense of the scale of the AWP fraud, and the ways in which phony pricing corrupted everything it touched, by examining the details of an $884 million settlement, which included a $290 million criminal fine, between TAP Pharmaceutical Products Inc. and the Department of Justice. The 2001 settlement was the largest payment in the history of health care fraud litigation at the time. TAP manufactured Lupron Depot, a prostate cancer drug. It gave doctors, primarily urologists, free supplies of Lupron with the understanding that they would bill patients and Medicare for the drugs as if the drugs had been purchased and dispensed. TAP also gave urologists other inducements to prescribe Lupron: off-invoice price discounts; free trips to expensive ski and golf resorts; "educational grants" and "consulting fees" that were really cash payments running into the tens of thousands of dollars with no strings attached; payments of bar tabs and holiday expenses; financial support for advertising expenses; and debt forgiveness.[41] The federal investigation commenced after TAP sales representatives effectively offered a bribe—a $65,000 "education grant" plus the opportunity to exploit Medicare—to the director of pharmacy programs at Tufts Health Plan in Massachusetts. The director called the cops. Many other doctors accepted TAP's bribes, however, and sales of Lupron soared.

Why did TAP stoop to buying physicians' loyalty? Partly because a competitor, AstraZeneca, was doing the same thing. AstraZeneca produced Zoladex, a drug that was functionally similar to Lupron but significantly cheaper. AstraZeneca was using the same tactics to win business.[42] In 2003, AstraZeneca paid $335 million to settle with the Justice Department. The settlement included a criminal fine of almost $100 million and a guilty plea.

TAP and AstraZeneca engaged in shady dealings not only because enormous sums were at stake but also because third-party payment means there is almost never anyone minding the store. From 1991 through 1998, Medicare shelled out more than $2.5 billion for Lupron treatments plus another $513 million for Zoladex.[43] Private insurers and patients contributed about $1 billion more.[44]

The lure of easy money seduced many physicians. By the time the Justice Department concluded its prosecutions of TAP and AstraZeneca, six practicing urologists had pled guilty to crimes and two more faced prosecution.[45] Altogether, hundreds of urologists pocketed millions of dollars by charging for thousands of doses of Lupron and Zoladex that TAP and AstraZeneca gave them for free and by receiving AWP-based payments from Medicare and patients that greatly exceeded their actual costs.

In market economies, producers profit by selling products more cheaply. Lower prices pull consumers away from competing products that cost more. Medicare and Medicaid reversed the normal relationship between price and quantity, enabling drug manufacturers to increase sales to doctors and pharmacists by charging government programs *more*. Higher prices brought higher profits, instead of the reverse. Companies competed for market share by offering doctors and pharmacists more and more of the taxpayers' money. Worse, each company had an incentive to raise its phony AWPs faster than its competitors raised theirs. Only a government spending other people's money could create so perverse an arrangement and stick with it long after the predictable consequences came home to roost.

### It Is Not Fraud If You Knew We Were Lying

Not all drug companies that were involved in the AWP scheme admitted wrongdoing. Most conceded that *Redbook* prices were grossly inflated, but even so many denied that they committed fraud. They contended, first, that doctors and pharmacies got the extra money, not them, so they shouldn't be on the hook for any overpayments. Second, they claimed that public officials knew for years that *Redbook* prices were unreliable and still chose to pay. For example, in 2003, GlaxoSmithKline (GSK) issued the following statement:

> Those who designed and administered the New York Medicaid and EPIC [Elderly Pharmaceutical Insurance Coverage] programs as well as the federal Medicare program have known for decades that tying reimbursements to AWP causes the programs to pay doctors and pharmacies more for certain drugs than the doctors and pharmacies paid for the medicines themselves. The federal government has urged state Medicaid programs for years not to reimburse for drugs at AWP (a price calculated and reported by third-party vendors) for that very reason.
>
> Now the Attorney General is trying to hold [GSK] and other pharmaceutical companies accountable for the state's own conscious decision to reimburse doctors and pharmacies more for drugs than they paid for them.[46]

GSK is not the only one singing this tune. Michael Greve and the late Jack Calfee, two scholars at the American Enterprise Institute, said the fraud charge is "a striking accusation to make, since the process has been well established, well known, and much debated for more than 30 years."[47] They repeated an old joke in pharmaceutical circles, that AWP actually stands for "ain't what's paid."[48]

The charge of government complicity raises an obvious question. Did federal and state officials know that *Redbook* prices were inflated? Yes, they did. In fact, they knew for years, even decades, that Medicare, Medicaid, and the patients they served vastly overpaid for covered drugs. Federal and state program auditors had been investigating AWP-based drug pricing since the 1980s.[49] One source reported that at least 15 reports criticizing the use of AWPs by state Medicaid agencies were released between 1984 and 1997.[50]

Here are some examples of what federal officials knew:

- Reports issued by the Office of Inspector General (OIG) for the U.S. Department of Health and Human Services in 1984 and 1989 concluded that the *Redbook* and other wholesale price guides overstated "the true cost of drugs" to pharmacists and physicians by almost 16 percent.[51]
- A series of OIG reports released in 1996 and 1997 showed that *Redbook* prices for albuterol and certain other drugs administered to patients with breathing difficulties were grossly inflated. By reimbursing doctors' and hospitals' actual average costs instead of published AWPs, Medicare could have saved $94 million dollars from January 1994 to February 1995, 35 percent of the $269 million Medicare actually paid for these drugs.[52]
- A 1997 OIG report showed that, in 1996, Medicare paid $447 million above cost for 22 covered drugs, often shelling out more than double the actual wholesale prices paid by physicians.[53]
- A 2000 OIG report shows Medicare and Medicaid patients would jointly have saved $155 million per year by paying prices charged by internet pharmacies.[54]
- In 2001, the General Accounting Office reported that, in 2000, Medicare payments for physician-billed drugs were at least $532 million higher than providers' acquisition costs.[55]

As an article published in 2001 reported, "Repeated federal investigations have shown that the average wholesale prices (AWP) reported by manufacturers to Medicare . . . are way above what they actually charge physicians. The companies inflate AWPs as a way of inducing physicians . . . to buy their drugs."[56] Using the amounts paid by the Veterans Health Administration, which did not rely on AWPs, as comparisons, Medicare and Medicaid overpaid by $1.6 billion and $1.1 billion per year, respectively.[57]

Even members of Congress knew that drug companies used inflated AWPs as a means of "market[ing] their drugs to physicians and pharmacies based on this windfall profit which in reality is nothing more than a government funded kick-back to the provider." Rep. Pete Stark, the author of these remarks, which he sent to the president of the Pharmaceutical Research and Manufacturers Association (PhRMA) in 2000, had a chart of examples in which "the Medicare beneficiaries' 20% co-payment exceeds the entire costs of the drug."[58] Congress, whose members are supposed to assure that taxpayers receive good value for their dollars, knew that AWP-based payments inflated the amounts that Medicare, Medicaid, and the programs' beneficiaries paid for drugs. But they let the practice continue.

In fact, Congress prevented Medicare and Medicaid from switching from AWPs to any other arrangement that would have brought payments more nearly into line with providers' actual costs. Despite all the reports critical of AWPs that had been issued before, Congress enacted the Balanced Budget Act of 1997 (BBA), which set Medicare payments for drugs at 95 percent of AWP. When doing so, it ignored pleas from members of the Clinton administration, who protested that AWPs are like sticker prices for cars, which few people actually paid.[59] The legislative history of the BBA even notes an OIG report that AWP-based payments by Medicare for 10 oncology drugs exceeded providers' actual acquisition costs by anywhere from 20 percent to 1,000 percent.[60] In later years, Congress repeatedly refused to act on bills that would have based payments on actual acquisition costs.

Congress even frustrated the Clinton administration's unilateral attempt to stop using AWPs. In mid-2000, Donna Shalala, the secretary of Health and Human Services, informed Congress that the Health Care Financing Administration, which then oversaw Medicare, was preparing a regulation that would switch from published AWPs to AWPs based on providers' actual acquisition costs. Congress enacted a statute preventing her from doing that later that year.[61] A few years later, Congress again mandated the use of AWPs in the Medicare Prescription Drug Improvement and Modernization Act of 2003, although it reduced the baseline from 95 percent of AWP to 85 percent.

Could it be any clearer that Congress insisted upon the retention of AWP-based payments for prescription drugs even though its members knew that AWPs were inflated, often massively? Congress aided and abetted the waste of taxpayers' dollars and the pillaging of patients, whose copays were inflated to satisfy the demands of big industry players.

One could hardly want better evidence that political control of the health care economy is a core driver of medical spending. But if you do, you need only visit your local drugstore or shop for over-the-counter drugs online. You will see hundreds of real prices, all set as low as possible in hope of gaining your business. When consumers buy medicines in markets without "help" from the government, the only way to profit is by offering them what they want at prices they are willing to pay.

### You Say Avastin, I Say Lucentis

Avastin and Lucentis are two different medicines that contain the same active component and are made by the same company, Genentech. If you think they sell for the same price, you have much to learn. Lucentis is almost 40 times as expensive as Avastin. Understanding how both medications came into existence and came to be priced so differently shows yet another way in which pharmaceutical companies are adept at creating and exploiting marketing exclusivity.

Avastin is a cancer treatment that works by slowing the growth of blood vessels that feed tumors. After it was approved, some enterprising ophthalmologists thought that it might work on an entirely different illness: wet macular degeneration, a vision impairment caused by the excessive growth of blood vessels at the back of the eye. They tried it out by injecting very small doses of Avastin directly into patients' eyes. (Physicians can use products approved by the U.S. Food and Drug Administration [FDA] as they wish, even if the FDA approved the drug for use with a different disease. We discuss "off-label" use of drugs in Chapter 6.) The results were terrific, and the use of Avastin to treat wet macular degeneration quickly caught on.

Because only a small amount of Avastin was needed to treat patients' eyes, the drug was very inexpensive when used for this purpose. It cost about $60 per injection. Of course, that meant Genentech didn't make much money. A large vial designed to treat a cancer patient went a very long way when used in small doses by ophthalmologists.

When Genentech learned that the active ingredient in Avastin worked on wet macular degeneration, it created and obtained FDA approval for a new drug, Lucentis, to treat this condition. Lucentis was far pricier than Avastin. It sold for $2,300 a dose—38 times as much as Avastin. Genentech didn't try to show that Lucentis worked any better on wet macular degeneration than Avastin, and "when the National Eye Institute tested Lucentis against Avastin, it found essentially no difference."[62] Six randomized clinical trials have found Avastin and Lucentis are largely equivalent.[63]

Because of the price difference, many ophthalmologists kept using Avastin instead of switching to Lucentis. Genentech countered by discouraging ophthalmologists from using Avastin, raising bogus safety concerns and announcing that it would stop selling the drug to the repackaging firms that were cutting it into eye-appropriate doses.[64] When ophthalmologists responded by threatening to sue, Genentech backed down.[65]

Lucentis is still a big seller for Genentech, however, accounting for more than $1 billion in domestic sales for four years in a row. In 2015, Medicare alone shelled out that much for the drug.[66] Why do so many eye doctors use pricier Lucentis when cheaper Avastin is available? You guessed it: Medicare pays physicians a lot more for using Lucentis. A 2013 *Washington Post* article explained the finances.

> Under Medicare repayment rules for drugs given by physicians, they are reimbursed for the average price of the drug plus 6 percent. That

means a drug with a higher price may be easier to sell to doctors than a cheaper one. In addition, Genentech offers rebates to doctors who use large volumes of the more expensive drug.[67]

Got that? Medicare pays doctors far more for administering Lucentis than Avastin to patients with wet macular degeneration *because* Genentech charges more for the former than the latter. Six percent of $2,300 is $138; 6 percent of $60 will barely buy you a white chocolate mocha at Starbucks. Genentech then sweetens the deal by giving doctors who use large amounts of Lucentis discounts that the doctors get to keep. It's easy to see how Medicare put taxpayers and seniors on the hook for $1.2 billion in payments for Lucentis in 2012.[68] The hard part is explaining why many doctors, to their credit, continue to use Avastin. The cost to taxpayers and elderly patients could be much higher.

If you are wondering why Medicare does not simply pay the same amount for Lucentis and Avastin or require physicians to use Avastin, the answer is that the law forbids the government from doing either. Medicare is a price taker, not a price setter. It pays the prevailing rates for drugs, the prevailing rates being whatever manufacturers want to charge for them. In the case of patented drugs, this means that manufacturers can effectively set prices as high as they want and Medicare has to pay. Medicare also has limited ability to dictate which treatments it will pay for, lest it be seen as preventing doctors from recommending or using whatever medications will work best for their patients. In combination, this means that Lucentis will keep on generating billions of dollars in sales for Genentech for the foreseeable future, even though Avastin is a far cheaper substitute.

If you are wondering how this crazy state of affairs came about, the answer is that political control of health care gives pharmaceutical companies, pharmacists, and physicians the incentive and the power to bend the rules to suit them, while individual taxpayers have little incentive, and even less power, to fight back.

Chapters 1–3 have focused on misconduct involving prescription medications. There are deep, structural problems in this sector, including the proliferation of sales monopolies; terrible incentives created by the payment system and, especially, by government programs; and the impossibility of effective government monitoring of the tens of thousands of profit-seeking businesses and money-grubbing people who are connected to the distribution system. Welcome to the dark side of the American health care system. Unfortunately, there is much more to come. The next three chapters examine the practice of medicine by physicians.

# CHAPTER 4: DON'T GO BREAKING MY HEART

## FULL METAL JACKET

When the actress, comedienne, and blonde bombshell Mae West observed that "too much of a good thing can be wonderful," she was talking about sex, not stents. But, unlike sex, "too many stents can kill you," as Shirlee Peterson observed after her husband, Bruce, died with 21 of them in his chest.[1]

Surprisingly, 21 stents is not even close to the record. Another patient treated by the same physician—a Texas cardiologist named Dr. Samuel DeMaio—had 31 stents implanted.[2] In this patient, the stents reportedly ran more than two feet in length.[3] That's what, in a bit of dark humor, interventional cardiologists call "a full metal jacket."[4] According to Dr. Ralph Brindis, a past president of the American College of Cardiology, the average number of stents per patient is 1.2 to 1.4.[5]

A stent is a cylinder of fine metal mesh that helps keep open a blood vessel that was previously blocked by cholesterol plaque. Typically, a cardiologist snakes a balloon-tipped catheter to the site of the blockage and then inflates it to compress the plaque. This procedure opens the artery but also weakens it. To prevent the weakened artery from collapsing, the cardiologist then inserts a stent. There are different stents for different places in the vascular system—from the coronary arteries in the heart to the peripheral arteries spread throughout the body. Typically, cardiologists work on the blockages involving the heart, whereas interventional radiologists handle the peripheral arteries. After patients receive stents, they must take blood thinners for the rest of their lives. Otherwise, blood clots may form causing heart attacks and strokes. In the medical literature, the process of inserting a stent is known as percutaneous cardiac intervention (PCI).

## THE DOCTOR'S DILEMMA:
## THE RIGHT TREATMENT OR THE MOST LUCRATIVE ONE?

The Petersons relied on Dr. DeMaio to determine whether Bruce needed a stent and to insert one if he did. This created a conflict of interest. Dr. DeMaio stood to make more money—a lot more—by recommending an aggressive treatment (stenting) rather than by advising Bruce to use diet, exercise, or medications. The low-tech approach might have been the right strategy for Bruce, but it would have required Dr. DeMaio to pass up a lucrative opportunity.

This conflict of interest did not distinguish Dr. DeMaio from the tens of thousands of other doctors who diagnose patients and then treat them. All physicians who perform both services can have conflicts. What distinguishes Dr. DeMaio and other interventional cardiologists from other doctors is that the financial stakes in their conflicts are much larger. "Stenting belongs to one of the bleakest chapters in the history of Western medicine," says Nortin Hadler, a professor of Medicine at the University of North Carolina at Chapel Hill, because "the interventional cardiology industry has a cash flow comparable to the GDP of many countries."[6]

Most of the revenue that stenting generates goes to the hospitals where the procedures take place. The doctors who perform these procedures receive a separate fee that averages about $1,000.[7] That may not sound like much, but it is roughly four times the fee a physician receives for advising a patient to use diet, exercise, and medication.

The monetary incentive to overtreat does not end there. Because cardiac procedures are so lucrative, hospitals use directorships, consultancies, and other made-up arrangements to reward doctors who refer patients or perform these procedures.[8] In combination with the base payment, this creates a large incentive for cardiologists to implant stents, even when they are not necessary.

## AN EPIDEMIC OF UNNECESSARY STENTINGS

Don't think that doctors would stick devices into people who don't need them? Think again. According to a *Bloomberg News* article, "Two out of three elective stents, or more than 200,000 procedures a year, are unnecessary."[9] The article cited Dr. David Brown, a cardiologist at Stony Brook University School of Medicine in New York, as authority, and he should know. In 2012, Brown coauthored a meta-analysis of eight clinical trials that collectively compared over 7,000 patients with stable coronary artery disease (CAD), some of whom received stents while others received only much cheaper medicines. The conclusion? In patients with stable CAD, there was no evidence that stents were superior to medical therapy for preventing death, nonfatal heart attacks, unplanned revascularizations, or angina.[10]

In 2014, Dr. Brown published a second study. This one assessed the relative efficacy of stents plus medication versus medication alone for patients with stable CAD and reduced blood flow to the heart, a problem known as ischemia. The 2014 meta-analysis examined the results of five clinical trials that collectively involved over 4,000 patients. Again, stents conferred no benefit. Ischemic patients who received stents weren't less likely to die or suffer nonfatal heart attacks, unplanned revascularizations, or angina, compared to those who only took medication.[11] The COURAGE study, published in 2015, which tracked ischemic heart disease patients for 15 years, confirmed these findings.[12]

The financial cost of implanting stents in hundreds of thousands of patients who don't need them reportedly runs to about $2.4 billion a year.[13] That's just for the stents. To calculate the total cost, you'd have to add in the millions upon millions of dollars spent on blood thinners and medical monitoring, and then subtract the (far more modest) cost of medical management of those who did not receive stents. If we count only the direct costs, $2.4 billion isn't that large a number in the scheme of overall spending on health care—but, as Sen. Everett Dirksen (R–IL) famously observed, "a billion here, a billion there, and pretty soon you're talking about real money."[14]

To their credit, interventional cardiologists have begun to get the overuse of stents under control. From 2009 to 2014, the number of inappropriate nonacute PCIs declined.[15] But problems persist. For example, every year thousands of asymptomatic patients undergo PCI as a precaution before being operated on for noncardiac maladies, even though mounting evidence shows that the procedure does them no good.[16]

Shirlee Peterson claimed that an excessive number of stentings killed her husband. Dr. DeMaio disagreed and claimed to have treated Bruce appropriately. Their dispute figured in an investigation by the Texas Medical Board (TMB). Initially, the TMB filed a complaint asserting that the many "unneeded stents" caused various complications, and ultimately resulted in Peterson's death.[17] The TMB's complaint alleged that Dr. DeMaio had mistreated an additional eight patients during the same time period (2008–2009) by placing multiple stents in areas of insignificant or moderate disease; that he performed multiple angiograms in patients who were asymptomatic and had normal stress tests; and that he had unnecessarily implanted cardiac defibrillators in two patients.[18]

The TMB ultimately walked back most of its allegations. According to a news report, it found that DeMaio "placed multiple, elongated, overlapping drug-eluting stents in areas of insignificant or only moderate disease, and that his 'reading of angiography film as it relates to percentage of arterial occlusion was flawed.'"[19] However, the board did not revoke Dr. DeMaio's medical license. Nor did it impose much of a penalty. Instead, Dr. DeMaio agreed to undergo 30 hours of continuing medical education (including 5 hours on ethics) and 2 years of oversight by another physician, plus a $10,000 penalty.[20] The TMB did not report DeMaio to the National Practitioner Data Bank, which tracks doctors who commit malpractice or are disciplined. In the end, Dr. DeMaio was left free to continue practicing cardiology in Texas.

When it comes to stenting, the worst offenders fill a rogues' gallery. In 2011, a jury convicted Dr. John R. McLean of defrauding Medicare, Medicaid, and private insurers by inserting unnecessary cardiac stents, ordering unnecessary tests, and making false entries in patients' medical records. Investigators alleged McLean performed more than 200 unnecessary stent procedures at the Peninsula Regional Medical Center (PRMC) and falsified patients' records to cover up the fraud. Dr. McLean surrendered his medical license and was sentenced to a prison term of eight years. PRMC paid $2.8 million to settle federal claims stemming from McLean's actions.[21]

McLean was one of two Maryland cardiologists who were under investigation at the same time. The other was Dr. Mark G. Midei, a staff cardiologist at the St. Joseph Medical Center (SJMC) in Towson. Like McLean, he pulled in an enormous income by performing hundreds of unnecessary heart procedures and falsifying medical records to cover his tracks. After his misdeeds were discovered, SJMC suspended his practice in May 2009. Then, in January of the following year, SJMC sent letters to almost 600 patients, informing them that they might have been stented unnecessarily. The disclosure precipitated a flood of lawsuits, most of which SJMC and Colorado-based Catholic Health Initiatives (CHI), its former parent company, eventually settled.[22] According to one news report, CHI agreed to pony up $37 million to settle a class action that may have included as many as 273 former patients, after having previously settled 242 pending cases for an undisclosed amount.[23] Some cases appear to have been resolved individually as well. SJMC also agreed to pay $22 million to resolve claims that it had paid kickbacks to MidAtlantic Cardiovascular Associates, the private medical group that employed Midei before SJMC lured him away.[24]

Midei's story is interesting for other reasons. Between 1984 and 2009, Midei performed 40,000 cardiac procedures but was never sued by a patient for performing an unnecessary implantation. The malpractice system completely failed to identify him as a bad actor, much less to deter him. So much for the claim that patients and their greedy contingent-fee lawyers will sue doctors over even the tiniest mistakes.

The government agency in Maryland that licenses physicians also recognized the problem far too late. Although it began receiving complaints about Midei in November 2008, it didn't revoke his medical license until 2011, a full year after the scandal broke.[25] In context, this tardiness isn't all that surprising. State medical boards rely on complaints from patients, malpractice settlements, and disciplinary actions by other states to signal the need to investigate bad doctors. Midei's patients weren't complaining or suing—because they didn't know their stents were unnecessary—so he flew under the radar.

The case also illustrates how valuable doctors like Midei are to the hospitals at which they practice. SJMC recruited Midei in 2008 by *tripling* the $600,000 salary he was pulling down at MidAtlantic Cardiovascular Associates. That's how lucrative interventional cardiology can be. SJMC wouldn't have paid Midei almost $2 million a year unless he was generating revenues far in excess of that for the hospital. After Midei's suspension was publicized, the volume of implanted drug-eluting stents dropped by 45 percent at SJMC, and by 6–20 percent at other hospitals in Baltimore.[26]

Midei also had a cozy relationship with stent-maker Abbott Laboratories, which spent over $2,000 for a barbeque at his house that included "a whole smoked pig and other fixings." The cause for celebration? Midei had implanted 30 of Abbott's stents in one day, "perhaps setting the single day implant record," according to an unnamed Abbott official.[27] If that's not a clear conflict of interest, nothing is. Abbott also displayed its gratitude by hiring Midei as a consultant after SJMC let him go.[28]

Another scandal involving unnecessary stents occurred at a second St. Joseph Hospital (SJH) that was also owned by CHI but located in London, Kentucky. This time, the surgeries at issue were performed by a team of cardiologists led by Dr. Sandesh "Sam" Patil. After hundreds of patients filed lawsuits accusing Patil of inserting stents they did not need, the Kentucky Medical Licensure Board examined the records for five patients and found that he "plac[ed] stents without justification in three of them." Eventually, Patil pled guilty to criminal charges, admitting that he had made false statements about patients' medical conditions so he could be paid for inserting stents in them. His plea deal called for a prison term of 30 to 37 months.[29]

As in Baltimore, the number of stenting procedures that were performed at SJH dropped dramatically after the scandal became public. According to University of Louisville professor emeritus Dr. Peter Hasselbacher, before news of the lawsuits broke, SJH did more angioplasties with stents than either of Kentucky's two major teaching hospitals. Subsequently, "the number of invasive procedures dropped by one-third, which [Hasselbacher] called 'the most persuasive evidence that too many cardiac catheterizations with placement of stents might have been performed.'"[30]

If two of every three elective stents are implanted needlessly, it should come as no surprise that many more physicians than we can mention here have been accused of overstenting. Skipping over many convicted offenders, we award the Worst-of-the-Worst to Dr. Najam Azmat and the folks at the Satilla Regional Medical Center who hired him.[31] When the two cardiologists who formerly did stenting procedures at Satilla started taking their patients elsewhere, Robert Trimm, Satilla's CEO, brought in Azmat by offering him a guaranteed salary of $600,000 in his first year plus a signing bonus of $25,000.[32] The compensation was lavish, supposedly because surgeons had to be paid extra to move to tiny Waycross, Georgia, the bit of Okefenokee swampland that Satilla called home.

Azmat had completed a surgical residency, but he had almost no experience with stents. When he applied for the position at Satilla, "his only hands on training in stents consisted of two weekend courses practicing on cadavers and pigs."[33] After accepting the job, he attended a two-day class during which he implanted at least two stents in the renal arteries of live humans.

Things went badly from the start. Nurses who worked with Azmat saw that he didn't know which catheters to use, what their names were, or how they worked. After her second surgery with him, nurse Lana Rogers told both Trimm and Harmon Raulerson, the manager of Satilla's Heart Center, that Azmat's lack of training was obvious. Hospital administrators had no interest in stepping in; when one "nurse asked a hospital official if 'someone was going to have to die before we can stop Azmat,' the official responded, 'yes' or 'probably'. . . ."[34]

Unfortunately, Azmat didn't learn on the job either. A former patient who was a professor of radiology at Duke University sued Azmat for placing a stent in the wrong leg.[35] Quality experts call that type of "wrong-site surgery" a "never event," because it's *never* supposed to happen. It took four attempts for Azmat to insert a stent into the leg of another patient, Norman Copeland.[36] Even when he eventually succeeded, Azmat used the wrong stent and caused the patient considerable pain. There were also serious questions about whether the procedure was necessary in the first place.[37]

The cascade of mistakes led the nurses to revolt. They threatened to quit if they were asked to work with Azmat again.[38] The hospital suspended Azmat's privileges for 10 days, but he returned to implanting stents thereafter.

Azmat subsequently treated Ruth Minter, a mother of five who had been suffering from pain in her back and stomach. He recommended a stent to improve the flow of blood to her kidneys. During the procedure, he botched the insertion and penetrated the wall of her right kidney. This led to internal bleeding and an airlift to a Florida hospital, where Minter underwent emergency surgery. To no avail. Seventeen days later, she died of hemorrhagic shock and multiple organ failure. According to the Department of Justice, which intervened in a whistleblower lawsuit filed by nurse Rogers, the procedure that Azmat performed on Minter "was not medically indicated," meaning it should never have been performed.[39]

Her case was hardly unique. "Federal investigators found more than 30 patients who received 'worthless,' poor or unnecessary care from Azmat, according to experts' case reviews and other documents filed in federal court."[40] A U.S. Department of Justice lawyer reportedly said in open court that Satilla's "administrators knew Azmat wasn't qualified, yet allowed him to keep working, 'profiting all along the way with the lucrative hospital service claims it received in connection with those procedures.'"[41] Satilla paid $840,000 to resolve the federal case. The hospital also settled for undisclosed amounts with Minter's family and seven other patients who sued for medical malpractice.[42]

As for Azmat, his privileges were eventually suspended by Satilla, and he resigned from the hospital after his professional liability insurer wisely refused to renew his malpractice coverage.[43] He then took up work at a pain clinic in Lexington, Kentucky, where he reportedly earned $7,500 a week prescribing narcotics. He was suspended from participating in Medicare and other federal health insurance programs in May 2012. In 2013, he was arrested for running a pill mill in Garden City, Georgia. He was convicted in 2014 and sentenced to 11 years and 1 month in prison. He was nicknamed "Dr. Hazmat" in the federal indictment.

Azmat's case exemplifies the inability of state licensing boards to protect patients from dangerous physicians.[44] Although he began harming patients in the mid-1990s, Azmat wasn't convicted and punished for his crimes until 2014. In 1997, the Hardin Memorial Hospital in Elizabethtown, Kentucky, where Azmat worked early in his career, restricted his privileges after finding that patients involved in 23 percent of his surgeries experienced intraoperative or postoperative complications.[45] Azmat had also been named as a defendant in three different malpractice cases before he joined Satilla's staff in 2005. As noted above, Satilla suspended his privileges for 10 days in 2006. Next there was a flood of fraud allegations and malpractice suits relating to Azmat's actions at Satilla. Despite the many warning signs, however, all three of the states in which Azmat was licensed—Indiana, Kentucky, and Georgia—let him continue treating patients.

Kentucky finally yanked Azmat's license in 2012, when a local emergency room doctor ratted him out for prescribing dangerous drugs.[46] Indiana followed suit the same year. But Georgia, the state where all the dangerous and unnecessary stenting occurred, didn't do anything until 2013, and its medical board acted only after an article published in *Modern Healthcare* lampooned the board for letting him keep his license after he was arrested and jailed.[47]

It is clear there is an epidemic of unnecessary stenting, but it is equally clear that there are also millions of patients whom stents have helped, many by saving their lives. For example, a 2013 study that focused on high-risk CAD patients concluded that those who received PCI plus

medical treatment died far less often than those who received medical treatment alone.[48] The problem of distinguishing between necessary
and unnecessary stenting is simple to state but hard to solve. The line
between appropriate and inappropriate treatments doesn't draw itself.
It depends on the expected benefits of a treatment and whether they
exceed the expected costs, and the answer will vary from patient to
patient. Unfortunately, our politically controlled, third-party payment
system leaves most of that information with cardiologists and hospitals,
on whom the system lavishes money only when they perform aggressive procedures and regardless of the consequences for patients. Stented
patients may experience no improvement or even die; our politically
controlled, third-party payer system cuts the checks regardless. The
predictable result is that many doctors overstent and too many patients
wind up with full metal jackets.

## NOTHING NEW HERE

Paying for every service a physician recommends has served the medical profession well in financial terms, but it has also led to waste, fraud,
and abuse. In too many cases, it has led to injury and death too. We've
focused on stents, but problems with excessive cardiac treatments are
very old news. "Long before the first unnecessary-stent charges started
making headlines across the [United States], cardiology leaders ha[d]
been warning their peers that if they didn't start policing their own
'appropriate use' of devices and procedures, someone else was going to
step in to do it for them."[49]

Outsiders took over the job of policing misconduct at the Redding
Medical Center (RMC) in Redding, California. Acting on a tip from
a patient who claimed that physicians at the hospital were performing
unnecessary angiograms, cardiac artery bypass graft surgeries (CABG—
pronounced "cabbage"), and heart-valve replacements, the FBI raided
the hospital in October of 2002.[50] The evidence gathered then and
during subsequent lawsuits supported allegations that two RMC doctors,
Chae Hyun Moon and Fidel Realyvazquez Jr., performed unnecessary
but highly profitable cardiac procedures on over 750 patients. Medicare

reportedly paid RMC more than $300,000 for each CABG surgery. The surgeries were thought to have killed at least 94 patients and to have caused many others to suffer strokes, paralysis, and heart attacks.[51]

The scandal at RMC received substantial press attention, including an expose on *60 Minutes*, and was eventually covered at book length.[52] The doctors contested the allegations and neither went to jail, but the U.S. Department of Health and Human Services told Tenet Health Care Corporation, the owner of RMC, that it would discontinue federal funding unless Tenet sold the facility. Tenet complied and forked over $369 million to settle with 769 patients who claimed to have been victims of unnecessary cardiac surgeries, plus another $54 million to resolve fraud investigations by public regulators.[53] At the time, the latter was the largest penalty for overbilling in history.

As for the surgeons, Dr. Moon's cardiology group kicked in $24 million to the civil settlements, and Moon himself stopped practicing medicine. Realyvazquez entered into a deal with the California Medical Board pursuant to which his license was revoked then immediately reinstated with a three-year probationary period, during which he was required to receive training in ethics and medicine and to be supervised by other physicians.[54]

It's hard to know which is more shocking: that so many people were mistreated at RMC or that Medicare and other payers just kept on paying for procedures that were harming patients. At the height of its operations, RMC's cardiac surgery unit was performing procedures at a fantastic rate. In one 12-month period, Moon charged Medicare for 876 left-heart catheterizations, four times the rate of the next-highest cardiologist in Northern California. Medicare paid Moon more than every other cardiologist in Northern California except one.[55]

RMC benefited greatly from Moon's stellar work ethic. In the fiscal year that ended June 30, 2002, RMC generated pretax net income of $94 million, the most of any of Tenet's 40 California hospitals.[56] Over the same period, the Mercy Medical Center, a larger hospital located near RMC, generated pretax net income of only $5 million. Even so, the bureaucrats who run the Medicare program sat on their hands. Their job was to pay claims, not to second-guess providers' actions.

## Sometimes Less Is More

Having discussed the overuse of stents and other interventional cardiac procedures, we should also mention two recent studies, the first of which showed that "less is more" for seniors in a way that would be comical if it weren't so sad. Cardiologists have two big conventions a year: the annual meetings of the American Heart Association and the American College of Cardiology. Because so many physicians attend these meetings, hospitals have fewer doctors available to serve patients who come in with acute cardiac conditions like heart attacks and cardiac arrest when the conventions are in progress.

A clever group of researchers compared the 30-day all-cause mortality rates for Medicare recipients with these problems who were admitted to hospitals during the conventions to those for patients who were admitted three weeks before and three weeks after the conventions. The latter groups were treated when the hospitals' staffs were at full force. The researchers "hypothesized that mortality would be higher . . . during the cardiology meeting dates" and "that differences in outcomes would be largest in teaching hospitals, where a disproportionately larger fraction of cardiologists may attend cardiology meetings."[57]

To their surprise, patients suffering from heart failure or cardiac arrest who showed up at major teaching hospitals while the conventions were underway fared *better* than those who arrived on other dates. Their 30-day mortality rates were *lower*, not higher, when fewer doctors were in town. Why? Although the researchers qualified their answers carefully, the most plausible explanation was "that the intensity of care provided during meeting dates [was] lower and that for high-risk patients with cardiovascular disease, the harms of [more intensive] care may unexpectedly outweigh the benefits."[58] High-risk patients fared better when doctors at teaching hospitals were off at meetings because they received *less* care.

The second study, known as ORBITA, appeared just as we were wrapping up this book. Wanting to quantify the impact of stents on patients with stable angina (ischemic chest pain) and severe single-vessel stenosis (narrowing) of a cardiac artery, ORBITA divided 200 patients randomly into two groups. One group received stents. The other under-went a "sham procedure," which fooled people into thinking they had stents implanted, even though they did not. This enabled the researchers to control for placebo effects. When researchers tested members of both groups six weeks after their procedures, they found no discernible dif-ferences between the two groups in terms of chest pain, ability to exer-cise on a treadmill, or a host of other measures.[59] Stated differently, in patients with stable angina and single vessel disease, the placebo worked as well as the stents.

In a commentary on the study, Drs. David L. Brown and Rita F. Redberg observed:

> First and foremost, the results of ORBITA show unequivocally that there are no benefits for PCI compared with medical therapy for stable angina, even when angina is [resistant] to medical therapy. Based on these data, all cardiology guidelines should be revised to downgrade the recommendation for PCI in patients with angina despite use of medical therapy.

Brown and Redberg titled their piece "Last Nail in the Coffin for PCI in Stable Angina."[60] At least one cardiologist got the message. The *New York Times* reported that Dr. Brahmajee K. Nallamothu, an interventional cardiologist at the University of Michigan, coincidentally had a stenting procedure to open a blocked artery scheduled for the day he happened to read the study. Nallamothu found the study's results so convincing that he canceled the procedure. "I took him off the table," Nallamothu said.[61]

Despite Nallamothu's example, we wish we shared Brown's and Redberg's optimism that cardiologists will stop performing PCI for sta-ble angina now that ORBITA has made it crystal clear that less can be more. So long as cardiologists have an economic incentive to use (and overuse) stents, we expect many of them will continue to do so, despite the fact that those stents increase the risk of "death (0.65%), myocardial infarction (15%), renal injury (13%), stroke (0.2%), and vascular compli-cations (2–6%)."[62] If we want cardiologists to change their behavior, we should change their incentives.

### We Love Cardiologists, but Not Their Conflicts

It may seem like we have something against cardiologists. Not so. We admire cardiologists and owe them dearly. A few years ago, a cardiologist who specializes in electrophysiology saved one of our lives. We are grateful and have no wish to seem otherwise.

We had an abundance of specialties from which to choose. Instead of concentrating on cardiologists, we could've written about unnecessary back surgeries,[63] or the efforts orthopedic surgeons made to close down the Agency for Health Care Policy and Research when it came out with treatment guidelines that would have required fewer lucrative interventions and more "watching and waiting" for patients to heal.[64] We could have focused on dentists, some of whom have conducted unnecessary "mass production" procedures on poor children to maximize Medicaid payments.[65] We could have examined doctors who treat cancer patients, many of whom perform unnecessary tests and procedures on seniors who are too old to benefit.[66] They also prescribe drugs that cost tens of thousands of dollars to administer but that have never been shown to extend or improve patients' lives.[67] We could have focused on physicians who admit patients to intensive care units (ICUs) because, in one study, more than half the patients at an academic public hospital's ICU could have been cared for in a less expensive setting and were unlikely to benefit from ICU care.[68] We could have reported on the fact that physicians who treat patients for stenosis of the carotid artery perform surgery far more often than guidelines recommend, and far more often when compensated on a fee-for-service basis than when paid a salary.[69] The subtitle of a 2017 article copublished by *ProPublica* and the *Atlantic* tells the story of excess in American health care: "Years after research contradicts common practices, patients continue to demand them and doctors continue to deliver. The result is an epidemic of unnecessary and unhelpful treatment."[70]

We focused on cardiologists for the reason we identified at the start. Compared to most other physicians, they have larger conflicts of interest because they recommend and perform big-ticket procedures that generate enormous revenue flows. The "cath labs" and operating theaters where cardiac procedures are performed generate substantial fractions of many hospitals' net profits. This is why hospitals pay interventional cardiologists fabulous salaries[71] and enter into sweetheart deals that compensate outside cardiology groups for referrals.[72] Not surprisingly, the pressure to perform procedures is intense. It is to the profession's credit that cardiologists resist the pressure as often as they do; but, given the strength of the incentive to overtreat, a high rate of unnecessary procedures is inevitable. Bad incentives corrode good judgment.

Let there be no mistake: doctors have plenty of freedom to recommend unnecessary treatments. The vast majority of medical decisions involve subjective judgments. Sanjaya Kumar, chief medical officer at Quantros, and David B. Nash, dean of the Jefferson School of Population Health at Thomas Jefferson University, explain:

> Reams of research point to the same finding: physicians looking at the same thing will disagree with each other, or even with themselves, from 10 percent to 50 percent of the time during virtually every aspect of the medical-care process—from taking a medical history to doing a physical examination, reading a laboratory test, performing a pathological diagnosis and recommending a treatment. Physician judgment is highly variable.
>
> Give a group of cardiologists high-quality coronary angiograms (a type of radiograph or X-ray) of typical patients and they will disagree about the diagnosis for about half of the patients. They will disagree with themselves on two successive readings of the same angiograms up to one-third of the time. Ask a group of experts to estimate the effect of colon-cancer screening on colon-cancer mortality and answers will range from five percent to 95 percent.
>
> Ask fifty cardiovascular surgeons to estimate the probabilities of various risks associated with xenografts (animal-tissue transplant) versus mechanical heart valves and you'll get answers to the same question ranging from zero percent to about 50 percent. (Ask about the 10-year probability of valve failure with xenografts and you'll get a range of three percent to 95 percent.)
>
> Give surgeons a written description of a surgical problem, and half of the group will recommend surgery, while the other half will not. Survey them again two years later and as many as 40 percent of the same surgeons will disagree with their previous opinions and change their recommendations. . . .[73]

Given the uncertainty that attends medical assessments, it is critical for doctors to be unconflicted when diagnosing patients and recommending treatments—particularly when they will perform the treatments they recommend. But existing compensation arrangements create strong conflicts that incline doctors to recommend more treatments than patients need. The result is an epidemic of overuse that kills tens of thousands of patients, injures hundreds of thousands of others, and wastes perhaps a trillion dollars a year. And the blame rests with a politically controlled third-party payment system, which is designed to move as much money as possible to health care providers and won't let qualms about corrupting doctors' integrity stand in the way.

# CHAPTER 5: MONEY MATTERS

## It Was Good for Me. Was It Good for You?

"The Completely Honest OB/GYN" is a character created by The Second City comedy troupe. He shoots straight no matter how awkward or unpleasant the truth may be. When a pregnant couple complains that he's 45 minutes late for their appointment, he responds, "Those times are for patients, not for doctors." When the wife says she wants a natural delivery, he asks, "Are you sure? Because a C-section would be way easier for me."[1]

Might OB/GYNs really encourage cesarean sections (C-sections) for their own convenience? The folks at the Childbirth Connection think so. In a detailed discussion replete with citations to the public health literature, they point out that "a planned cesarean section is an especially efficient way for professionals to organize their hospital work, office work and personal life."[2] Like cars coming off an assembly line, C-sections are more predictable than natural deliveries, which can take unexpected twists and turns. C-sections are also significantly more profitable than vaginal deliveries, particularly on a per-hour basis. Does this explain why the C-section rate is so high? Thirty-two percent of deliveries are by C-section, but the optimal rate is estimated to be less than one-third of that number.[3]

Medical professionals deny that financial considerations influence their treatment recommendations. For many doctors, physician assistants, and other providers, this is true. For others, it is not. The evidence that financial compensation affects many providers' medical practices is solid. Two economists found that, on average, a 2 percent increase in Medicare's payment rate for a procedure generates a 3 percent increase in volume. The effect on elective procedures was especially pronounced. Higher Medicare payments also drove investments in technologies like magnetic resonance imaging scanners. Patients seem not to have benefited from more intensive, high-tech treatments: the measurable health benefits were negligible.[4]

Urology provides a case study of the connection between compensation and choice of treatments. In the 1990s and early 2000s, men with prostate cancer had several options, including two treatments designed to slow the growth of tumors by inhibiting the production of testosterone. One option was surgical removal of the testicles (orchiectomy). The other was a drug regimen known as androgen deprivation therapy (ADT). Because the two treatments were equally effective, one would have expected the choice of procedures to be driven by considerations such as side effects, quality of life, or differences in recovery time.

In fact, men overwhelmingly chose ADT over orchiectomy. In 2003, Medicare shelled out at least $1 billion for ADT while spending a paltry $1.5 million on surgeries.[5] The difference in the number of procedures was vast.

Because ADT was 10–20 times more expensive than orchiectomy, the preference for it inflated Medicare's costs. But that was not the real problem. The problem was that ADT drugs were so profitable that urologists prescribed them to many men who did not need them. A study published in the *New England Journal of Medicine* found that 40 percent of the patients who received ADT should not have.[6] "Hundreds of thousands of men were chemically castrated for no reason; that's the biggest scandal of all," said Anthony Zietman of Harvard Medical School, who directs the radiation-oncology program for residents at Massachusetts General Hospital. "The money was too irresistible."[7] Medicare overpaid doctors for ADT drugs, so doctors prescribed them too often.

How profitable were these medicines? By prescribing them, urologists could make as much as $5,000 per patient.[8] For some doctors, drug-related payments generated up to 50 percent of their revenues.[9]

ADT drugs were excessively profitable partly because of the phony average wholesale prices, discussed in Chapter 3, that two companies, TAP Pharmaceutical Products Inc. (TAP) and AstraZeneca LP, submitted for them. In some instances, urologists received even more money through hidden deals with these companies, which rewarded them for using their products and discouraged them from switching to a different brand. These deals were illegal, and heads rolled when they came to light. TAP and AstraZeneca collectively paid more than $1 billion in settlements, and several urologists went to jail.[10]

The scandal involving ADT drugs helped occasion the enactment of the Medicare Modernization Act (MMA) in 2003. The MMA greatly increased health care spending overall, but it took a nip out of payments for cancer drugs. By 2005, urologists were receiving less than half as much as they once did for administering the two most popular ADT drugs, Lupron and Zoladex.

Treatment practices turned on a dime. The frequency of ADT sharply declined while surgeries suddenly became more common. Yes, once reimbursement for ADT drugs dropped, urologists physically castrated their patients more often, making it clear that financial incentives for physicians had helped determine the treatments that patients received. And, because many men who would have been given ADT before now received no treatments at all, inappropriate use fell by 44 percent in a mere two years.[11]

## RADIATING FOR DOLLARS

With the end of massive overpayments for cancer drugs, urologists went looking for new ways to make money. They were upfront about their reasons. In 2004, *Urology Times*, a trade publication, ran an article under the title "New ventures may help make up for lost reimbursement," the point of which was that urologists were "turn[ing] to a variety of non-traditional income producers" in an effort to recoup revenues lost as a result of declining payments for ADT.[12]

Most of the new ventures involved invading other health care providers' turf. For example, instead of sending a patient needing a computed tomography (CT) scan to a radiology lab, a urologist could buy a scanner, hire a radiologist, provide the service in-house, and capture the profit.

> Since urologists routinely order CT scans for diagnosis of stones in kidney and ureters, with as few as three studies a day, an in-house CT scanner would pay for itself in about a year. In a hypothetical example of a pelvic scan without contrast, three studies a day would generate more than $163,000 over 5 years.[13]

The article encouraged urologists to consider performing lab work on blood tests and tissue samples in-house too.

Tucked inside the *Urology Times* article was another one with a punning lead: "IMRT may provide new stream for urologists."[14] This second article reported that "[u]rologists' search for new revenue streams has led them to join forces with radiation oncologists in a venture aimed at capitalizing on the anticipated growth of intensity modulated radiation therapy (IMRT) as a treatment for early-stage prostate cancer."[15] IMRT is fancy and expensive. Just what the doctors needed.

IMRT attacks prostate tumors with X-rays delivered in big doses from multiple angles. But it is not clearly superior to other prostate cancer treatment options, including active monitoring, surgical removal of the prostate, drug therapy, implantation of radioactive seeds, or external beam radiation therapy—a different radiation treatment. In fact, published studies suggest that for men with newly diagnosed, nonmetastatic prostate cancer, no therapy or approach is uniquely better than the others.[16] All have pluses and minuses.

IMRT is, however, very expensive, as shown in Figure 5-1.[17] In the words of Jean Mitchell, an economist at the McCourt School of Public Policy at Georgetown University who authored a leading study of IMRT usage, "Medicare is paying a lot of money for aggressive treatment of prostate cancer where it's basically not going to change anything in terms of giving a patient more years of life."[18]

The profitability of IMRT didn't matter much to urologists when they had to refer patients needing it to radiation oncologists. The law

**Figure 5-1.** Cost of Alternative Treatments for Clinically Localized Prostate Cancer (2005)

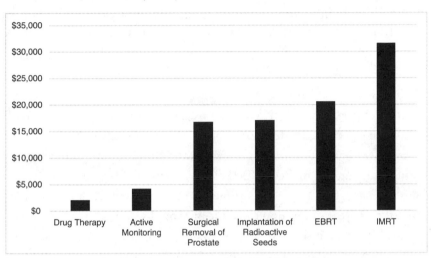

Source: Jean M. Mitchell, "Urologists' Use of Intensity-Modulated Radiation Therapy for Prostate Cancer," *New England Journal of Medicine* 269, no. 17 (2013): 1629–37, http://www.nejm.org/doi/full/10.1056/NEJMsa1201141.
Note: EBRT = external beam radiation therapy; IMRT = intensity modulated radiation therapy.

prohibited oncologists from paying kickbacks for referrals, so urologists had relatively little financial interest in recommending IMRT. This changed when urologists hired oncologists and began offering IMRT in-house. Now, every IMRT treatment put money in a urologist's pocket.

> This side business pays doctors up to $40,000 per patient from Medicare, or 645 times what a urologist gets for a standard office visit, and as much as 20 times what the federal insurance program pays a surgeon to remove a cancerous prostate gland, according to published studies. Reimbursement from private insurers for IMRT can be even higher.[19]

As of 2010, about one in every five urologists offered IMRT in-house. The incentive to push patients into IMRT was obvious.

So was the effect on treatments. Doctors at Chesapeake Urology Associates in Baltimore, Maryland, referred about 12 percent of new prostate cancer patients for IMRT before the practice acquired its own machine in 2007. IMRT referrals then jumped to 43 percent. "In Horry County, South Carolina, IMRT referrals nearly doubled after the Myrtle Beach area's main urology practice merged with the region's largest IMRT clinic."[20] Overall, Mitchell found that, "[w]hen urologists have a financial stake in IMRT, the portion of patients referred for it roughly triples within about two years."[21]

The consequences were predictable. First, the cost of treating prostate cancer patients skyrocketed. Second, many patients received IMRT who didn't need it. In the words of urologist and researcher Matthew Cooperberg, who teaches at the Medical Center at the University of California, San Francisco, "IMRT is overused, period."[22] Cooperberg estimates that about 25,000 men with prostate cancer who receive IMRT each year either don't need it or would fare just as well if given cheaper alternative therapies. "Doctors do what they're paid to do," he said. "If you tell them they can earn $2,000 for surgery or $37,000 for IMRT, what do you think will happen?"[23] The financial cost? About $1 billion annually in overspending.[24]

## WHAT'S MINE IS MINE, AND WHAT'S YOURS IS MINE TOO

Unfortunately, turf wars between competing specialty groups often muddy the evidence that doctors' financial interests influence treatment recommendations. In 2012, Professor Mitchell published a study showing that urologists who offered laboratory services in-house billed Medicare for more prostate biopsies than urologists who did not, but detected fewer cases of cancer—a clear indication of overuse.[25] How did urologists react? By accusing the competing professionals—pathologists and radiation oncologists—who helped fund Mitchell's research of making "a money grab."[26] Dr. Deepak A. Kapoor, president of the Large Urology Group Practice Association, said that Mitchell's study "simply furthers the political agenda of its sponsors to recapture lost market share and does not deserve credible recognition."[27] He also found it "offensive" to suggest that urologists "were performing extra and unnecessary pathology work for their own remuneration" and criticized the methodology Mitchell employed.[28]

It matters little whether, in this particular instance, Mitchell or Kapoor has the better argument. The point that incentives influence both the means by which medical treatments are delivered and physicians' treatment recommendations is beyond dispute. When bringing ancillary services like IMRT and pathology labs in-house, urologists admitted that they were expanding their practices to make money. They wanted to replace revenues they lost when ADT stopped being a profit center. Nor is there any point in denying that physicians respond to economic incentives, just like other people, or in being ashamed of the fact that they do. Every business owner has to worry about revenue flows. Urologists run (health care) businesses, so they have to worry about revenues too. Better to admit that incentives matter and focus on getting them right than to pretend that they don't.

Besides, urologists are hardly alone. After the MMA cut payments for chemotherapy agents, oncologists altered their practices too. They shifted away from drugs whose payments were reduced and switched to more profitable ones. They also gave drugs to more patients.[29] Why? Because oncologists wanted to replace the income they lost. In the words of leading health care researcher and Harvard professor Joseph Newhouse, "hospitals and doctors will respond to changes in how they are paid."[30] That is not (or at least should not be) surprising—particularly when the "markups were a substantial portion of their income."[31]

Having taken it on the chin when Congress passed the MMA, oncologists were loaded for bear when the U.S. Center for Medicare and Medicaid Innovation recently announced its intention to experiment with a new way of compensating them for administering infusion drugs. Instead of paying the average sales price plus 6 percent—an arrangement that, as we discussed in Chapter 3, encourages providers to choose expensive medications over cheaper ones—it proposed a 2.5 percent bonus plus a flat payment of $16.80 per drug per day. Because the cost of infusing drugs doesn't vary with their sales prices, the arrangement has intuitive appeal.

But the experiment, which had the potential to reduce Medicare's drug-related payments by all of 0.7 percent, went nowhere—because oncologists teamed up with pharma companies and killed it. Paul

Gileno, founder and president of the U.S. Pain Foundation, a not-for-profit organization funded by Pfizer and GlaxoSmithKline, said that the demo "would have severely undermined the quality and availability of care for patients suffering from cancer."[32] It is a curious objection, given that providers never complain when *over*payments undermine the quality of care for cancer patients. And, of course, if the experiment had actually reduced the quality of care, the idea could have been scrapped. The real risk was that it might have proved that Medicare could pay oncologists less without endangering patients at all. Oncologists would not have liked that.

### RENAL FAILURES

When it comes to gaming Medicare's payment rules, kidney dialysis providers are among the worst offenders. Dialysis is big business. Medicare spends over $30 billion annually on treatments and medications for patients with end-stage renal disease. Until 2011, Medicare used a hybrid payment model that paid a flat rate for the basic dialysis service plus additional amounts for injectable medications and lab tests. The flat rate was known as "prospective payment" and the payments for medicines and tests were known as "separate billables."

Dialysis companies couldn't easily manipulate the prospective payment, but they did control the separate billables. This arrangement enabled them to inflate their revenues by pumping dialysis patients full of drugs and by using more expensive drugs (like erythropoietin) instead of cheaper ones to manage patients' anemia. "Over time, separately billable services became the primary profit center for most dialysis units, and [erythropoietin became] Medicare's largest drug expense."[33] Many patients suffered, because the high blood cell counts caused by excessive use of erythropoietin were associated with cardiovascular problems, including heart attacks and blood clots.[34]

One company, DaVita Health Care Partners, Inc., the country's largest provider of dialysis services, was especially ingenious. It figured out how to make money by throwing medicines away. The scam was set out in a whistleblower complaint filed by Dr. Alon Vainer and

Mr. Daniel Barbir, respectively, and formerly the medical director and a nurse at a Georgia dialysis center. The Department of Justice joined the case after it was filed.

The lawsuit focused on Venofer, an injectable drug that helps prevent iron deficiency anemia, and Zemplar, a vitamin D supplement. Until 2011, Medicare paid for these drugs on the basis of the amount dispensed. For example, if a pharmacist dispensed a 100 milligram (mg) vial of Venofer, Medicare might pay $30. Importantly, it paid $30 even if the provider injected only 25, 50, or 75 mg into the patient. The leftover portion was deemed to be unavoidable waste.

The whistleblowers charged that DaVita turned the drug payment system to its advantage by increasing the amounts of Venofer and Zemplar that it wasted. Venofer came in 100 mg vials, and the accepted treatment protocol was to give a dialysis patient an entire vial once or twice a month. This produced zero waste. DaVita didn't do that. Instead, DaVita clinics gave 25 mg doses more frequently. But because the drug came only in 100 mg vials, each 25 mg dose of Venofer produced 75 mg of waste, which DaVita threw out. Then DaVita billed Medicare for the full average sales price of the 100 mg vial, plus 6 percent.[35] In a two-month period, a DaVita clinic in Roswell, Georgia, allegedly threw out 19,750 mg of Venofer while administering only 9,625 mg to patients. Because Medicare paid DaVita on the basis of the number of vials that were used, the more medicine DaVita wasted, the more money it made.

DaVita tried to defend its practice of administering Venofer in small doses on medical grounds. Experts interviewed by a *New York Times* reporter were not persuaded. Dr. Michael Auerbach of Georgetown University said that "no clinical reason" and "no safety reason" justified giving Venofer in 25 mg increments.[36] According to the reporter, "Dr. Daniel Coyne, a nephrologist at Washington University School of Medicine who treats some patients at DaVita clinics, said it was 'absolutely true' that the iron drug was given a bit at a time to make more money."[37] Dr. Coyne also asked rhetorically, "How could it be that patients in DaVita facilities were getting so much more iron than patients in other facilities and not getting iron overload?"[38] "The answer," he continued, "is the iron wasn't going into them. It was being thrown away to make a profit."[39]

The whistleblowers' complaint also contended that DaVita stopped wasting drugs when Medicare changed payment approaches in 2011. Under the new rules, Medicare paid dialysis clinics a flat rate of $230 per treatment. No longer were injectable medicines billed separately. "For the dialysis centers, that instantly transformed the expensive drugs from a profit center to a drain on profits."[40] According to the whistleblowers, DaVita quickly switched its Venofer regimen from four 25 mg injections to one 100 mg injection, thereby reducing the number of vials dispensed and eliminating the waste. The change in injection protocols was "an instant case study of how financial incentives can influence treatment choices."[41]

But DaVita did more than just eliminate waste. Drugs now hurt its bottom line, so it cut back on them and substituted cheaper medicines for more expensive ones. Other providers did the same. A study published in the *American Journal of Kidney Diseases* in 2013 found that erythropoietin use started to decline a few months before Medicare rolled out the new payment system and continued to fall throughout 2011.[42] Vitamin D use also fell, and "there was a dramatic shift away from" a pricey drug to one that cost less.[43] Finally, "the mix of iron products changed" again as clinics cut back on "expensive formulations."[44] These drug conservation measures saved providers so much money that their profits rose under Medicare's new payment model, even though Medicare's outlays fell.

Really, though, we didn't need a peer-reviewed study to figure out that treatment practices changed radically. Epogen, manufactured by Amgen, is the most popular erythropoietin-stimulating agent. In the first quarter of 2011, "Amgen's sales of Epogen, all of which are for use in dialysis in the United States, decreased 14 percent."[45] Dialysis patients no longer had to worry about getting too much erythropoietin.

Instead, they had to worry about getting too little. As "the average dosage of anti-anemia drugs taken by dialysis patients decreased by 18 percent from 2010 to 2011," anemia occurred more often and more patients required blood transfusions.[46] "[I]n each of the first nine months of 2011, the share of dialysis patients covered by Medicare who received blood transfusions increased by 9 to 22 percent over the corresponding months in 2010. . . . There had been virtually no change in transfusion rates between 2009 and 2010."[47] This was bad news for hopeful kidney transplant recipients. "[B]ecause transfusions . . . can change body chemistry and make it more difficult to find a compatible organ," dialysis patients who receive them are "more likely to be among the 4,500 Americans who die each year while waiting for kidney transplants."[48]

Once again, these findings indicate how important it is to design payment incentives properly, and to recognize that physicians and health care businesses can and will respond immediately and dramatically to the incentives that are created. Unfortunately, political control of health care spending makes it hard to get the incentives right. Providers who are overpaid (relative to the true market value of their services) will not volunteer that fact. Instead, they will lobby aggressively to maintain the excess payments. And, when the government pays too little, they will vigorously lobby for more, arguing that patients are unable to access needed care. Finally, when the government pays for the wrong thing or pays for the right thing in the wrong way, many providers will happily deliver the specified services and pocket the money. In our politically controlled system, it takes a long time for mistakes to be identified and corrected.

By contrast, when services are sold in competitive markets to patients who pay directly, providers are automatically encouraged to figure out what works best and deliver it. Markets reward providers who outperform their competitors by sending them more business. We discuss direct payment for medical treatments further in Chapter 17.

Nearly all health care providers whose scams are discovered deny having done anything wrong. DaVita was no exception. It defended against the whistleblowers' lawsuit by claiming that Medicare approved its treatment protocol. But the house of cards began to fall in 2012, when DaVita settled a similar case involving Epogen in Texas for $55 million— while also proclaiming its innocence.[49] Then, in 2013, DaVita reserved $300 million "to settle criminal and civil anti-kickback investigations by the Department of Justice," which claimed, among other things, that DaVita paid nephrologists in the Denver area to refer patients to its facilities.[50] The final collapse came in 2015, when the feds announced that DaVita would pay $450 million to resolve allegations that it sought to make money by intentionally wasting drugs.[51]

It may seem like providers—OB/GYNs, urologists, oncologists, and dialysis clinics—are the villains of this chapter. They are not. By pointing out that they respond to incentives, we are not suggesting that they differ from other people or businesses. The truth is that we admire health care providers enormously. One of us is a doctor and the other is married to a physician assistant. How could we not?

The real villains of this chapter are governmentally administered compensation arrangements that cause the interests of providers and patients to diverge. Once one recognizes that providers respond to incentives, one should immediately appreciate the importance of making it financially advantageous for providers to do what is best for patients. Compensation arrangements designed by regulators and elected officials only do that by accident, if ever. In every one of the examples discussed in this chapter, persons exercising governmental powers created compensation arrangements that rewarded providers for mistreating patients. The blame lies with them, or, more accurately, with the system that puts them in charge.

It is perfectly predictable that payment arrangements designed by government officials will cause the interests of providers and patients to conflict. Not only do these regulators lack the information needed to design compensation arrangements correctly, but their incentives are also defective. They neither gain when they design payment arrangements correctly nor lose when they incentivize providers to do harm. The combination of deficient information and defective incentives reminds us of the old gag, "What's the difference between ignorance and apathy? I don't know and I don't care."

Worse still, the project of aligning the interests of providers and patients is intrinsically hard. No compensation arrangement can motivate an agent to serve a principal well in all circumstances and, because technologies, knowledge, and other important factors change over time, an arrangement that works well today may perform poorly tomorrow. Markets deal with both problems by creating always-present incentives for sellers to take buyers' interests to heart. Providers that serve patients well and adapt quickly to changes win customers and thrive. Those that serve patients poorly or seek to exploit them for financial reasons lose customers and fail. Markets do automatically what regulators don't do at all.

## CHAPTER 6: INTEGRITY

The Foundation for a Better Life creates public service ads supporting values like honesty, optimism, courage, and integrity. One of its billboards features Mike Masiello, a mechanic on Long Island. After spending almost three hours trying to fix a car, he realized the problem was unfixable. When the customer asked about the bill, Mike demurred, "I couldn't fix it. I won't take your money."[1]

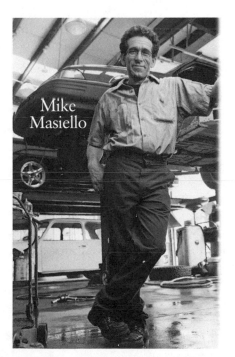

# Couldn't fix it. Refused money.

**INTEGRITY**

*Pass It On:*

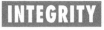

In the private sector, service providers who can't solve customers' problems often go unpaid. Trial lawyers are famous for this. They get paid only when they recover money for their injured clients. The payment arrangement they use is known as the contingency fee. It encourages them to choose clients with good cases and to do only things that are likely to make their clients' claims more valuable. (Defendants complain that contingent-fee arrangements make plaintiffs' lawyers too aggressive in service of their clients. But then again, plaintiffs' lawyers don't work for defendants.)

Health care providers don't work on contingency. Every day, they get paid for treating illnesses they can't fix. The most obvious example is "futile" care, which provides no benefit to patients. A recent study by critical care specialists at University of California at Los Angeles (UCLA) found that 11 percent of the patients treated in their own intensive care unit "received aggressive treatment the doctors considered futile." Another 8.6 percent "probably" received futile care.[2] But UCLA doubtless billed and was paid for providing such care.

The difficulty of denying medical treatment to patients in critical condition must be obvious to any caring person. We do not mean to criticize doctors for being human. But treatments for intensive care unit patients who can't be saved are the expensive tip of a much larger iceberg. Health care providers regularly dispense services that are unlikely to help patients and that may actually harm them. Some providers take this behavior to extremes, but these outliers are responsible for a small fraction of both the costs and the injuries that these treatments entail. The real problem is that the delivery of services of unproven value is business as usual in health care.

### Antibiotics for All

Consider sore throats. There's not much doctors can do about them. The vast majority don't even warrant an office visit because the recommended treatment is rest and fluids. Only the few patients that have strep throat require antibiotics, and a quick test can show whether a given patient falls into that small group. Even so, 60 percent of the roughly

15 million Americans who go to the doctor every year with a sore throat come home with prescriptions for antibiotics, even though antibiotics have no effect on the viruses that cause most sore throats. What about acute bronchitis, also known as a chest cold? The national antibiotic prescribing rate for acute bronchitis should be close to zero because it too is usually viral, but it is actually 73 percent.[3] Then there's the flu. About half of all flu patients treated at outpatient clinics receive antibiotics even though the flu is viral too.[4]

Antibiotic overuse is as old as antibiotics. The Centers for Disease Control and Prevention has discouraged the unnecessary prescribing of antibiotics for decades. But the campaign to change doctors' prescribing habits has failed so badly that some inappropriate prescriptions are now more common than ever before. Zithromax, which was introduced in the United States in 1991, is one example. During 1997–1998, it was hardly ever used for the treatment of adult patients with sore throats. By 2009–2010, doctors were doling it out to 15 percent of these patients.[5]

The volume of inappropriate prescribing of antibiotics is staggering. Every year, doctors prescribe more than 133 million courses of antibiotics to nonhospitalized patients. Depending on the source, between one-third and one-half of these prescriptions are unnecessary.[6] That's somewhere between 44.3 and 66.5 million useless prescriptions per year, counting only antibiotics.

One conservative estimate put the price at $500 million a year but noted that the actual cost could be 40 times as much, or $20 billion. The report added that 5 percent to 25 percent of patients given antibiotics experience diarrhea or other side effects, and many require follow-up treatments. Indeed, "[m]ore than 140,000 people, many of them young children, land in the emergency room each year with a serious reaction to an antibiotic. Nearly 9,000 of those patients have to be hospitalized."[7] Unnecessary prescriptions also contribute to the rise of antibiotic-resistant bacteria.[8]

Antibiotic resistance, diarrhea, trips to the emergency room, hospitalizations, and somewhere between $500 million and $20 billion poured down the drain. That's the tally of unnecessary waste and injury for just one type of medication. What explains this persistent problem?

The conventional wisdom is that patients want their doctors to do some-thing, so doctors write prescriptions. As Shannon Brownlee wrote in *Time* magazine, "Most [doctors] do it out of habit or to make their patients happy. A mother brings her sick child to the pediatrician and expects to walk out with a prescription. It takes time for the doctor to explain why antibiotics won't do any good and might in fact do her child harm."[9] If Brownlee's right, doctors are contributing to antibiotic resistance, sending kids to emer-gency rooms, and wasting enormous amounts of money because it's easier to hand out drugs than to deal with overly demanding moms.

Is that really the reason? There is another possibility. Doctors may prescribe antibiotics and other medications too often because insurers pay them extra when they prescribe drugs. In 2008, Medicare paid $63.73 for a low-complexity office visit (Current Procedural Terminol-ogy [CPT] code: 99213), but $96.01—almost 50 percent more—for a visit that involved "a new diagnosis with a prescription, an order for lab-oratory tests or X-rays, or a request for a specialty consult" (CPT code: 99214).[10] The premium that private insurers paid was nearly the same.[11] The incentive to dole out drugs should be apparent. If you're thinking that the same incentive system could drive overuse of specialty consults, lab tests, and X-rays, you're catching on. A 2008 medical journal article titled "10 Billing & Coding Tips to Boost Your Reimbursement" noted that just one additional 99214 code per day could net a physician "as much as $8,393 over the course of a year."[12]

A big problem with the American health care system is that it pays providers well for doing things that don't actually help patients. Dr. Rita F. Redberg, a professor of medicine at the University of California, San Francisco, and the chief editor of *JAMA Internal Medicine*—whom we met in Chapter 4—provides more examples, all drawn from Medicare:

- In 2009, Medicare shelled out more than $100 million for 550,000 screening colonoscopies. About 40 percent were for patients over 75, even though the United States Preventive Ser-vices Task Force (USPSTF), an independent panel of experts financed by the Department of Health and Human Services, advised that these tests provided no net benefit.

- In 2008, Medicare spent more than $50 million on screenings for prostate cancer in men 75 and older and on screenings for cervical cancer in women 65 and older who had a previous normal Pap smear, again in the face of contrary recommendations by the USPSTF. Medicare spent millions more on unnecessary procedures that followed these tests.

- Two recent randomized trials found that patients who received two popular procedures for vertebral fractures, kyphoplasty and vertebroplasty, fared no better than those who received a sham procedure. Besides being ineffective, these procedures also exposed patients to considerable risks. "Nevertheless, Medicare pays for 100,000 of these procedures a year, at a cost of around $1 billion."

- One-fifth of all implantable cardiac defibrillators are placed in patients who are unlikely to benefit from them. The cost to Medicare is $50,000 to $100,000 per implantation.

The total tally for unnecessary tests and procedures is staggering. Citing the chief actuary for Medicare, Redberg reported that Medicare's 2010 budget could have been reduced by "$75 billion to $150 billion . . . without reducing needed services," simply by withholding payments for things that don't work.[13]

Redberg focused on studies of the Medicare program, but the problem of paying for things that don't work extends well beyond medical treatments for seniors. Consider three examples supplied by Dr. David Newman.[14]

- Back surgeries to relieve pain are, in the majority of cases, no better than nonsurgical treatment. Yet doctors perform 600,000 of these surgeries each year, at a cost of over $20 billion.

- Despite studies showing that arthroscopic surgery to correct osteoarthritis of the knee is no better than sham surgery and is much more expensive and invasive than physical therapy, doctors perform the procedure on more than a half million Americans per year, at a cost of $3 billion.[15]

- Administering beta-blockers to heart attack patients "does not save lives, and occasionally causes dangerous heart failure." Even so, "the medical community has continued to strongly recommend immediate beta-blocker treatment."[16]

Dr. Newman thinks these practices persist, despite evidence of ineffectiveness, because elegant theories support them.[17] He might have added that they also generate billions of dollars in revenue for health care providers. Many "comparative effectiveness" researchers think money is the primary driver. When trying to explain why providers keep delivering services shown to be ineffective or inferior, they observe, "Economic incentives, including the pervasiveness of both fee-for-service reimbursement and generous insurance coverage, are among the most commonly cited" causes.[18]

### Big Money for Ineffective Tests and Treatments

Many big-ticket items could be added to these lists. Consider medical imaging. Radiologists perform more than 95 million high-tech scans each year, at a cost of more than $100 billion. One problem is that many scans, perhaps as many as half of them, are useless because their quality is poor. Health insurers pay for them anyway, because they don't know whether the scans are good.[19]

A second problem is that doctors who purchase their own imaging equipment or own interests in imaging centers have incentives to order lots of unnecessary scans. "Studies have found that up to 3.2 times as many scans are ordered in such cases."[20] Self-referral is "tempting," according to Dr. Bruce Hillman, a radiology professor at the University of Virginia, because "[i]t's all profits." A group of doctors "can reportedly make an extra $500,000 to $1 million a year simply by acquiring a scanner."[21]

Other widely used treatments that don't work, in the sense of either improving health or savings lives, are routine prostate-specific antigen (PSA) tests for prostate cancer in asymptomatic men and routine screening mammograms for breast cancer in healthy, middle-aged women.

Start with PSA tests. Dr. Richard J. Ablin, the researcher who first isolated the prostate-specific antigen, coauthored a book, *The Great Prostate
Hoax: How Big Medicine Hijacked the PSA Test and Caused a Public Health
Disaster*, about the widespread and knowing misuse of PSA tests.[22] He is
palpably angry with the responsible members of the medical-industrial
complex, many of whom he identifies by name.

Ablin's basic point is straightforward and persuasive: PSA is a
*prostate*-specific molecule, not a prostate *cancer*–specific molecule. In lay
language, a PSA test shows only that some amount of a chemical produced by the prostate gland can be found in a sample of a patient's blood.
A high PSA score therefore provides an unreliable basis for diagnosing
prostate cancer. Such an inference would be justified if the molecule was
prostate *cancer* specific, but as Ablin explains it is not:

> PSA levels are affected by a host of factors unrelated to cancer. For
> example, if a long-haul truck driver barreling over the Grand Tetons
> at night stops in a clinic the next morning to have a blood test, the
> jostling ride over the mountains could have elevated his PSA level. An
> amorous motel romp that evening could further elevate the level. So
> might [other relatively common conditions]. . . . The list of possible
> offenders goes on, but the outcome of PSA testing remains the same:
> the level is affected by numerous stimuli and the numbers do not nec-
> essarily indicate cancer.[23]

Even so, every year 30 million healthy men receive routine PSA tests
as screens for cancer, a million men with high PSA scores are subjected
to needle biopsies of the prostate gland, and more than 100,000 men
undergo radical prostatectomies, "most of which are unnecessary."[24]

For many men, the consequences of an elevated PSA test range from
unpleasant to devastating. Eighty percent of the time, men with high PSA
levels who get prostate biopsies turn out not to have cancer. The biopsies
often cause pain, bleeding, and infections; some men die. All of these side
effects stem from a test that is not very reliable in the first place.

What about the remaining 20 percent of the men with high PSA
levels? They do have prostate cancer, but studies show that most of them
would die from something else because most prostate tumors grow

slowly. Dr. Peter B. Bach, of the Memorial Sloan-Kettering Cancer Center, framed the matter this way: Suppose that, in 2009, a man had a positive PSA test followed by a biopsy revealing prostate cancer, for which he was treated. "There is a one in 50 chance that, in 2019 or later, he will be spared death from a cancer that would otherwise have killed him. And there is a 49 in 50 chance that he will have been treated unnecessarily for a cancer that was never a threat to his life."[25] As the saying goes, lots of men die *with* prostate cancer; relatively few die *of* prostate cancer. And treating prostate cancer has many potential serious side effects, including incontinence, erectile dysfunction, pain, bleeding, infection, and death.

Because PSA tests are not specific to prostate cancer, the results of several major studies are unsurprising. According to a review of the evidence conducted by researchers at the Oregon Health and Science University, "After about 10 years, PSA-based screening results in small or no reduction in prostate cancer-specific mortality and is associated with harms related to subsequent evaluation and treatments, some of which may be unnecessary."[26] PSA tests do discover some cancers serendipitously, and for that reason they do save some lives. But in return they exact a staggering toll in dollars and impairment of quality of life.

Why are so many men subjected to blood tests, biopsies, and surgeries they would be better off without? Money. We get what we pay for. We pay urologists for delivering PSA tests and performing surgeries, so we get both by the boatload irrespective of how often they actually benefit patients.

The analysis for mammograms is similar. Mammograms do detect breast cancers, but according to researchers at Dartmouth, only 3–13 percent of women whose breast cancers are found by mammograms are actually helped by the test.

> Translated into real numbers, that means screening mammography helps 4,000 to 18,000 women each year. Although those numbers are not inconsequential, they represent just a small portion of the 230,000 women given a breast cancer diagnosis each year, and a fraction of the 39 million women who undergo mammograms each year in the United States.[27]

In other words, "of the 138,000 women found to have breast cancer each year as a result of mammography screening, 120,000 to 134,000 are not helped by the test."[28] That's 87–97 percent. But many of these women have surgeries, radiation treatments, and chemotherapy, all of which are unpleasant, risky, and expensive. In an article published in the *New England Journal of Medicine* in 2014, leading researchers wrote that a "review of 10 trials involving more than 600,000 women showed there was no evidence suggesting an effect of mammography screening on overall mortality."[29]

Sometimes, doctors understandably think that they are helping patients by delivering treatments and prescribing drugs that later evidence suggests don't work. They are naturally confused when early studies report promising results that later and more reliable studies contradict. This happens so often that an entire field of research, known as medical reversals, focuses on it. The most recent addition to this literature appeared in late 2017, when the *Lancet* published a randomized study that compared arthroscopic subacromial decompression—a common surgery for shoulder pain in which bone spurs and soft tissue are removed—with sham surgery (a placebo) and no treatment at all. The researchers found no clinically significant differences among the patients in the three groups. The invasive surgery was no better than the sham surgery, and neither procedure was significantly better than doing nothing at all.[30]

You might think that, when better studies show that treatments don't work, doctors would stop recommending those treatments. The problem is that the early, less reliable studies spawn whole industries because doctors rush to perform services and prescribe medications that they expect to help patients. Years later, when better research reverses the initial study, shutting down the industry is hard because so many providers depend on it for their livelihoods.

Ablin discusses this in *The Great Prostate Hoax*. He quotes a Canadian physician who posits, "Without radical prostatectomies, more than half of all the urology practices in the United States would go belly-up." Ablin agrees that financial considerations often account for inappropriate behavior: "many urologists defend PSA screening because without the test they would be pushed to the edges of irrelevance and . . . to bankruptcy."[31]

Urologists are far from the only doctors in this position. Medical reversals have the potential to cut into other doctors' practices too. In 2011, researchers at the Mayo Clinic found that almost half of the established medical practices they reviewed were no better than alternatives that were less expensive, simpler, or easier.[32] In 2013, the same group produced a second report finding that 146 articles published in the prestigious *New England Journal of Medicine* from 2001 to 2010 reversed older studies, casting doubt on the effectiveness of 128 medical practices.[33] But, because providers made money delivering them, the practices didn't go away. In the words of Dr. Vinay Prasad, an oncologist with the National Cancer Institute and lead author of the report: "[W]hen we learn in certain cases that we were wrong, it's much harder to stop doing something that we have been doing, especially when there's money involved, and especially when the finances of the person making the recommendation are tied to the patient going through [with the recommended care]."[34]

## BLAME INSURANCE

How did we get into this fix? By basing insurance payments for services on providers' assessments of "medical necessity."[35] For much of the 20th century, doctors enjoyed great freedom to decide which treatments patients should receive. When they recommended treatments, patients went along. In effect, physicians controlled the level of demand for the services they supplied, constrained only by the state of medical science and patients' ability to pay.[36]

The rise of third-party payment, including Medicare and Medicaid as well as private insurance, accelerated the pace of medical science and reduced patients' incentive to scrutinize physicians' recommendations. This disabled whatever brakes there were on health care spending. Predictably enough, demand went through the roof. Physicians made money and gained prestige by treating patients, so they gave their stamp of approval to many procedures of unproven efficacy. Writing late in the 20th century, professors Mark Hall and Gerard Anderson noted that "most current medical procedures were adopted without ever having been tested rigorously" and that "some of the procedures commonly used today have limited or no medical value."[37] In support, they cited a 1990 report by the Bipartisan Commission on Comprehensive Health Care, which found that "only 10–20% of the medical procedures used today have been subjected to randomized clinical trials—the most conclusive method of determining if a procedure is medically effective."[38] This is still true today. "Only a fraction of what physicians do is based on solid evidence from Grade-A randomized, controlled trials; the rest is based instead on weak or no evidence and on subjective judgment."[39]

Clinical Evidence is a database that "showcase[es] the best available evidence on common clinical interventions" to support evidence-based medical decisionmaking. The folks who run it summarized what we know about 3,000 treatments in Figure 6-1.[40] No one knows whether

**Figure 6-1.** Effectiveness of 3,000 Treatments in Randomized Controlled Trials

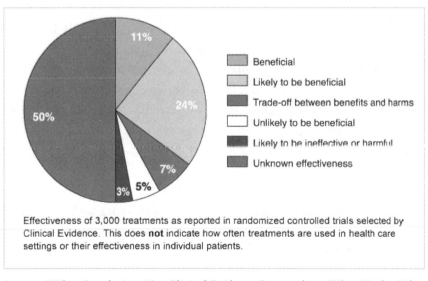

Effectiveness of 3,000 treatments as reported in randomized controlled trials selected by Clinical Evidence. This does **not** indicate how often treatments are used in health care settings or their effectiveness in individual patients.

Source: "What Conclusions Has Clinical Evidence Drawn about What Works, What Doesn't Based on Randomized Controlled Trial Evidence?" *BMJ Clinical Evidence*, accessed Oct. 7, 2017, http://clinicalevidence.bmj.com/x/set/static/cms/efficacy-categorisations.html.

half of the procedures work or not. Another 8 percent are either unlikely
to help patients or likely to harm them.

Some untested treatments eventually prove to be helpful. But many
turn out to be duds, and the duds generate billions of dollars in medical
bills. PSA tests again provide an example. When the USPSTF recommended against regular PSA screenings in 2012, urologists protested and
refused to abide by the new guidelines.[41] Their reaction was predictable.
PSA testing is a $30 billion industry.[42] Threaten to shut down something
that lucrative and providers will be angry.

## Providers Won't Regulate Themselves

Many professional associations know that their members deliver treatments that don't work or whose efficacy is unproven. But, instead of
providing solid leadership, they have dealt with the problem schizo-
phrenically, indirectly enabling their members to keep doing whatever
they want.

Consider how the cardiology profession dealt with the problem of
excessive stenting, which we discussed in Chapter 4. In hope of curb-
ing abuses, it promulgated appropriate use criteria (AUCs), which "are
developed to determine whether a particular approach to care is reasonable in a given clinical scenario."[43] In 2009, a consortium of organizations published AUCs for cardiac revascularization procedures,
including the insertion of stents. They sorted 180 possible treatment
scenarios into three groups: appropriate, uncertain, and inappropriate.[44]
The last category was meant to capture all cases in which stenting was
"not generally acceptable," was "not a reasonable approach for the indication," and was "unlikely to improve the patients' health outcomes or
survival." A recent study found that uniform adherence to AUCs would
save $2.3 billion.[45] Inappropriate and uncertain stentings are that com-
mon and that costly.[46]

But when it came to requiring cardiologists to abide by AUCs, which
many physicians derisively call "cookbook medicine," the associations
demurred. Pushback from practicing cardiologists led them to revise the
AUCs, even to the point of renaming the categories. The category once

called "uncertain" was rechristened "may be appropriate." The "inap-propriate" category is now "rarely appropriate."[47]

Why the new labels? The official explanation was that the AUCs were never intended to prevent patients from receiving the medical treat-ments recommended by their physicians. The backstory was that, when procedures were classified as inappropriate, insurers balked at paying. "The term 'inappropriate' caused such a visceral response," said Robert Hendel, a cardiologist at the University of Miami who reportedly pressed hard for the new terminologies. "A lot of regulators and payers were say-ing, 'If it's inappropriate, why should we pay for it, and why should it be done at all?'"[48] Good questions.

Even under the original category names, the AUCs left a huge amount of room for cardiologists to exercise discretion. Many treatment scenarios fell into the uncertain/may-be-appropriate zone. When doc-tors recommended these treatments, insurers covered them even though, given the state of medical knowledge, it was impossible to be confident that implanting a stent would help a patient. But cardiologists wanted guaranteed payment for even more questionable procedures. They want-ed insurance to cover all of their treatment recommendations, including those that would have been deemed inappropriate under the AUCs. This is the view that helped foster the epidemic of overstenting.

Isn't a better question why payers should cover anything other than treatments that the evidence shows will improve health? According to the AUC classification scheme, interventions are "appropriate" when the science shows that "coronary revascularization would likely improve a patient's health status (symptoms, function, or quality of life) or surviv-al." They are deemed "uncertain" when "more research, more patient information, or both [are] needed to further classify the indication."[49] In plain English, the label "uncertain" is chosen when the science doesn't show that a procedure will help given a patient's condition. But if there is too little evidence to conclude that a procedure will be beneficial, why should a cardiologist perform it? And why should Medicare, Medicaid, or a private insurer be expected to pay? Why not wait until we have enough information to be confident that the likelihood of helping a patient is strong?

### IS A MEDICAL LICENSE A LICENSE TO EXPERIMENT?

The same question can be asked about many of the prescriptions that cardiologists hand out. Like other doctors, cardiologists often prescribe drugs for "off-label" uses that the U.S. Food and Drug Administration (FDA) hasn't approved or found to be effective. A drug named Vascepa provides an example. The FDA approved Vascepa as a treatment for patients whose triglyceride levels were off the charts. Knowing that Vascepa reduced triglyceride levels in these patients, cardiologists started prescribing it to many others, including those whose triglyceride levels were merely elevated. They did this despite the lack of "clinical evidence affirmatively demonstrating that lowering triglyceride levels [in the broader group of patients] . . . ultimately reduces cardiovascular risk."[50] No one knows whether Vascepa helped the thousands of people in the broader group who took it.

Physicians have prescribed drugs for off-label uses millions or even billions of times.[51] No one knows how many of these prescriptions helped patients or how many harmed them. We know only that "'off-label' prescribing may place patients at risk of harm without adequate knowledge of the therapeutic risks and benefits."[52] Procedures that are classified as "uncertain" by AUCs do the same. No one can say whether they help patients or harm them because guesswork is all the science permits.

Although we are certain that most doctors who perform "uncertain" procedures or prescribe medications "off-label" have patients' best interests at heart, the cold, hard, and uncomfortable truth is that they are experimenting on people. This is surely appropriate in some situations, such as when a patient has a life-threatening illness and all approved treatments have failed. But in less dire circumstances, the calculus is more complicated. Do we really want to encourage doctors to experiment without the benefit of patients' informed consent, approved research protocols, rigorous data collection methods, control groups, and oversight by institutional review boards?

In fairness, many off-label uses are well established and apparently helpful, clinical trials are expensive and time consuming, and some experiments turn out well for patients. (We discuss ophthalmologists' inventive off-label use of a cancer drug to treat wet macular degeneration in Chapter 3.) The answer is not clear-cut. Our point is just that the payment system provides a clear and unambiguous signal, encouraging any and all off-label uses.

Not surprisingly, these massive experiments often fail. Time and again, clinical research has shown that commonly prescribed procedures and drugs either confer no benefits on patients or actually harm them. Consider a recent example. Since the late 1960s, cardiologists and other doctors have implanted filters in patients who are at risk of suffering from blood clots in their veins. The filters are supposed to keep clots from reaching the lungs, where they often prove fatal. But no study showed that the filters benefited patients who are also receiving anticoagulants—medicines that prevent clots from forming. And the filters have known side effects. Finally, in 2015, the *Journal of the American Medical Association* published a randomized, controlled study of the issue. It found that the filters "conferred no benefit whatsoever" over anticoagulant medication alone.[53]

The result wasn't altogether surprising. In 2013, the authors of a study of variation in treatment practices across hospitals observed that, although 50,000 patients received filters each year, "there [was] no evidence that inserting a [filter] improved survival."[54] Taking note of this fact, three doctors who commented on the 2013 study wondered, "How Could a Medical Device Be So Well Accepted Without Any Evidence of Efficacy?"[55]

We offer three reasons. First, doctors had a theory suggesting that the filters should work. Second, once the practice of using filters gained a following, doctors simply "assumed that there was strong evidence for their use."[56] Why else would so many doctors have put so many filters in so many patients? Third, Medicare, Medicaid, and other payers covered the procedures. In hospital settings, Medicare paid $3,300 for filter insertion, $2,600 for filter repositioning, and $2,600 for filter removal. When these procedures were performed in a doctor's office, the fees were $2,800, $1,800, and $1,750, respectively.[57] Treatment patterns got well ahead of the science. When the science finally caught up, there was a large financial incentive not to reverse course.

AUCs and other professional guidelines are pointless unless they limit practitioners' discretion and prevent them from recommending aggressive treatments too often. The tendency to overprescribe reflects a confluence of factors: physicians' strong desire to help, their belief in the efficacy of their tools, and, of course, the strong financial incentive to perform procedures. As Dr. Redberg put it when discussing the epidemic of overstenting, "It's like asking a barber if you need a haircut. To an interventional cardiologist, stents are good for almost everyone."[58]

## The Politics of Waste

Many doctors still offer their male patients routine PSA tests, including elderly patients for whom the tests are a complete waste of time.[59] Insurers still pay for the tests too. They're reluctant to cut back on benefits because they risk being caught in a political firestorm when they do. Government agencies run the same risk. Consequently, many are loath to recommend against unnecessary medical services.

Consider the fate that befell the Agency for Health Care Policy and Research (AHCPR) when it issued recommendations discouraging the use of surgery for the treatment of lower back pain. AHCPR convened a panel of experts who, after conducting a comprehensive review of the clinical literature, concluded that there was no evidence that surgery should be the first-line treatment for lower back pain.[60] They also concluded that there was no evidence that spinal-fusion surgery was superior to other surgical procedures but that it did lead "to more complications, longer hospital stays and higher hospital charges than other types of back surgery."[61] Acting on these findings would have required orthopedic surgeons to curtail these treatments, thereby reducing their income.

Instead of complying, disgruntled surgeons joined forces with congressional critics of the Clinton health plan and attacked the AHCPR.[62] The agency ultimately survived, but Congress dramatically reduced its budget, rescinded its authority to issue treatment guidelines, and gave the agency a new name: the Agency for Healthcare Research and Quality.

The AHCPR issued those findings in 1994. Since then, little has changed. "[T]here are still no rigorous, independently funded clinical trials showing that back surgery is superior to less invasive treatments," but orthopedic surgeons keep on operating and insurers keep on paying, even for spinal fusions. In fact, the number of those procedures has grown, "from about 100,000 in 1997 to 303,000 in 2006."[63]

Nor have the politics of waste changed. Fifteen years after the brouhaha surrounding the AHCPR, the USPSTF was overwhelmed when it recommended that healthy women in their 40s should not have routine annual mammograms.[64] The guideline reflected the USPSTF's assessment of the evidence that, for normal women in this age group, the expected health benefits of frequent mammograms are so small and the expected health costs are so large that the procedure would probably do more harm than good. The balance tilted negative because mammograms generated false positive findings, which caused women to undergo unnecessary treatments for tumors that posed no risk to their health. Financial costs did not enter the picture—federal law prohibits the USPSTF from considering the dollars that might be saved by reducing the frequency of mammograms. Had financial considerations been taken into account, the USPSTF's conclusion would have been even stronger.

Congress deliberately attempted to insulate the USPSTF from politics, so its members can focus solely on whatever the evidence says. But because the USPSTF had not consulted the relevant interest groups, its members were unprepared for the firestorm its recommendation against mammograms unleashed. No sooner were the new guidelines announced than trade associations accused the USPSTF of trying to save a few bucks by putting women's health at risk. "Leaders of the American College of Radiology and the Society of Breast Imaging issued statements . . . that the new recommendations looked like an effort to cut costs."[65] Prominent doctors piled on. *Time* magazine quoted Dr. David Dershaw, the director of breast imaging at Memorial Sloan-Kettering Cancer Center in New York City, as saying that he was "appalled and horrified. There is no doubt that mammography screening in women in their 40s saves lives. To recommend that women abandon that is absolutely horrifying to me."[66]

Patient advocacy groups followed the industry's lead. When the American Cancer Society announced its rejection of the new treatment recommendation, Dr. Otis Brawley, its chief medical officer, took advantage of the public's ignorance and stood its logic on its head. "With its new recommendations, the [USPSTF] is essentially telling women that mammography at age 40 to 49 saves lives; just not enough of them."[67] As it happens, that's exactly right: the procedure does not save enough lives to make up for the damage it inflicts. Brawley just left out the second part.

As always, politicians tried to use the uproar to their advantage. The recommendation came in the midst of a debate over whether to enact health care reform. Republicans used the issue to accuse Democrats of wanting to ration care. Representative Marsha Blackburn's (R-TN) comments were typical: "This is how rationing begins. This is the little toe in the edge of the water. This is when you start getting a bureaucrat between you and your physician. This is what we have warned about."[68] Then-representative Candice Miller (R-MI) called the recommendation "'a huge step backward' that puts the nation on a 'slippery slope' to discouraging screening for other diseases based on cost rather than medical need."[69] Then-representative Michele Bachmann (R-MN) played the gender card and stoked unspecified fears: "Women . . . may lose a great deal of clout in decision making. . . . We don't know how far government will go in this bureaucracy."[70] Bachmann would later run for president.

A few Democrats tried to defend the recommendations,[71] but President Obama's Secretary of Health and Human Services Kathleen Sebelius was not one of them. Instead of backing the USPSTF, she pointed out that President George W. Bush had appointed its members. Then she disavowed the new guideline, expressing her personal opinion that women in their 40s should have annual mammograms. She also asserted that annual mammograms would still be covered by private and public insurance, no matter what the Task Force said.[72] As far as we know, Sebelius had no training in medicine, statistics, or anything else relevant to the issue in question. But, she had been a politician, and she knew which way the wind was blowing.

The following year, Sebelius confirmed that, under Obamacare, annual mammograms would be covered—for free. The new insurance plans in which people enroll, she wrote, "will be required to cover recommended preventive services without charging you a copayment or deductible. This includes annual screening mammograms for women starting at age 40."[73] Free is in the eye of the beholder, of course. Mammograms run about $200 apiece, and the total cost of screening the cohort of women in their 40s has been pegged at $2.24 billion.[74] Someone's going to pay, just not patients at the point of service. They'll get millions of mammograms that are more likely to harm them than help them. But at least they'll be "free."

The decision to require coverage of mammograms for women in their 40s actually ran counter to a provision of Obamacare. The law requires Medicare and private health insurance plans to bear the entire cost of preventive services to which the USPSTF assigned a grade of A or B, both of which meant that the USPSTF "recommends the service."[75] But the USPSTF came out *against* diagnostic mammograms.[76] So why did Obamacare cover them?

Because Congress overrode that part of the law. When the controversy erupted, members of both parties worried that women would blame the USPSTF's decision on them. So they amended Obamacare by grandfathering in the old 2002 guideline, which favored annual breast cancer screenings for women in their 40s.[77] Republicans abandoned their commitment to reduce federal spending the instant an opportunity arose to shower money on an important voting bloc. Democrats abandoned their commitment to letting science guide policy. Both parties' actions bring to mind Groucho Marx's famous quip: "These are my principles. If you don't like them . . . well, I have others."

The mammogram debacle made it clear that we can't (and shouldn't) trust Congress to control health care spending. It taught the USPSTF a lesson too. When the parties submitted their proposals to undo its 2009 ruling, the GOP's bill included a provision stripping the USPSTF of its power to make binding recommendations. Having endured that brush with death after being attacked from all sides, the USPSTF will presumably avoid controversy going forward. We can't expect it to stem the growth of health care spending either.

What about Obamacare? Although Obamacare put some money into outcomes research, it explicitly focused the responsible entity (the Patient-Centered Outcomes Research Institute, or "PCORI") on comparative effectiveness research—that is, whether different treatments

work better than each other—not cost-effectiveness research, a more
rigorous way of evaluating medical tests and treatments. And the law
significantly constrains the ability of the federal government to use the
results of PCORI's work to make coverage or reimbursement decisions. Professor Nick Bagley, who believes that Obamacare's statutory
language actually provides PCORI with a lot of flexibility, nevertheless acknowledges that "it would be foolish—maybe suicidal—for the
institute to dwell on cost concerns."[78] If PCORI decides to disregard
Bagley's assessment, we expect the result will be déjà vu all over again.

## Why Do Private Insurers Keep Paying for Treatments that Don't Work?

If we can't depend on the federal government to keep doctors from wasting money and hurting patients, what about private insurers? Won't they
leap at the opportunity to save a buck by denying coverage for things
that are shown not to work?

Unfortunately, in many cases, the answer appears to be "no." First,
private insurers typically get paid a small percentage of the amount of
money they pay out. The more money they pay out, the more money
they make. When private insurers cut back on the stream of payments,
they lower their own take. Just like everyone else in the health care
system, their incentives point in the wrong direction. Second, the last
time insurers did try to step up to the plate (in response to pressure from
employers), they got their heads handed to them. During the 1990s, private insurers tried to use managed care to clamp down on the provision
of unnecessary services by requiring pre-approval for some treatments,
limiting the facilities at which doctors could provide certain procedures, and denying coverage for extended hospitalizations. The resulting "managed care backlash" was real—and it made it clear to insurers
that there would be real costs in trying to reduce health care providers'
revenue streams.

Consider how private insurers handled the problem of percutaneous vertebroplasty. This procedure, which we mentioned briefly above,
involves injecting bone cement into the spine to treat vertebral fractures.

Medicare first covered the procedure in 2001, and most private insurers followed suit. In 2009, the *New England Journal of Medicine* published two randomized double-blind studies that compared it with a sham procedure that involved inserting needles into the spine without actually injecting the bone cement. Both studies showed no evidence that vertebroplasty performed any better than the sham procedure. Even so, private insurers continued to cover the procedure and physicians continue to perform it at will.[79] Even compelling new information indicating that a procedure is worthless cannot spur private insurers to act.

There's a TV commercial where the comedian Beck Bennett asks a group of school kids "Who thinks more is better than less?" All the kids raise their hands. That's what most Americans think about health care. But more is often worse. More can injure. More can kill. And more always costs more money. The AHCPR tried to tell us. Private insurance companies tried to tell us. The USPSTF tried to tell us. But we didn't want to listen, because it's all someone else's money anyway. And health care providers don't want *any* of it to stop coming to them. It's best for them if we think like the school kids: *more is better . . . more is better . . . more is better. . . .*

# CHAPTER 7: PROVIDERS AND POLITICIANS

## WELCOME TO COLLEGE

If you're like us, you were taught in high school civics class that law-makers care about the interests of the general public and will spurn those who seek to exploit public power for private ends. Like us, you were snookered.

In reality, health care politics is a constant and unremitting fight to the death over who will pocket the trillions of dollars we spend every year. Contrary to the high-school-civics view, lawmakers are not trying to restrain providers and insurers. In reality, politicians and providers are co-conspirators against the public interest.

Consider the case of Dr. Salomon Melgen. Our story begins in the mid-1970s, when the Carter administration released the names of physicians and group practices that received more than $100,000 in Medicare payments. Providers didn't want anyone to know how much money they were making, so the AMA and the Florida Medical Association persuaded a federal district court judge that disclosing this information invaded physicians' privacy interests. Their argument should have been laughed out of court. Information about government payments to public contractors and employees is disclosed as a matter of course. Only top-secret programs are exempt from the public's right to know.

For some strange reason, the court issued the injunction that organized medicine wanted. Then something even more surprising happened. Instead of appealing, seeking corrective legislation, or otherwise
attempting to limit the impact of the injunction, the U.S. Department
of Health and Human Services (HHS) did a complete reversal. It abandoned all efforts to make Medicare's payment information public and
spent the next 30-plus years relying on the injunction as a basis for treating all provider-level payment information as top secret. Stated differently, for more than three decades the federal government and health
care providers worked together to conceal an ocean of waste, fraud, and
abuse from the taxpayers who were footing the bill.

The injunction was finally lifted in 2011 thanks to a lawsuit filed by
*The Wall Street Journal* (WSJ). The WSJ had obtained limited data from
Medicare and used it to produce a series of reports on fraud, waste, and
abuse. However, the injunction prevented the WSJ from revealing the
names of the involved physicians and from calling attention to HHS's
persistent failure to adequately address these problems. So the WSJ sued
to have the injunction set aside—the exact thing that HHS had refused
to do. The WSJ won, and after a two-year delay, HHS released information on all Medicare payments to physicians in 2012.

The impact was immediate. In 2014, the WSJ identified a raft of
physicians with suspicious billing patterns. One who stuck out was
Dr. Salomon E. Melgen, an ophthalmologist who practiced in North
Palm Beach, Florida.[1] Dr. Melgen was Medicare's heaviest hitter, with
$21 million in payments in 2012 alone. Most of Dr. Melgen's billing was
for Lucentis, a drug used to treat macular degeneration in the elderly.
(We explained the financial incentive he had to use expensive Lucentis
instead of much cheaper Avastin in Chapter 3.) But Dr. Melgen's charges
for Lucentis were way out of line with that of his peers. What happened
next offers a case study of the politics of fraud control.

## THE POLITICS OF FRAUD CONTROL

How on earth did Melgen make so much money from Medicare? In
fairness, he didn't pocket the full $21 million. For physician-dispensed

pharmaceuticals, Medicare pays the physician the acquisition cost of the drug plus a 6 percent administration fee. A sizable chunk of the $21 million represented the acquisition cost of the Lucentis Melgen dispensed. But Melgen allegedly charged Medicare four times for each vial of Lucentis he used. The vials contained enough medicine to treat four patients, but standard medical policy was to use a fresh vial for each patient and discard the excess. Melgen had a different idea. He used the same vial to treat multiple patients and then billed Medicare as if he had purchased a new vial for each person. As a result, he was "reimbursed $6,000 to $8,000 for a vial that cost him $2,000," plus the 6 percent fee he was also entitled to. Could the use of the word "reimburse" be less apt?[2]

Melgen's $21 million one-year haul was not his first brush with over-billing. Years before, HHS had pegged him as an outlier and concluded that he had overbilled Medicare by $9 million during 2007–2008. Melgen had actually billed $13.5 million for Lucentis during that period, but HHS sought to recoup only two-thirds of that amount. HHS did not try to throw Melgen out of the Medicare program for ripping it off to the tune of $9 million, or even scrutinize his subsequent billings before paying them. It says something about the government's interest in punishing bad actors and its interest in protecting taxpayers that HHS kept paying Melgen's Medicare claims for new patients at a feverish pace while his 2007–2008 case went through multiple levels of appeal.

As was his right, Melgen put on a full defense. He hired the former head of the Department of Justice's Medicare fraud task force as his attorney. He called on his political protectors, enlisting the aid of Sen. Robert Menendez (D-NJ) and Sen. Harry Reid (D-NV), who was then the Senate majority leader. In 2009, Menendez "called Jonathan Blum, the Medicare director at CMS [U.S. Centers for Medicare and Medicaid Services], to express concern. . . . Menendez brought up Melgen's case . . . in the context of broader concerns about [Medicare's billing] guidelines." A Menendez staffer also contacted a CMS official and allegedly pressured him to back off, stating, "bad medicine is not illegal. Medicare should pay these claims." The point is worth repeating. One federal employee told another that the taxpayers should pay for what both of them understood to be "bad medicine."[3]

In 2012, Menendez "raised Melgen's case again at a meeting with CMS Acting Administrator Marilyn Tavenner."[4] Frustrated that he was getting nowhere, Menendez asked Reid to arrange a meeting with HHS Secretary Kathleen Sebelius. That meeting was held on August 2, 2012, in Reid's office. Secretary Sebelius brought along Jonathan Blum. At that meeting, Menendez again pushed for Medicare to drop the overbilling charges, allowing Melgen to keep the disputed $9 million.[5]

Menendez claims not to have known that Melgen was under ongoing investigation and insists he did not request any specific action. But why on earth did a senator from New Jersey feel the need to intervene on behalf of a Florida doctor? And why did the Senate majority leader, who was from Nevada, feel the need to help? Perhaps it had something to do with the fact that Melgen donated more than $700,000 to Reid's political action committee, a fair chunk of which was reportedly spent on Menendez's reelection campaign. Melgen donated additional money to Menendez directly. Plus, Melgen threw in several flights to the Dominican Republic on his private jet, where Menendez had stayed at Melgen's seaside mansion.[6]

In 2015, a federal grand jury indicted Menendez, charging that he "accept[ed] gifts from" Melgen "in exchange for using the power of his Senate office to benefit Melgen's financial and personal interests."[7] According to the U.S. Department of Justice, Menendez "accepted up to $1 million worth of lavish gifts and campaign contributions from Melgen" and sought to influence "the outcome of Medicare billing disputes worth tens of millions of dollars." Bribery charges were also filed against Melgen, who was subsequently indicted on additional grounds by a second grand jury.

Both Melgen and Menendez asserted their innocence. At a press conference, Menendez complained that federal prosecutors "don't know the difference between friendship and corruption." That remark led the famously cynical novelist Carl Hiaasen to pen a column entitled, "It Wasn't Corruption—It Was a Bro-Mance."[8]

At Melgen's criminal trial, federal prosecutors contended that he'd stolen up to $105 million from Medicare.[9] About $41 million was attributable to his practice of billing for the same drug vials repeatedly. The rest was connected to a different type of fraud. Melgen, they contended, intentionally misdiagnosed patients' medical conditions so he could bill Medicare for treating them. According to Dr. Adam Berger, who testified as an expert witness for the prosecution, Melgen reported "almost every patient he saw" as having wet age-related macular degeneration ("wet AMD"). "But in the courtroom, experts called by federal prosecutors saw no signs in the scans to confirm Melgen's diagnoses of wet AMD, and even the defense's own witnesses who looked at the same images struggled to find evidence of the disease." The diagnosis of wet AMD is also easily and cheaply made by means of an optical coherence tomography machine—a machine that Melgen "did not even own . . . despite the fact that virtually every retina specialist in the country uses this technology to diagnose their patients and make sure they are responding to treatment." Melgen also used "a highly controversial and unapproved laser procedure" to treat patients for wet AMD, then disguised what he was doing by billing Medicare under a code for a different procedure—15,000 times. As Berger wryly remarked, "That explains the private jet."[10]

The jury found Melgen guilty on all counts and the trial judge sentenced him to 17 years. Menendez fared better at his bribery trial. After hearing evidence for 11 weeks, the jury deadlocked and the judge declared a mistrial.[11] After some post-trial maneuvering, federal prosecutors decided to drop the case. The line between bromance and bribery may always be blurry. The larger problem is that political control over health care spending increases both the incentives and the opportunities for bribery.

## INSTITUTIONALIZED CORRUPTION

Perhaps Melgen's example is just an isolated case about a single bad physician. Maybe Menendez was overzealous in aggressively advocating for Melgen. Maybe Reid shouldn't have facilitated the meeting at which Menendez pressured HHS employees to drop the case. Surely most politicians know better and will do everything in their power to ensure that the government buys the highest quality health care at the lowest possible price. Right?

Not even close. Both the political corruption of medicine and the medical corruption of politics are pervasive, long standing, and bipartisan. Providers ceaselessly lobby Congress and state legislatures to ensure that the flow of taxpayer money continues undiminished, and that no one holds them accountable for what they do with it. No matter how egregious the fraud, waste, or abuse, or the exploitation of consumers, providers and their lobbyists have a stock set of plausible-sounding justifications for leaving the payment and regulatory systems exactly as they are. They then plow much of that money into political contributions at both the federal and state levels. Melgen's sizable contributions to Reid and Menendez are chump change compared to the aggregate amount that health care providers spend on politics. These outlays help to ensure public officials will tinker with the payment and regulatory systems as little as possible. As the Melgen-Menendez bromance shows, they also buy protection in the rare event that bureaucrats try to clamp down on the worst excesses.

Consider spending by pharmaceutical companies and their lobbyists. Between 1997 and 2015, the pharma sector "donated" $3.3 billion (in nominal dollars) to congressional campaigns—43 percent more than the second-largest contributing industry.[12] Hospitals and nursing homes contributed another $1.4 billion. Physicians and other health professionals added still another $1.2 billion. All in, that works out to about $735,000 per legislator per year.

One way to view these payments is as kickbacks or bribes, where providers grease politicians to keep the money flowing. Another interpretation is that contributions are protection payments made because politicians use their control of providers' revenue streams to extract money from them.[13] Still another possibility is that political contributions are a form of speech. On this account, providers sincerely believe they are doing the right thing by supporting politicians who favor their industry. All three things could be happening at the same time, of course.

Either way, what emerges is an unholy alliance between providers and politicians against the common good. Examples abound. Consider one from 2009, when President Obama was busily selling his health reforms and telling everyone that his proposal would bend the cost curve downward. According to the WSJ, Peter Orszag, the White House budget director, went to meet with a small group of House Democrats:

> The meeting started well, with one lawmaker after another echoing his message that spending controls were critical to any health-care overhaul. . . . Then one member said her top priority was winning higher payments for oxygen suppliers, the officials say.
>
> Mr. Orszag was taken aback. Officials had been trying for years to cut payments to suppliers of oxygen and other medical equipment, which critics say are inflated. Yet when a new competitive bidding process was set to take effect last year, industry supporters in Congress were able to delay the plan. They are still fighting to block changes.[14]

Medicare's spending on oxygen and other durable medical equipment (DME) is small potatoes, but to DME suppliers and the members of Congress they support, those dollars matter a lot.

The negotiations that preceded the enactment of Obamacare provided plenty of opportunities to nurture the bromance between providers and politicians too. In one reported instance, the pharmaceutical industry offered to "give back" $80 billion out of its expected future sales and to sponsor up to $100 million in ads supporting Obamacare in exchange for the Obama administration's abandoning plans that would have cost the industry even more.[15] Michael Cannon described this, and other deals that were cut, as a "protection racket."[16] Stated differently: *nice place you got here—be a shame if anything happened to it.* Obamacare's architects cut special deals that protected or enriched providers and other businesses in multiple states.[17]

Another example shows how providers use their political muscle to keep payments flowing when the administrators at CMS try to cut back on waste and fraud. In 2011, the *Journal of the American Medical Association* published an article focusing on implantable cardiac defibrillators (ICDs). ICDs are used for the treatment of cardiac arrhythmias. Using a database of more than 100,000 ICD procedures, the study found that "roughly one-quarter of patients who had devices implanted did not meet guideline-recommended criteria for receiving them."[18] With more than 100,000 ICDs being implanted every year at an average cost exceeding $35,000 per procedure, HHS was blowing almost $800 million a year on just this one form of unnecessary cardiac surgery.[19]

HHS responded by announcing it would start auditing claims for "several big ticket cardiology and orthopedic procedures" in 11 states *before* paying them.[20] In Florida, Medicare would review all claims relating to stents, percutaneous cardiac intervention without stents, ICDs, pacemakers, and other vascular and circulatory-system procedures before paying the claims to ensure they "complied with all Medicare payment rules," including medical necessity. This is exactly what credit card companies do when they identify questionable charges: block payments and investigate. But for Medicare, which normally pays claims first and asks questions later, if ever, this was a radical change. Because prepayment review would greatly decrease cardiac care spending, stock prices for affected health care companies dropped by up to 10 percent.[21]

But Wall Street misjudged the political power of the medical profession. Industry groups representing cardiologists, orthopedists, hospitals, and device manufacturers mobilized their members to pressure the government to back down. And they succeeded. First, HHS delayed the start date for prepayment review by about half a year. Then it reduced the fraction of Florida claims that would undergo prepayment review from 100 percent to 30 percent.[22] Then it dramatically limited how many cardiac-related categories would be subject to prepayment review. Finally, it cancelled the entire project in 2013—a full and unconditional surrender before the health care industry. As far as we could discover, no prepayment reviews ever occurred. If any did, the results were never published.

HHS backed down because the industry mounted a brutal multifront counteroffensive.[23] The AMA pressured HHS directly to drop the audit plan, claiming that it would jeopardize seniors' access to medical services by discouraging doctors and hospitals from treating them. The American Hospital Association pursued relief in federal courts, claiming that HHS was refusing to pay for medically necessary care. In Congress, the industry sought to clip the wings of the recovery audit contractors (RACs) that Medicare uses to screen claims for improper payments. The RACs had irritated hospitals, cardiologists, and other health care providers by recouping over $5 billion in overpayments on Medicare claims from 2009 to 2013. The medical propriety of claims for cardiac procedures was consistently one of the reasons most often identified by the RACs as a reason for rejecting claims. The industry convinced lawmakers in the House and Senate to introduce bills changing the way RACs were paid and limiting their ability to demand records from hospitals. It got more than 100 members of Congress to sign a letter to HHS Secretary Kathleen Sebelius denouncing abuses by RACs and demanding they be brought under control. Faced with this kind of overwhelming political opposition, is it any surprise that HHS caved?

GIVING DOCTORS THEIR FIX

That was hardly the only time the federal government attempted to restrain health care spending, only to surrender to the industry. In 1997, Congress revised the way Medicare pays doctors. The new formula, known as the sustainable growth rate (SGR), provided that, if Medicare spending on physician services grew more slowly than GDP, doctors would automatically receive more. But, if payments to doctors grew faster than GDP, payments to physicians would automatically be reduced.[24] The object was to prevent the deficit from exploding by ensuring that Medicare spending on doctors grew at the same rate as the rest of the economy.

In 2002, the SGR formula triggered a payment cut of 4.8 percent. Physicians were not happy. They responded with substantial campaign contributions and aggressive lobbying, both peaking in intensity around the time the SGR cuts were scheduled to occur. Physicians wanted to eliminate the cuts and repeal the SGR. That would have caused the deficit to mushroom, however, so Congress was not willing to go that far.

Instead, it responded with a temporary measure that became known as the "doc fix."[25] Rather than eliminate the payment reductions that were due to occur, Congress rolled them over into the next year. Then, when 2003 arrived and the SGR required additional cuts, Congress enacted another doc fix and rolled all of the prior years' cuts into 2004. This process repeated itself year after year. Congress delayed the SGR cuts 17 times, and in many years, it sweetened the doc fix by giving doctors a raise.

As Congress kept delaying the cuts and stacking them up, the potential impact on both doctors and the deficit became huge. By 2015, the delayed cuts and the new cost growth would have required Medicare to reduce payments to physicians by 25 percent. A cut of that magnitude would have had catastrophic effects. Thousands of doctors would have immediately withdrawn from Medicare, leaving elderly patients scrambling for access to care. Angry seniors would have besieged Congress and voted against anyone who didn't fix the problem immediately. Congress went through that experience with the Medicare Catastrophic Coverage Act in the late 1980s, and it had no interest in repeating the experience.[26] So, Congress had to fix the SGR—but how? The AMA wanted Congress to repeal the SGR in its entirety. Once that happened, the cuts would vanish and money would continue to flow.

But there were two big hurdles. One was the enormous cost of swallowing the accumulated deferred cuts. In 2012, the Congressional Budget Office put the cost of repealing the SGR at $316 billion. No one knew where that money would come from, but the AMA did not care. Its object was to make doctors richer. Whether the money came from college loan programs, food stamps, environmental protection, or deficit spending didn't matter. But conservative members of Congress wanted a plan to pay for the SGR repeal, so the repeal was stalled for years.

The second obstacle was that the annual doc fix was a "bell ringer" that generated substantial campaign contributions for politicians and huge fees for K Street lobbying firms.[27] Physicians needed a new fix every year, and they had to bribe Congress to get it. Both Congress and the lobbyists had an interest in making the repeal process as profitable for themselves as possible, which they did by forcing the medical profession to live with a series of one-year bills.

Doctors finally triumphed when Congress passed MACRA (the Medicare Access and CHIP [Children's Health Insurance Program] Reauthorization Act of 2015) with bipartisan support. The SGR was gone. Instead of facing a future filled with payment cuts, doctors were guaranteed raises through 2019. The beast was fed, as everyone knew it would be eventually. The money needed to pay for MACRA was never found. Ninety-seven percent of the cost of repealing the SGR was plowed into the deficit.

The fight over the doc fix demonstrates all of the pathologies we have discussed in this chapter. Health care providers feel entitled to lots of money—the more the better. From their perspective, government exists to make that happen. Occasionally, Congress will make a half-hearted attempt to keep the annual spending increases at some reasonable level— say, growing only as fast as the rest of the economy—and providers will promptly crush it. They will pay handsomely to eliminate any impediments to the continued flow of taxpayer dollars. Given how the battle over the SGR turned out, it is unlikely that Congress will soon gin up the courage to fundamentally reform the health care payment system. The more money the government spends on health care, the more dependent the health care sector becomes on the government. And, the more dependent the health care sector is on the government, the more aggressively it lobbies to ensure that the flow of money continues—and increases.

## Isn't Bromance Wonderful?

If we assume that politicians are running a business and that health care providers are some of their best customers, it quickly becomes clear why there is an epidemic of unnecessary medical treatment. Unnecessary treatments are the reward for the health care sector's lavish political spending. And the reward is enormous. In 2015, health economist Paul Keckley and his coauthors observed that unnecessary medical care, "usually associated with excess testing, surgical procedures or overprescribing[,] accounts for up to 30% of what is spent in health care."[28] With total spending now north of $3 trillion, this means Americans waste $1 trillion on health care in just one year. That's $400 billion more than the U.S. government spends on national defense.

Keckley's 30 percent figure is an all-in number. It includes things like fraud losses and costs stemming from failures to deliver appropriate medical services, as well as overtreatment. It's a conservative estimate too. In 2012, the *Journal of the American Medical Association* published an article by Donald Berwick, the former acting CMS administrator, and Andrew Hackbarth, a researcher at RAND. They concluded that a reasonable *midpoint* estimate of the all-in total for waste was 34 percent of national health care spending.[29] Berwick and Hackbarth put the high end of the range at 47 percent, a shocking $1.4 trillion in 2015. The Institute of Medicine put it this way:

> Unnecessary health care costs and waste exceed the 2009 budget for the Department of Defense by more than $100 billion. Health care waste also amounts to more than 1.5 times the nation's total infrastructure investment in 2004, including roads, railroads, aviation, drinking water, telecommunications, and other structures. To put these estimates in the context of health care expenditures, the estimated redirected funds could provide health insurance coverage for more than 150 million workers (including both employer and employee contributions), a number that exceeds the 2009 civilian labor force. And the total projected amounts could pay the salaries of all of the nation's first response personnel, including firefighters, police officers, and emergency medical technicians, for more than 12 years.[30]

The only way to waste that many dollars is by overusing just about everything the health care sector has to offer. As ludicrous as that sounds, that's what we do. Overuse is so widespread that Robin Hanson, a clever health economist who also has degrees in physics and philosophy of science, has seriously argued that we could reduce medical spending by 50 percent without doing damage to our collective health. "Our main problem in health policy," he contends,

> is a huge overemphasis on medicine. The U.S. spends one sixth of national income on medicine, more than on all manufacturing. But health policy experts know that we see at best only weak aggregate relations between health and medicine, in contrast to apparently strong aggregate relations between health and many other factors, such as exercise, diet, sleep, smoking, pollution, climate, and social status. Cutting half of medical spending would seem to cost little in health, and yet would free up vast resources for other health and utility gains. To their shame, health experts have not said this loudly and clearly enough.[31]

Later in the same article, Hanson reiterates this claim in boldface, stating, **"we could cut U.S. medical spending in half without substantial net health costs.** This would give us the equivalent of an 8% pay raise."[32] Cutting medical spending in half would mean saving $1.7 trillion *every year.* Imagine the good that could be done with that amount of money.

Even associations of medical professionals, which exist mainly to promote their members' interests, admit that medicine is overused and have been shamed into calling for cutbacks. In connection with the ABIM Foundation's "Choosing Wisely" campaign, 70 societies of medical specialists issued lists of procedures that their members should perform *less* often. The America Urogynecologic Society discouraged OB/GYNs from removing ovaries during hysterectomies performed on premenopausal women with normal cancer risk. The American Society for Reproductive Medicine discouraged fertility doctors from prescribing testosterone to men attempting to initiate pregnancy. The Society for Post-Acute and Long-Term Care Medicine discouraged gerontologists from prescribing anti-psychotic medications to patients with dementia and from recommending screenings for various forms of cancer in patients whose life expectancy is less than 10 years. The variety of recommendations on the Choosing Wisely website reflects the pervasiveness of overuse in the medical sector.

Prestigious medical journals have lent their support to the movement. In 2010, *JAMA Internal Medicine* launched its "Less Is More" campaign, which emphasizes that patients often do better when treated less intensively. In other words, unnecessary medical services do more than cost money. They kill and injure patients too. The deaths of 30,000 Medicare recipients each year have been attributed to overly aggressive medical treatments.[33] Think about that: almost 100 seniors a day die from medical procedures they didn't need and shouldn't have received.

Neither the Choosing Wisely campaign nor the Less Is More campaign has done much to discourage overuse.[34] Shannon Brownlee, whose book *Overtreated* focused attention on the problem in 2004, was still lamenting in 2015 that "rampant overuse deprives the health care system of money"—hundreds of billions of dollars, she believes—"that could be better spent making sure patients have care they *do* need. . . . Overuse perpetuates the status quo—a system devoid of transparency, in which clinicians are paid to do more, not better."[35] Exhortations to do less have little effect when the economic incentives encourage providers to do more.

The contrast between medicine and other service sectors is striking. No one contends that plumbers install more toilets than homeowners need, that electricians install too many light fixtures or ceiling fans, or that lawn care companies fertilize or mow their customers' yards too often. Nor are associations of lawyers, accountants, insurance adjusters, engineers, or other professionals calling upon their members to cut back. The medical sector is the only one in which there is an epidemic of overuse. Not coincidentally, it is also the only one in which control over spending rests mainly with government officials and other third-party payers.

The project of moving as many taxpayer dollars as possible into the health care sector is a joint undertaking in which the repeat players all conspire against the public. Government and medical providers are on the same side. The lesser cheats, by which we mean the criminals who commit the most blatant frauds, simply see the doors to the treasury unguarded and decide to join the raid. The conspiracy between public officials and health care providers has already cost the public trillions of dollars. It will not stop on its own.

SECONDARY CONDITIONS OF PRIMARY INTEREST

Most epidemics are caused by infectious diseases such as influenza, malaria, HIV, dengue fever, or Ebola. But America's politicized third-party payment system has also caused a few. Acute heart failure, which involves a dangerous and often deadly breakdown in the heart's abil ity to pump blood, is one of them. From 2008 through 2010, Chino Valley Medical Center (CVMC) in San Bernardino County, California, claimed that 35.2 percent of its Medicare patients suffered from acute heart failure as a secondary condition to other problems for which they were hospitalized.[1] This seems to have been untrue. Rather, CVMC appears to have created a seeming epidemic by inflating its billings.

In a 2011 exposé, investigative journalists from California Watch discovered that CVMC had "billed Medicare for the costs of confronting what appear[ed] to be a cardiac crisis of unprecedented dimension." CVMC's patients were experiencing acute heart failure at a rate that was six times the statewide average. The epidemic hit CVMC's Medicare patients with septicemia (a life-threatening blood infection) particularly hard; almost 8 percent of the Medicare patients treated by CVMC had both septicemia and acute heart failure—more than 15 times the statewide average.[2]

Was there really an epidemic of heart failure among elderly patients in San Bernardino County? If so, it is hard to explain why other hospitals in the area missed it. They too had cardiac care units, but they didn't experience a similar rise in heart failure cases. Either CVMC was a statistical anomaly or something else was going on.

Given what California Watch found, that "something else" appears to have been "upcoding"—an industry term meaning that CVMC was manipulating patients' records to trigger larger payments from Medicare and other insurers. Medicare pays more for treating patients with major complications. By making patients seem sicker than they were, CVMC was able to game Medicare's payment system and reap substantially larger payments.

Medicare pays a fixed amount for the hospitalization of a patient with a particular illness. To make things concrete, let's say the fee is $5,500 for a hospitalized patient with Legionnaires' disease. If the patient also has a secondary condition, like acute heart failure, Medicare pays more, because the patient requires additional services. In the case of our imaginary patient with Legionnaires' disease, adding acute heart failure as a secondary condition might trigger a bonus payment of almost $6,000 more—bringing the total payment up to $11,400.

Upcoding is possible because Medicare doesn't know whether a given patient has acute heart failure as a secondary condition. Medicare doesn't even know whether a patient has the coded *primary* condition. As Medicare's failed experiment with prepayment review (discussed in Chapter 7) demonstrates, Congress doesn't much care, either. Medicare relies on hospitals to bill honestly. Unfortunately, many hospitals take advantage and boost their revenues and profits by making up secondary conditions that don't exist.

That certainly seems to be what CVMC did. CVMC didn't report *a single* acute heart failure case as a secondary condition in 2006, before bonus payments were available. By contrast, after bonus payments were introduced in 2007, California Watch found that CVMC treated "1,971 Medicare patients for acute heart failure" between 2008 and 2010, and "in 88 percent of the cases, [acute heart failure] was listed as a secondary diagnosis that typically would trigger bonus payments."[3]

California Watch interviewed two heart specialists who said they found CVMC's heart failure rate implausible. Dr. Gregg Fonarow, the director of the Ahmanson–UCLA Cardiomyopathy Center and the associate chief of the Department of Cardiology at the David Geffen School of Medicine at UCLA, stated, "You don't see (hospitals) where 35 percent of the Medicare population has heart failure." Dr. Steven Shayani, a cardiologist and president of the New York Heart Research Foundation, observed that CVMC's acute heart failure complication rate "doesn't make any sense" and wondered why Medicare officials weren't investigating.[4] Both experts suspected that doctors or billing personnel at CVMC were exaggerating patients' illnesses.

## PRIME'S NUMBERS

CVMC was owned by Prime Health Care Services, which operates a chain of hospitals, including 13 in Southern California. In a shocking coincidence, of the 10 California hospitals with the highest reported rates of acute heart failure, Prime owned 8. Prime's hospitals also reported unusually high rates of other dire and rare conditions. One of these was kwashiorkor, an extreme form of malnutrition most often experienced by starving children in sub-Saharan countries that are stricken by droughts or embroiled in civil wars.[5] The kwashiorkor secondary diagnosis entitled Prime to $6,000 extra per patient. At one Prime hospital in Shasta County, California, fully 16 percent of Medicare patients were suffering from kwashiorkor—70 times the statewide average. Overall, Prime reported that 25 percent of its Medicare patients were malnourished, compared to a statewide average of 7.5 percent. In another shocking coincidence, of the 10 California hospitals with the highest reported rates of malnutrition, Prime owned 8.

Here's another way to look at the same numbers. Prime hospitals treated 3.6 percent of Medicare patients in California, but they accounted for 12 percent of the state's malnutrition cases and 36 percent of its kwashiorkor cases. If Prime's billing figures were right, the elderly population in California was extremely malnourished.[6] The mystery, again, was why other hospitals missed the epidemic. Their Medicare bills rarely

**Figure 8-1.** Incidence of Listed Illnesses per 1,000 Medicare Patients at California Hospitals (2009–2010)

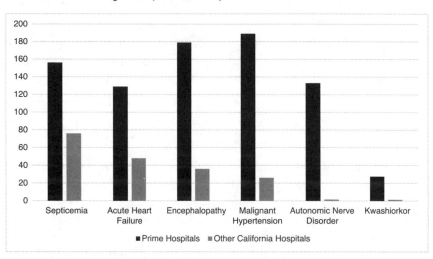

Source: Adapted from California Watch, "Prime Healthcare Reports Outsized Rates of Unusual Conditions," December 16, 2011, http://static.apps.cironline.org/prime-health-care/.

mentioned kwashiorkor. Either Prime's doctors were unusually adept at spotting sub-Saharan malnutrition or something else was happening.

Prime's billing records indicated it was also experiencing epidemics of other diseases that its competitors were failing to treat. Figure 8-1 shows how illness rates reported at Prime's hospitals differed from those at other California hospitals, as reported by California Watch. If Prime's bills were right, medical personnel at other hospitals were systematically failing to detect serious illnesses.

Did real illnesses explain these extraordinary differences, or was Prime systematically defrauding Medicare? One important piece of evidence: the kwashiorkor epidemic at Prime ended right after California Watch published its story.[7] At the Prime hospital in Shasta County, the rate of kwashiorkor plummeted overnight, from 16 percent of admitted Medicare beneficiaries to zero. Similar results were observed at other Prime hospitals. Either the media can work miracle cures or Prime stopped billing for kwashiorkor as a phony secondary condition the minute it got caught.

## UPCODING EMERGENCY CARE

If Prime hospitals were upcoding, they weren't alone. After Medicare implemented bonus payments for secondary conditions in 2007, "63 other hospitals that had reported no [cases of] acute heart failure in 2006 also began recording cases of the ailment."[8] Prime hospitals even had company in other states when it came to reporting elevated frequencies of kwashiorkor. In 2012, the Good Samaritan Hospital of Maryland settled claims that, from 2005 to 2008, it inflated its Medicaid bills by falsely reporting that its patients suffered from this ailment. Two Catholic hospitals, Christus St. Vincent Regional Medical Center in Santa Fe, New Mexico, and Mercy Medical Center in Des Moines, Iowa, "each billed Medicare for more than 100 cases of kwashiorkor between 2010 and 2011." All of these diagnoses were found to be unwarranted. (The hospitals blamed faulty billing software.) "All told, the federal health care program paid more than $700 million in 2010 and 2011 for patients diagnosed with kwashiorkor."[9]

There's more to the upcoding story than phony secondary conditions, however. The Center for Public Integrity (CPI) published a series of "Cracking the Codes" investigative news reports in which it found widespread overcharging by hospitals for treatments delivered to Medicare patients.[10] For example, the bills submitted by the Baylor Medical Center in Irving, Texas, indicated that its patients were "among the sickest in the country." "In 2008, the hospital billed Medicare for the two most expensive levels of care for eight of every 10 patients it treated and released from its emergency room—almost twice the national average. . . . Among those claims, 64 percent of the total were for the most expensive level of care."[11] According to CPI's published account, a Baylor spokesperson conceded that the hospitals' bills for emergency room (ER) treatments were out of line with industry standards.

That may not have been true. Upcoding is so widespread that it may be the industry standard. Studying the first decade of the 21st century, CPI found that hospitals added more than $1 billion to the cost of Medicare by using the most remunerative billing codes more often. "Use of the top two most expensive codes for emergency room care nationwide nearly doubled, from 25 percent to 45 percent of all claims, during the time period examined."[12] In many instances, the patients for whom these codes were used were not seriously ill. "Often, they were treated for seemingly minor injuries and complaints" and sent home without being admitted to the hospital.[13]

How did hospitals account for the increase in the severity of illness reported? By claiming that sicker patients were coming to their ERs. Dr. Stephen Pitts, an emergency physician and associate professor in the Emory University School of Medicine who examined data on ER visits, dismissed this explanation. "It's total nonsense," according to Dr. Pitts.[14]

The CPI attributed the billing surge to "lax government oversight, confusion about proper billing standards, and widespread payment errors that have plagued Medicare for more than a decade. And the data suggest that some hospitals are working the billing system—and its flaws—to maximize payments." Dr. Donald Berwick, a former Medicare administrator, agreed, saying, "They are learning how to play the game." Barbara Vandegrift, a health care consultant, was even blunter: "It's 'wait until we get caught and we'll fight it at that point.'"[15] This attitude makes sense because the risk of being caught is small. Medicare lets hospitals establish their own billing policies, offers little guidance, and rarely audits.

### PAYMENT-INDUCED CURES

The payment system doesn't just cause epidemics. It sometimes cures them too. The most famous example involves pneumonia, a respiratory infection that can be deadly. Between 2003 and 2009, the medical establishment seemed to have pneumonia on the ropes. Hospitalizations for pneumonia dropped by 27 percent and the death rate fell by a third. The reason for these stunning improvements was not entirely clear. Doctors were treating pneumonia the same way they had been for years.

Most people know better than to look a gift horse in the mouth. Why question a victory in the endless war against infectious diseases? But academic researchers were curious, so they looked into hospitals' coding practices. Their findings, which appeared in the *Journal of the American Medical Association*, showed that credit for the victory belonged to the payment system, not to hospitals or physicians.[16] Although admissions with a *primary* diagnosis of pneumonia fell from 2003 to 2009, hospitalizations with a primary diagnosis of sepsis and a *secondary* diagnosis of pneumonia rose by an almost equal amount. The rate at which patients with pneumonia were hospitalized hadn't declined at all. The reduction in death rates was phony as well. Patients whose primary diagnosis was pneumonia were dying less often, but when researchers combined those patients with the patients who had pneumonia coded as a secondary diagnosis, they found that the death rate hadn't budged. Pneumonia was just as common and as deadly as always. Public health officials were using billing records to track infection rates—and they were deceived by a change in the billing practices of hospitals. The triumph over pneumonia was a paper victory, not a real one.

Why had hospitals changed their coding? The lead author of the study observed that "there's a strong financial incentive for coding based on sepsis versus pneumonia" because hospitals get paid more for doing so. There was also a national campaign to raise awareness about sepsis. The combination made it easy for providers to change their coding practices.[17]

The payment system also created a false victory over avoidable hospital readmissions, which are thought to occur when hospitals provide shoddy care, release patients too soon, or provide inadequate services postdischarge. Wanting to encourage hospitals to do better, Medicare began a "pay-for-performance" initiative that included financial penalties for hospitals that readmitted too many patients within 30 days of discharging them. The initiative, known as the Hospital Readmissions Reduction Program (HRRP), seemed to be successful. Readmission rates fell by about 70,000 cases the year it took effect.

In fact, the quality of care delivered by hospitals had not improved. They reduced their readmission rates by gaming the payment system. Instead of admitting patients who appeared to be at risk for premature readmission, they put them on observational status or treated them in their emergency rooms. When these patients later returned for additional treatments, they could be admitted without causing problems because they had not been formally admitted the first time around. Hospitals also used these tactics to avoid readmitting patients who returned within 30 days of being discharged. They'd put these patients on observational status or treat them in ERs too, so they wouldn't count as readmissions either. More than two-thirds of the decline in readmissions had nothing to do with quality of care and everything to do with gaming the payment system.[18]

Not only did the HRRP not cause hospitals to treat patients better, the initiative may have actually cost thousands of patients their lives, according to a study published in *JAMA Cardiology* in 2017. Since heart failure (HF) is "the leading cause of readmissions among Medicare beneficiaries," researchers decided to study the relationship between the HRRP and mortality in patients with HF. They found that as the HRRP drove down the 30-day and 1-year readmission rates for HF patients, the 30-day and 1-year mortality rates for these patients increased.[19] Dr. Gregg Fonarow, one of the researchers involved in the study, estimated that "10,000 patients a year with heart failure [were] losing their lives as a consequence of [the HRRP], an absolutely devastating level of potential harm."[20] Wanting to avoid the financial penalties they stood to incur by readmitting patients too often, hospitals and doctors were treating HF patients in ways that shortened their lives.

## TURBOCHARGED BILLING AND OUTLIER PAYMENTS

Few people associate hospitals with greed. Most consider them "good guy" community organizations that differ fundamentally from other businesses of similar size. The fact that many are nonprofit organizations adds to the halo effect. But the truth is that hospitals are big businesses and are run as such. Like the other businesses that operate in the health care sector, they are adept at taking patients and their insurers (both public and private) to the cleaners.

Consider the amounts that hospitals charge for their services. These figures are found on "chargemasters"—lists of charges (i.e., prices) that all hospitals maintain. At one point, these charges may have been closely related to hospitals' actual costs, but over time they took on a life of their own. A study published in *Health Affairs* found that chargemaster prices are, on average, 3.4 times the actual cost of patient care. At the 50 greediest hospitals, charges are more than 10 times actual costs.[21] Into the 1980s, Medicare paid hospitals on a cost-plus basis, so hospitals profited by inflating their costs. Medicare no longer uses that arrangement, but hospitals still gain by exaggerating.

One reason is that they have learned how to use inflated chargemasters to extract additional dollars from insurers and patients. These effects were quantified in a 2017 study by Michael Batty, an economist at the Federal Reserve Board, and Benedic Ippolito, a researcher at the American Enterprise Institute. Combining national data on hospitals' list prices with data from California on payments, they found that "an additional dollar in the price set by the hospital chargemaster was associated with an extra 15 cents in payments from a commercially-insured patient."[22] The effect on uninsured patients was larger: a 20-cent increase in payments for every extra list-price dollar. The researchers also learned that the effect on uninsured patients disappeared after 2007, when California's Hospital Fair Pricing Act kicked in. The act allows hospitals to charge uninsured patients only as much as Medicare pays. (Although this section focuses on prices, it is worth noting that Batty and Ippolito found no correlation between hospitals' chargemaster prices and the quality of care they delivered, as measured by 30-day readmission rates. Pricier hospitals weren't better than cheaper ones.)

It is easy to see how inflated chargemaster prices enable hospitals to extract extra dollars from uninsured patients. Many uninsured patients pay all or part of their bills, and the amounts they pay correlate with what they are charged. Charge them more, and they pay more. It is as simple as that.

When it comes to obtaining payments from insurers, the role of chargemasters is both less obvious and more complex. One possibility is that hospitals set their list prices high so as to be able to bargain down from them in negotiations with insurers, stopping when the discounts are just large enough to get insurers to agree. This "flea market" strategy helps hospitals price-discriminate, just as drug companies do (see chapters 1–3), and it is consistent with the fact that hospitals' negotiated prices are industry secrets. By negotiating different discounts from their list prices for different payers, hospitals can charge each payer the most it is willing to pay—that's price discrimination. But the strategy works only if the discounts that hospitals are willing to accept remain hidden. Otherwise, all insurers will know how low hospitals are willing to go.

Another theory offered by Batty and Ippolito is that hospitals use high list prices to gain leverage over insurers. They do this in a surprising way: by exposing patients to high out-of-network charges unless their insurers include them in their networks. Suppose that a city has two hospitals—Hospital A and Hospital B—but only Hospital A is in a patient's insurance network. If the patient is involved in an accident or the patient's doctor has admitting privileges only at Hospital B, there is a risk that the patient will have to be treated there and will be balance billed for the out-of-network charge. Wanting to eliminate that risk, the patient may go looking for a new insurer that has both Hospital A and Hospital B in its network. And the higher Hospital B's list prices are, the more the patient will want to avoid the risk by finding a new insurer. The desire to retain subscribers will therefore exert pressure on insurers to strike deals with all major providers in their areas, enhancing the providers' leverage in price negotiations.

Even though Medicare no longer pays on a cost-plus basis in most situations, high chargemaster prices still help hospitals extract dollars from it too. When an elderly patient's treatment ends up costing a hospital a lot more than Medicare normally pays, hospitals can claim extra "outlier" payments. And, when determining whether an outlier payment is warranted and how large it should be, Medicare uses chargemaster prices as proxies for hospitals' costs. Once again, political control of the payment system lets providers set the prices they receive from Medicare. By inflating their chargemaster prices, hospitals can increase both the likelihood of receiving outlier payments and the amounts they are paid.

The practice of using chargemasters to obtain outlier payments by inflating costs is known as "turbocharging." Many hospital companies have played this game. Tenet Health Care Corporation (discussed in Chapter 4) allegedly collected more than $1 billion in outlier payments by inflating its prices to an average of 477 percent of costs. Tenet's outlier payments went from $351 million in fiscal year 2000 to $763 million in fiscal year 2002.[23] At most hospitals, outlier payments generated 4–5 percent of Medicare revenue, but at Tenet they accounted for 23.5 percent of Medicare revenue in 2003. Eventually, Tenet was forced to clean house and modify its chargemaster. When it did so, its outlier payments plummeted. Tenet ultimately paid more than $900 million for misconduct involving turbocharging, upcoding, and paying kickbacks to physicians. It also paid another $10 million to resolve securities fraud claims relating to turbocharging.[24]

Beth Israel Medical Center (BIMC) also got caught turbocharging and admitted guilt as part of a $13 million settlement.[25] BIMC inflated its charges by 200 percent between 1996 and 2003, even though its costs for treating Medicare patients grew by only 10 percent. In dollar terms, from 1996 to 2003, BIMC's Medicare inpatient costs increased by only $17.4 million, while its Medicare inpatient charges increased by more than $285 million.[26]

Usually, wrongdoers refuse to confess culpability when settling with the feds. Why did BIMC choose to come clean? We suspect that the feds insisted on a confession because the evidence was so damning. There were many memoranda and emails in which hospital executives embraced the turbocharging strategy. For example, in 2000, a vice president for patient financial services at the company that owned BIMC wrote that the hospital would "keep the charges high even at the lowest levels of service in the E.R."[27] Another executive wrote of "feeling a bit giddy" at the thought of "getting $10 million of outlier revenue." A third advised caution because she feared that BIMC's turbocharging would be detected.

The Lenox Hill Hospital, which gained considerable fame when Beyoncé went there to deliver her daughter, also pled guilty to turbocharging. It "admitted, acknowledged, and accepted responsibility for having increased its charges based on revenue models that did not directly take into account the costs of the services provided, and as a result obtaining Medicare outlier payments it would not otherwise have received."[28] Federal prosecutors claimed that from February 2002 through August 2003, Lenox Hill intentionally raised its room and board charges and manipulated its overall charge structure to make it appear as though its treatment of certain patients was unusually costly, when in fact it was not. The settlement required Lenox Hill to pay $11.75 million. Beyoncé and Jay-Z, who spent an estimated $1.3 million on their maternity suite and delivery, may not have known about Lenox Hill's deliberately inflated chargemaster prices, or they may have negotiated themselves a better deal. We should not assume the same for Lenox Hill's other patients.

Medicare changed its payment rules in 2003 to make it harder for hospitals to game the system. It subsequently discovered that hundreds of hospitals had turbocharged. How many did so without being caught, we will never know. Turbocharging has also resurfaced in the last few years. A *Wall Street Journal* article published in 2015 gave four examples:

1.  Somerset Medical Center in New Jersey had an increase in outlier payments in 2010 and 2011 six times higher than each of the five previous years. The payments in 2010 and 2011 together totaled $13.6 million. About $10.5 million of those payments were due to increased list prices.
2.  Christ Hospital in New Jersey collected $2.93 million in 2013 in special payments from Medicare, a 60 percent markup over 2012.
3.  Cedars-Sinai Medical Center in Los Angeles, one of the largest recipients of Medicare outlier payments in the country, had an increase in outlier payments of about $18 million due to list price increases in the 2013 fiscal year.
4.  Health Management Associates Inc. raised the list prices of a hospital chain it acquired in Florida in 2011. Medicare payments for outlier claims jumped from $150,000 to $6.2 million, of which $5.2 million was found to be due solely to list price increases. [29]

Continued turbocharging led Tom Scully, the former head of the U.S. Centers for Medicare and Medicaid Services (CMS) who implemented the change in payment rules in 2003, to remark that "efforts to curb excess payments are 'like Whac-a-Mole.'"[30] That's such a good analogy that we chose it as the title for our chapter on policing health care fraud (Chapter 12).

## OVERBILLING ELECTRONICALLY

The latest upcoding scams involve electronic health records (EHRs). The federal government tried to get providers to use EHRs for decades, claiming that they would improve quality and save money. Providers finally got on board when the federal government offered them $30 billion in bribes.[31]

The main thing EHRs appear to have improved was providers' ability to commit fraud. First, the EHR program itself was hit by providers who wanted to be paid for adopting EHRs, even though they had not. According to the *Dallas Morning News*, a chain of six small-town hospitals in Texas run by Dr. Tariq Mahmood received almost $16 million in bonus payments for implementing EHRs.[32] To get the money, the hospitals had to certify that they met various measures of "meaningful use" of electronic records. However, instead of actually using EHRs, the hospitals kept paper records and hired an outside vendor to manually input data into electronic form after patients were discharged. So much for "meaningful use."

Second, EHRs make providers much more efficient upcoders. Merely by clicking a button or a menu or copying information from one patient's records to another's, a provider can enter a condition, treatment, or other factor that triggers a high payment.

In 2012, the *New York Times* reported, "the move to electronic health records may be contributing to billions of dollars in higher costs for Medicare, private insurers and patients by making it easier for hospitals and physicians to bill more for their services, whether or not they provide additional care."[33] At Faxton St. Luke's Health care in Utica, New York, the fraction of patients treated in the emergency room who were supposedly treated at the highest level of service intensity (thereby triggering higher payments) rose by 43 percent in 2009, the year the hospital switched from paper records to EHRs. At the Baptist Hospital in Nashville, the portion of emergency patients who were supposedly treated at the highest level of service climbed 82 percent in 2010. This was the year Baptist switched to EHRs too. And at Methodist Medical Center of Illinois in Peoria, "billings for the highest level of emergency care jumped from 50 percent of its emergency room Medicare claims in 2006 to more than 80 percent in 2010, making the 353-bed hospital one of the country's most frequent users of high-paying evaluation codes."[34]

The perversity of subsidizing EHR adoption becomes even clearer when one compares hospitals that received subsidies with hospitals that didn't get the cash: "Over all, hospitals that received government incentives to adopt electronic records showed a 47 percent rise in Medicare payments at higher levels from 2006 to 2010 . . . compared with a 32 percent rise in hospitals that have not received any government incentives."[35] In 2010, 54 percent of emergency room claims were in the two highest-paying categories, up from 40 percent in 2006.[36] Congress literally paid hospitals to find ways to charge taxpayers more.

Multiple peer-reviewed studies and governmental reports show that upcoding and other forms of gaming are pervasive.[37] According to Dr. Donald W. Simborg, who chaired a federal panel on EHR fraud, "It's like doping and bicycling. Everybody knows it's going on."[38] In 2012, Kathleen Sebelius, secretary of the U.S. Department of Health and Human Services, and Eric Holder, the attorney general, sent the American Hospital Association and other industry groups a sternly worded letter urging them to discourage hospitals from using EHRs to game the system.[39] They might as well have asked scorpions not to sting frogs.[40]


ROBIN HOOD, M.D.

Doctors are surprisingly open about their willingness to game the payment system. In 2000, Dr. Matthew Wynia, the director of the AMA's Institute for Ethics, and coauthors published a study in the *Journal of the American Medical Association* reporting that 39 percent of physicians admitted to deceiving insurers within the previous year.[41] In 2002, *Medical Economics* asked doctors, "Have you ever exaggerated or misstated a patient's diagnosis to a third-party in order to secure authorization for a treatment, procedure, or hospital stay that might otherwise have been denied?" Twenty-one percent answered "Yes."[42] Internists reported fudging diagnoses more often than other specialties; 32 percent admitted using this tactic. Almost a decade later, another journal published a study finding "strong evidence" that the possibility of obtaining larger payments by charging for more intensive services than were actually delivered "influences physician's coding choice[s] for billing purposes across a variety of specialties."[43] "For general office visits," the study reported, "Medicare outlays attributable to upcoding may sum to as much as 15% of total expenditures for such visits."[44]

Physicians' openness about their willingness to commit fraud reflects a variety of beliefs that make it easy for them to rationalize cheating. First, many doctors believe that public and private insurers shortchange them routinely. Insurers pay too little, refuse to cover important services, and often deny coverage entirely for reasons that doctors find arbitrary and unfathomable. Second, physicians believe they are ethically obligated to help their patients. Deceiving insurers helps both doctors (who get paid) and patients (who get the services they need). In a society where TV shows like *ER*, *Scrubs*, and *Grey's Anatomy* portray doctors who defraud insurance companies as heroes saving patients from evil corporations, it's easy to rationalize gaming.

Consider the case of former gynecologist Neils H. Lauersen, whom Geraldo Rivera dubbed the "dyno gyno." Lauersen "was convicted in 2001 of billing insurance companies for gynecological operations when he was really giving fertility treatment for women he said could not afford it."[45] Gynecological procedures were covered by insurance. At the time, fertility treatments were not. So, Lauersen used codes for the former when performing the latter, manufacturing insurance coverage out of thin air.

Lauersen treated C. C. Dyer, then Geraldo Rivera's wife, who subsequently bore two children. She thought him a hero. "To me, he was Robin Hood, taking from the big bad companies and giving to the poor just trying to have a baby," Dyer said.[46] Lauersen was no Robin Hood. He lined his pockets by deceiving insurers. In his criminal trial, he was accused of collecting $5 million by intentionally miscoding procedures.[47]

His prodigious billings helped him maintain a fancy Park Avenue office and move about in the loftiest of social, artistic, and political circles.

Dozens of Lauersen's patients attended his trial and insisted, like Dyer, that he was a hero. A contemporaneous profile gives a sense of the arguments that were offered at trial:

> Although his defense hinges on the line that Lauersen did not perform infertility treatments at the expense of unwitting insurance companies, there's a steady undercurrent to it that says, *So what if he did*? "The government's calling me Robin Hood, robbing from insurers and giving to my patients," Lauersen says, smiling at the characterization. "Insurance companies should be paying for these women."[48]

The first trial ended with a hung jury. Press reports indicated that "one juror in particular said later that she simply did not believe insurance companies."[49] Then, New York's medical licensing board concluded that Lauersen was a danger to his patients and suspended his license to practice medicine. Court records indicated he had been sued 26 times, more than 6 times the lifetime average for OB/GYNs. Lauersen was then retried on the fraud charges, convicted, sentenced to seven years in prison, and ordered to pay $3.2 million in restitution.

Lauersen's actions were illegal. Even so, many people regard what he did as either desirable or, at worst, a petty offense. People hate insurers. A large segment of the public thinks they are greedy, bloodsucking parasites, and that insurance fraud is necessary to even the score.[50] Many of Lauersen's patients belonged to that group. They were happy to have their health care carriers pay for fertility-related services that their policies didn't cover, and for which they had never paid. Doctors find it easy to rationalize insurance fraud too. When asked about upcoding, they often shrug off the suggestion that suspect billing patterns indicate fraud and claim instead that their patients are unusually sick.

Thousands of self-declared, white-coated Robin Hoods are bleeding the federal treasury dry. According to a 2012 Office of the Inspector General report, 5,000 physicians "consistently billed for high level" codes when applying for payments from Medicare.[51] They get away with it partly because upcoding is easy. If a doctor selects one code when treating a new patient, Medicare will generate a check for about $37. If the doctor chooses a different code instead, Medicare will pay $190. Slight changes in billing codes can trigger bigger payments from private insurers too.[52] Payers' ability to monitor the accuracy of doctors' bills is limited, so as a practical matter, doctors can pick the codes they want. Not surprisingly, thousands pick the codes that generate the highest payments. With about one billion visits to doctors' offices a year, the aggregate financial impact of these small retail-level instances of cheating is staggering.

## BILLING FROM THE GRAVE

Upcoding is probably the most common form of overbilling, but there are many other types. Dr. Farid Fata, a Michigan oncologist, provided a recent and truly stomach-turning example of a different technique.

Fata told healthy patients that they had cancer so he could make money by giving them chemotherapy they didn't need. Fata reportedly "gave one of his patients 155 chemo treatments over two-and-a-half years—even though the patient was cancer-free."[53] He is said to have pumped other patients full of unnecessary blood therapies and iron treatments. Even though Dr. Fata was busy ripping off Medicare and his patients, a Detroit magazine named him one of the "Top Docs" in 2006, 2007, 2008, 2009, 2011, and 2012. In 2015, he was found guilty and sentenced to 45 years in prison after abusing the trust of more than 550 patients and receiving more than $17 million through fraudulent billings.[54] He dreamed of living out his life in a $3 million castle in Lebanon, but he is now, fortunately, rotting away in jail.[55] Dr. Fata may not be seeing patients anymore, but the Detroit magazine still has him listed on their website as a "Top Doctor."

When we read about Fata's misdeeds, we initially thought he was unique. We now know better. Dr. Salomon Melgen, whose story is discussed in Chapter 7, falsely diagnosed patients as suffering from wet age-related macular degeneration, then charged Medicare for treating them. Dr. David Ming Pon, who was sentenced to 10 years in prison, performed laser surgery on hundreds of patients whom he falsely diagnosed as having glaucoma. He too was convicted of Medicare fraud.[56]

With three such cases having popped up in a short span of years, we are forced to wonder how many more monsters are out there who have so far avoided discovery.

Other doctors make up claims out of whole cloth. In 2014, federal prosecutors charged Syed Imran Ahmed with submitting more than $85 million in Medicare claims for services he never delivered.[57] The feds also sought to seize his ritzy Long Island home, worth approximately $4 million. But they were too late to get all the loot. Ahmed wired $2 million out of the country immediately after being interviewed by the FBI.[58] Amazingly, Ahmed is thought to have committed the fraud over a period of just two short years—proof that a corrupt doctor can bleed the system of large sums quickly.

The feds win most Medicare fraud prosecutions, so Ahmed's conviction came as no surprise.[59] Still, most doctors who overbill are never even arrested, let alone tried. Many mix a limited number of fraudulent claims in with a larger volume of legitimate ones, making their fraud essentially invisible. Fata, the overmedicator, was a notorious overbiller, but his misdeeds were discovered after a nurse who once worked at his clinic turned him in. Despite the heinousness of his offenses, it still took the feds three years to arrest him after receiving the whistleblower's report.[60]

Fata and Ahmed can be punished because they're alive. But how are the feds supposed to deal with doctors who submit phony bills after they die? In 2007, Congress received a report showing that upward of 18,000 dead doctors had filed over 478,500 claims with Medicare. The report also revealed that Medicare had shelled out as much as $92 million to pay claims from dead doctors.[61] In 16 percent of the cases, the departed doctors had been dead for more than 10 years. But Medicare just kept on paying. Medicare opened for business in 1965, but almost 45 years later it still had "no reliable way to spot claims linked to dead doctors."[62] In 2009, 2,500 doctors who died before 2003 still had active identification numbers. In a model of understatement, Sen. Norm Coleman (R-MN) remarked, "When Medicare is paying claims and the doctor has been dead for 10 or 15 years, you know there is a serious problem."[63]

And, because every type of billing fraud that can occur does, there are also live doctors who bill for treating dead patients. One famous case involved Dr. Robert Williams, a Georgia physician. From 2007 to 2009, he submitted more than 50,000 claims to Medicare and more than 40,000 claims to Medicaid for group psychology sessions, many of which supposedly involved nursing home residents who were dead or hospitalized when the sessions were said to have occurred.[64] Medicall Physicians Group Ltd. ran a similar scam. In mid-2015, a Chicago jury convicted two people associated with Medicall of billing Medicare for physician services that were never delivered, including services that were supposedly rendered to patients who were dead, that were delivered by providers who were no longer employed by Medicall, or that were provided by professionals so industrious they worked more than 24 hours a day.[65]

How big a problem is this? No one knows. An Office of the Inspector General investigation found that, in a two-year period, Medicare "recovered $3 million in improper payments stemming from approximately 27,000 claims for services billed for deceased beneficiaries."[66] If CMS recovered that much, it undoubtedly paid out much more. But no one is keeping track.

### Rewarding the Guilty, Punishing the Innocent

CMS has tried to offset its losses from upcoding and other types of overpayment by reducing payments to providers in general. It did this in 1984 and 1985, when it cut hospital payments by 3.38 percent and 1.05 percent, respectively. It wanted to go after hospitals again in 2008, 2009, and 2010, but each time Congress intervened and prevented it from doing so. Upcoding also led CMS to whack payments to home health agencies by 2.75 percent each year from 2008 to 2010 and by 2.71 percent in 2011. Payments to inpatient rehabilitation facilities and long-term acute care hospitals have also been cut to offset this form of fraud.

Imposing across-the-board cuts rather than dealing with upcoding directly is counterproductive. It tempts honest providers to upcode. Otherwise, they get punished and lose money while the bad guys continue doing it. It therefore makes upcoding seem legitimate, reduces the stigma that normally accompanies illegal behavior, and destroys the norm of billing honestly.

It may help to see this point from another angle. When CMS reduces all providers' payments because of upcoding by some, it sends a clear signal that it can't tell the honest providers from the frauds. This means that it's smarter to upcode than to bill accurately because the odds of being singled out for punishment are small. It also makes providers who bill honestly look and feel like chumps. A government program that makes it more profitable to deceive regulators than to submit truthful bills is a program that sows the seeds of its own destruction, because it fosters attitudes and beliefs incompatible with the rule of law.

How much does all this upcoding cost? It's impossible to be sure, but a report from the HHS Office of the Inspector General found that, in just one year (2010), Medicare paid $6.7 billion too much for evaluation and management (E&M) services, a category that includes visits to doctors' offices, emergency room assessments, and inpatient hospital evaluations. To put the dollar figure in context, $6.7 billion was 21 percent of the total amount that Medicare paid for E&M that year.[67]

*ProPublica*'s study of Medicare spending data provides another look at the scope of the problem.[68] Using a five-level system with a score of 5 corresponding to the most expensive level of care, the watchdog group found that in 2012, 1,200 doctors and other health professionals billed at level 5 exclusively, while 600 more did so more than 90 percent of the time. Some 20,000 providers billed only at levels 4 and 5. Apparently, they never saw patients who required less complicated care, even though such patients appeared in other doctors' offices all the time. Of the more than 200 million office visits that Medicare paid for in 2012, only 4 percent commanded the most expensive rates—indicating something is almost certainly seriously awry with the billing practices of the 20,000 providers who billed only at levels 4 and 5.

How did the physicians who consistently used the most expensive codes explain their actions? When questioned by *ProPublica*, "[s]ome doctors . . . said that their patients were sicker than those of their peers and required more time and attention."[69] The Reverse Lake Wobegon Effect rears its ugly head again. Anyone want to bet on whether this is real or just another payment-induced epidemic?

# CHAPTER 9: OUT OF NETWORK, OUT OF LUCK

### Surprise! Here's Your Bill

McAllen, Texas, has attracted a lot of unwelcome attention. In 2009, surgeon and medical writer Atul Gawande pegged it as the highest-cost county in the United States for Medicare, with per-patient spending almost twice the national average. It was a mystery why spending there was so high. McAllen's population was similar to El Paso's, another border town in the same state, but Medicare's per-patient spending in El Paso was average.[1] Doctors and hospitals in McAllen simply delivered more services than providers anywhere else.

McAllen is America's capital of surprise medical bills too. These are bills that patients receive after being treated at hospitals that are in their insurance networks from physicians who are not in-network. According to a 2017 study published in the *New England Journal of Medicine*, 89 percent of the patients who were treated in emergency rooms at in-network McAllen hospitals received bills from doctors who didn't take their insurance.

These problems are not limited to McAllen. Complaints to the Texas Department of Insurance about surprise bills rose by 1,000 percent from 2012 to 2015.[2] Concern was so widespread that, in 2017, Texas enacted a new law that entitles patients to demand mediation for out-of-network bills.[3]

The law doesn't do much, but given Texas' pro-business slant, the legislation of any protection at all for consumers is remarkable.

The problem of surprise bills is nationwide. A Consumers Union survey found that about one-third of privately insured respondents had received an unanticipated bill within the preceding two years.[4] A survey conducted jointly by the Kaiser Family Foundation and the *New York Times* reported that, "among insured, non-elderly adults struggling with medical bill problems, charges from out-of-network providers were a contributing factor about one-third of the time."[5] According to a *New England Journal of Medicine* study, 22 percent of patients received a bill they did not expect.[6] A study in the health policy journal *Health Affairs* found that "20 percent of hospital inpatient admissions that originated in the emergency department, 14 percent of outpatient visits to the [emergency room, or ER], and 9 percent of elective inpatient admissions likely led to a surprise medical bill."[7] Another study of nine million ER visits from 2011 to 2015 found 22 percent of patients who went to an in-network hospital received a bill from an out-of-network ER physician.[8]

Surprise bills hit patients from many directions. They come from anesthesiologists, radiologists, surgical assistants, lab technicians, and other providers who, despite delivering services at hospitals that are in patients' insurance networks, are not in those networks themselves. In one reported instance, two parents were billed over $4,000 in out-of-network charges because, although the hospital where their infant son was born was in-network, its neonatal intensive care unit was not.[9]

When providers are out-of-network, they can bill patients at their own vastly inflated chargemaster prices instead of the discounted rates that insurers pay. If you've seen a bill from an in-network provider or the corresponding "explanation of benefits" from your insurer, you know what we mean. The hospital or physician may "charge" a chargemaster price of, say, $3,000 for a service. But the insurer will disallow a huge chunk of that—say, 75 percent. The real price is $750. The insurer will pay all, some, or none of that price, depending on the health plan's cost-sharing structure.

But, when a surprise bill from an out-of-network doctor comes in, it will demand $3,000 without the discount. The insurer then pays the same amount it would otherwise—that is, no more than $750. The patient is then on the hook for the rest—anywhere from $2,250 to $3,000. This is known as "balance billing." The patient is responsible for the difference because the doctor, being out of network, never agreed to accept the insurer's discounted rate.

Balance billing for out-of-network treatment is a scam. In almost every instance, the provider who is demanding the full rack rate routinely accepts far less as payment in full from in-network patients and from patients who are covered by Medicare or Medicaid. Those are the provider's real prices. As we discussed in the previous chapter, the rack rate or chargemaster price is simply a number pulled out of thin air to help providers extract as much as they can from each patient. Those numbers bear no relationship to providers' costs, either. On average, hospitals charge out-of-network patients 3.4 times, and the 50 worst offenders charge more than 10 times, the actual cost of the services they use.[10]

Hospitals are hardly alone in gouging patients. Aetna once sued an out-of-network New Jersey physician who treated a patient at an in-network hospital. Aetna claimed that the doctor charged $31,939 for services whose reasonable value was only $2,811, which Aetna paid. In a fit of generosity, the doctor then "balance billed" the patient just $10,635, rather than the entire $29,128 balance, a fact that itself indicates how inflated out-of-network rack rates can be.[11] Other doctors' rack rates are just as phony. According to a report published in the *Journal of the American Medical Association* in 2017, anesthesiologists, radiologists, and ER doctors regularly charge out-of-network patients four to six times more than they accept from Medicare for the same services.[12] Anesthesiologists were the worst offenders.

Balance bills are thought to average about $900, but providers often demand far more.[13] Peter Drier was told he had to have neck surgery. He researched his insurance coverage and thought he knew what to expect. But after the operation, he received a $117,000 surprise bill from an "assistant surgeon" he hadn't known about or met.[14] The bill was "20 to 40 times the usual local rate" and orders of magnitude larger than the $6,200 fee charged by the primary surgeon. Patricia Kaufman, who had surgery at a Long Island hospital for a chronic neurological condition, was victimized too. Two plastic surgeons charged more than $250,000 to sew up her incision, "a task done by a resident during [her] previous operations."[15] After Kaufman's insurer paid about $10,000, the surgeons balance billed her for the rest. John Elfrank-Dana, a 58-year-old father of three who worked as a public school teacher in New York City, needed a series of procedures after slipping on some steps and banging his head. His surprise bills tallied $106,000.[16] The list of examples of crippling surprise bills is endless—and they can wreak havoc with patients' finances, particularly if the provider sends the bill to a collection agency.

Rural residents, accident victims, and other persons who need to be airlifted to hospitals face especially great risks. Air ambulance services can charge whatever they want, so patients who use them can wind up on the hook for truly enormous sums.[17] Consider a representative example:

> When Amy Thomson's newborn daughter was in heart failure, Ms. Thomson had to use an air ambulance service in rural Montana for transport to a more capable facility. At the time, her insurance company, PacificSource, did not have an in-network air ambulance company near her family . . . . Ms. Thomson received a $43,000 balance bill from Airlift Northwest after PacificSource contributed a policy cap of $13,000.[18]

## Whose Fault Is It?

When one asks providers why balance billing occurs so often, they blame insurers. Rebecca Parker, the president of the American College of Emergency Physicians, provides a perfect example. When asked why ER doctors send out so many surprise bills, she replied: "This is insurance company bad behavior."[19] That seems like an odd thing to say, given that doctors, not insurers, send out the bills. But Dr. Steven Stack, who served as president of the American Medical Association, agrees. "The real crux of the problem," he says, "is that health insurers are refusing to pay fair market rates for the care provided."[20] Hospital administrators agree that insurers are the guilty parties, and should "pay more, expand their networks, and eliminate the problem."[21] If providers are right, the problem isn't that they're greedy. It's that insurers are cheap.

Naturally, insurers see things the other way around. They accuse doctors who balance bill for out-of-network charges of price gouging, and they accuse hospitals of being complicit. They contend that it is hospitals' "responsibility to ensure all physicians treating patients in their facility are covered by the same insurance contracts as the hospital."[22] Some insurers are steering people away from hospitals that refuse to do just that. Aetna encouraged its subscribers to avoid Allegheny Health Network hospitals in Pittsburgh when ER physicians there began to balance bill aggressively. UnitedHealthcare went one better—or one worse, depending on one's perspective. It announced that it would no longer cover any medical bills for members who unknowingly received out-of-network treatment by physicians at in-network hospitals.[23] The execs at UnitedHealthcare must have figured that administrators at in-network hospitals would be careful to assign only in-network doctors to patients if they knew that any contact with an out-of-network physician would eliminate insurance coverage for all of the bills.

Because all this finger-pointing leaves patients exposed, lawmakers have launched themselves into the breach. New York adopted a comprehensive approach that lets patients off the hook for out-of-network charges when they seek emergency medical treatments or are cared for at in-network hospitals. In these situations, providers have to accept insurers' in-network rates, but can use arbitration to try and get more. Altogether, about half the states have enacted laws that protect patients who need emergency medical treatments from surprise bills. But patients who receive scheduled procedures are still vulnerable. This is one reason why many health policy experts think federal regulation is necessary.[24]

The unanswered question is why so much surprise billing occurs. It isn't a problem in other contexts where people pay for things with insurance. If your car is damaged in an accident, the body shop will send you and your insurer a single, all-inclusive bill. You won't be charged a separate fee over and above what your insurer pays by the technician who does the paint job or the mechanic who replaces your dented fender. Body shops pay the workers whose services are required and bill for everything themselves. Market forces have pressured them to bundle services and charges into packages that are convenient for consumers and to accept compensation at rates that insurers and consumers are willing to pay.

Nothing prevents hospitals from doing what body shops do. They too could bring all service providers in-house and submit all-inclusive bills to patients and insurers. Then there would be no surprise bills. Hospitals could also allow doctors to remain independent but require them to have agreements with the same insurers the hospitals do, as a condition for treating patients. In fact, some hospitals do this.[25] Patients treated at these hospitals don't have to worry about being balance billed.

But many hospitals seem to go out of their way to create opportunities for surprise bills. Some have no doctors in their ERs who are in the same insurance networks they are. Literally every patient admitted to these hospitals' ERs is likely to end up being balance billed. The same fate awaits patients who undergo surgery at hospitals with no in-network anesthesiologists. After having her thumb operated on, Elaine Hightower was balance billed for $6,300. Her hospital and doctor were in-network but the anesthesiologist on duty that day wasn't.[26] Often, patients meet their anesthesiologists for the first time shortly before being wheeled into surgery. Those with the temerity to ask them whether they are in-network may discover the anesthesiologists themselves do not know. Then, the patient faces the Hobson's choice of risking a hefty out-of-network bill, or undergoing a procedure without anesthesia.[27] This is no way to run a railroad, let alone a hospital.

Why have some hospitals solved the problem of balance billing while others have not? And why are surprise bills from ER doctors, anesthesiologists, and a few others especially common?

## To Make or to Buy—That Is the Question

Anesthesiologists, radiologists, pathologists, and other doctors who send out lots of surprise bills tend to be independent contractors. They deliver services at hospitals, but they are not hospital employees. Their status differs from that of the many other doctors who *are* employees, a group that includes staff physicians of many types. In recent years, the number of staff physicians has exploded, as hospitals have brought on board thousands of doctors who formerly practiced independently. Over a three-year period ending in 2015, "Hospitals acquired 31,000 physician practices, a 50 percent increase."[28] The number of hospital-employed doctors now exceeds 140,000. By and large, these doctors don't balance bill because they are full-time employees. If the hospital is in-network, they are too.

Why did hospitals bring so many more doctors under their umbrellas while farming out their ERs to independent contractors and leaving other doctors, like anesthesiologists, radiologists, and pathologists, independent?

To understand the answer, it helps to know some basic economics. For a business, the decision to produce a good or service internally or to obtain it from an external supplier is known as a "make or buy" decision. Neither option is intrinsically better. When a business can profit more by making something itself than by buying it from someone else, it will choose the former option and acquire the resources needed to produce it. When it is more profitable to purchase a good or service from an external supplier, it will do that instead.

Today, for example, most businesses find it more economical to buy electric power from a utility than to generate it themselves. When deciding whether to "make or buy" electricity, they opt for the latter. As solar panels become cheaper and more efficient, though, the calculus is changing and some businesses are going off the grid. Some homeowners are doing so too. A transition from "buying" electric power from an external supplier to "making" it is underway because the costs and benefits of producing power are changing.

By bringing certain doctors in-house, hospitals are acting like other businesses that decide to make some services internally rather than buy them from an external source. Hospitals are trying to maximize their profits, which they think they can do by having some doctors become employees. By leaving other doctors outside, hospitals are implicitly saying that they are better off having customers separately buy the services those doctors provide. The same financial considerations that drive commercial firms to "make or buy" certain services also drive hospitals to make the same decisions.

How do hospitals profit by turning some (but not all) independent physicians into employees? When you look at the physicians who become hospital employees, two things stand out. First, many of these doctors provide services that generate payments known as "site-of-service differentials" that make it advantageous for hospitals to hire them. Second, many of these physicians refer patients to hospitals for profitable treatments. Some do both. The doctors that hospitals do not hire are those who offer neither site-of-service differentials nor patient referrals.

## A Migration of Wildebeests

Here's how site-of-service differentials affect hospital executives' thinking. Patients can receive medical treatments at different locations. For example, they can get colonoscopies in doctors' offices or at hospitals' outpatient departments, among other places. You might think that Medicare, Medicaid, and private insurers would pay the same amount for colonoscopies regardless of where they take place (also known as "site-neutral payment"). But you'd be very wrong. Payments vary considerably by location, and hospital-provided colonoscopies generate a lot more revenue.

In 2012, Medicare paid an average of $1,300 for colonoscopies performed in doctors' offices, but it shelled out $1,805—39 percent more—when these procedures were delivered at hospitals.[29] That is why only 4 percent of all colonoscopies were performed in doctors' offices that year.[30] By performing them in hospitals, doctors and hospitals were able to split the extra money. Because it is financially advantageous for hospitals to bring gastroenterologists (and other doctors who perform lots of colonoscopies) onto their staffs, colonoscopies don't generate lots of balance bills. (This is true for gastroenterologists' services. Anesthesia delivered in connection with colonoscopies may be a different story.)

The same was true for cardiologists. Consider an example discussed by the Medicare Payment Advisory Commission, or MedPAC, which studies and advises Congress on how to improve the government's payment systems. When a cardiologist in private practice provided a level II echocardiogram without contrast, Medicare paid $188. But, when a doctor connected to a hospital performed the same test in an outpatient context, the payment was $452.89.[31] That's an additional $265 that the hospital and doctor can share—including an additional $212 from taxpayers and $53 from the patient—to their mutual advantage. As Mark E. Miller, MedPAC's Executive Director, told Congress, site-of-service differentials like this one "giv[e] hospitals an incentive to acquire physician practices and bill for the same services at outpatient rates, increasing costs to [Medicare] and to the beneficiary."[32]

The incentive to "make" cardiac services in-house grew in 2009, when Medicare reduced payments to cardiologists with independent practices while raising payments to hospitals when staff cardiologists performed the same tests. Since then, the *New York Times* reports, "the number of cardiologists in private practice has plummeted as more and more doctors sold their practices to nearby hospitals that weren't subject to the new cuts." After one cardiology practice was bought by a hospital, its former chief operating officer likened the movement of doctors to "a migration of wildebeests."[33] One consequence of the migration was that cardiologists generated few balance bills. On the flip side, taxpayers ended up paying more to buy the same services, provided by the same physicians.

Site-of-service differentials exist for many medical treatments. In 2013, *Medical Economics* published a table showing site-of-service differentials for many routine visits to doctors' offices, also known as "evaluation and management services."[34] As shown in Figures 9-1 and 9-2, in every instance, the payments for hospital-based treatments were higher—often much higher—than when doctors performed these services independently.

There are also site-of-service differentials for cancer drugs. When a hospital gives a lung cancer patient a dose of Alimta, its fee is about $4,300 larger than a doctor with an independent practice would receive. For Herceptin, a drug given to women with breast cancer, the site-of-service differential is about $2,600. And for Avastin, when used to treat colon cancer, it is $7,500.[35] These site-of-service payment differentials

**Figure 9-1.** Medicare Payments for Identically Coded Evaluation and Management Services at Physicians' Offices vs. Hospital Outpatient Departments, New Patients (2013)

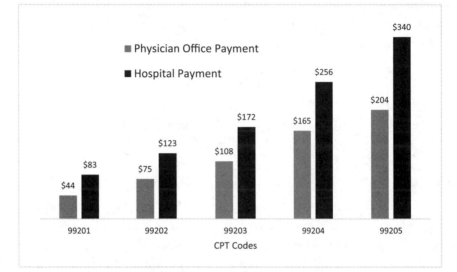

Source: Tammy Worth, "Hospital Facility Fees: Why Cost May Give Independent Physicians an Edge," *Medical Economics,* August 6, 2014, http://medicaleconomics .modernmedicine.com/medical-economics/content/tags/facility-fees/hospital-facility-fees-why-cost-may-give-independent-ph?page=full.
Note: CPT = Current Procedural Terminology.

help explain why hospitals have found it advantageous to bring cancer doctors in-house.[36]

The American Hospital Association and other industry groups contend that site-of-service differentials reflect hospitals' costs, which are higher than those of doctors in independent practice. That might be true in some instances. But, given that the same services are being provided in both settings, why are patients being treated at high-cost hospitals instead of low-cost doctors' offices in the first place? If patients were spending their own dollars, they wouldn't go to more expensive providers when cheaper ones were available, and just as good.

The American Hospital Association's argument also fails to explain why the higher rates apply when doctors who sell their practices to

**Figure 9-2.** Medicare Payments for Identically Coded Evaluation and Management Services at Physicians' Offices vs. Hospital Outpatient Departments, Existing Patients (2013)

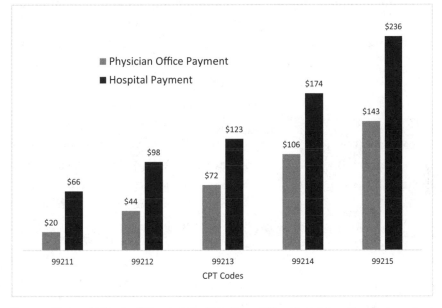

Source: Tammy Worth, "Hospital Facility Fees: Why Cost May Give Independent Physicians an Edge," *Medical Economics,* August 6, 2014, http://medicaleconomics .modernmedicine.com/medical-economics/content/tags/facility-fees/hospital-facility- fees-why-cost-may-give-independent-ph?page=full.
Note: CPT = Current Procedural Terminology.

hospitals keep on seeing patients at their old locations. When that happens, the costs of providing those services don't change at all.

> Imagine you're a Medicare patient, and you go to your doctor for an ultrasound of your heart one month. Medicare pays your doctor's office $189, and you pay about 20 percent of that bill as a copayment.
>
> Then, the next month, your doctor's practice has been bought by the local hospital. You go to the same building and get the same test from the same doctor, but suddenly the price has shot up to $453, as has your share of the bill. . . .
>
> Medicare . . . pays one price to independent doctors and another to doctors who work for large health systems—even if they are performing the exact same service in the exact same place.[37]

Gary Ziomek learned that location matters when he went in for physical therapy after spinal fusion surgery. The *Charlotte Observer* reports
that Ziomek's bill for a half-hour massage treatment was initially
$148. But after his provider "began billing as a hospital-based setting"
the price rose to $249.30—"even though he got the same therapy
from the same therapist in the same building." Ziomek was stuck with
a larger fraction of the higher bill too. Instead of a $20 copay for an
office visit, the encounter occurred in a "hospital-based setting," so
he had to meet a $250 deductible and cover 10 percent of the higher
price.[38]

We are not aware of any site-of-service differentials that would
induce hospitals to bring ER doctors, surgeons, or anesthesiologists
in-house. Because there is no incentive for hospitals to hire these physicians as employees, they remain independent and outside of hospitals'
networks. That's why they generate surprise bills.

Before leaving site-of-service differentials, we note that, after
being pressured by many sources for many years, Congress finally
took steps to eliminate them in the Bipartisan Budget Act of 2015
(BBA). But Congress exempted existing physician employment relationships and hospital outpatient departments from the new payment
policy."[39] In other words, site-of-service differentials for providers
who were already billing through hospitals before the BBA took
effect will continue indefinitely—even though everyone involved
recognizes that they are inappropriate. Even when health care providers lose, they win.


### Refer Them to Me

Hospitals make money by treating patients. But, except when patients
show up at their emergency rooms, they don't deal with patients
directly. They rely on physicians to send them patients who need
treatments that are delivered on the hospital's premises. Cardiac surgery and interventional cardiology generate large revenue streams for
hospitals, but the doctors who diagnose patients with heart problems
are often noninterventional cardiologists. To stay profitable, hospitals

need these noninterventional cardiologists to send patients to the hospital where they can be treated, whether in the operating room or cath lab.

When doctors practice independently, anti-kickback laws limit what hospitals can do to reward them for referring patients. They cannot pay for referrals, whether directly or indirectly. But nothing prevents hospitals from ensuring future patient flows by hiring doctors or acquiring their practices and paying them handsomely. So that is what hospitals do. Once that happens, doctors send their patients to the affiliated hospitals for care.

These employment relationships can have huge benefits for hospitals. Figure 9-3 shows the salaries that hospital-employed doctors draw versus the revenues they generate for the hospital.

On average, hospitals pay physicians 22 percent of the revenue they generate. Of course, the difference is not all profit, but it is clear that "physicians typically generate considerably more in 'downstream revenue' than they receive in the form of salaries or income guarantees."[40] And the surplus keeps rising. For all practice areas combined, the average net revenue in 2016 was $1,560,688, an increase of 7.7 percent over 2013. For specialty-care physicians, the increase was 12.8 percent.

Notice that Figure 9-3 does not include certain specialties. Anesthesiologists, radiologists, and pathologists are all missing, as are doctors who work in hospitals' ERs. That's because hospitals tend to treat these doctors as independent contractors, not employees. What do these disparate practice areas have in common? They do not refer many patients.

Neither anesthesiologists, nor radiologists, nor pathologists tend to have long-term relationships with patients. They are secondary members of teams that include other physicians whose relationships with patients are more direct. Because they do not bring patients to hospitals' doorsteps, hospitals have little to gain by hiring them as employees.

Emergency medicine physicians are in the same boat. Patients don't pick which ER to go to because they know the doctors that practice

**Figure 9–3.** Physician–Generated Revenue vs. Average Salaries

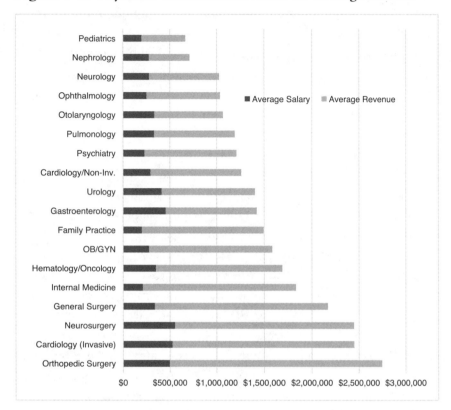

Source: Merritt Hawkins, "2016 Physician Inpatient/Outpatient Revenue Survey," 2016, https://www.merritthawkins.com/uploadedFiles/MerrittHawkins/Surveys/Merritt_ Hawkins-2016_RevSurvey.pdf.

there. They go to the closest or most convenient ER. For everyone but ER frequent-flyers, the visit to the ER is the first and last time these patients and physicians will meet. Any patient in the ER who needs to be hospitalized will be admitted to the hospital the ER is located in. For these reasons, hospitals can increase their patient volumes by having ERs, but they cannot gain referrals by bringing emergency medicine physicians in-house. (In fact, as we discuss further below, hospitals that contract with some ER staffing companies make more money by treating ER doctors as contractors.)

## THE ROOT CAUSE: PROVIDERS DON'T HAVE TO COMPETE FOR PATIENTS

The discussions of site-of-service differentials and referrals support a straightforward conclusion: balance billing continues to be a problem because neither doctors nor hospitals have a financial interest in ending the practice. A few exceptional hospitals do require all doctors to belong to the same insurance networks that they do, showing that hospitals could solve this problem if they wanted. But other hospitals haven't followed their lead because they see no upside to bringing in-house the doctors who send out balance bills. They cannot gain referrals or site-of-service differentials by doing so.

This is remarkable. Hospitals see no advantage in protecting patients from surprise bills, even though the bills worry patients greatly and saddle many of them with significant costs. In a competitive market, a seller that found a way to protect its customers from a significant financial risk to which other sellers deliberately left them exposed would advertise the fact and be rewarded with new business. Other sellers would then copy the innovation and offer it to their customers too, for fear of suffering financially if they didn't. In short order, most or all consumers would be protected. But hospitals don't compete for customers in free markets, so they worry much less than they should about attracting patients by adopting desirable innovations and about losing patients to innovative competitors. Surprise bills are a consequence of a lack of market competition.

The body shop that keeps your car in good repair would never think of letting one of its mechanics send out a surprise bill. It has to be customer friendly, so it packages all of the services it provides into a single bill and charges a competitive price. The body shop that keeps *you* running could do the same. It could require all of the providers who deliver services at its facilities to bill through its offices at rates that are acceptable to patients. It doesn't do that because it is confident that patients will keep coming through its doors, regardless of surprise bills.

The same goes for doctors who send out surprise bills. ER physicians, anesthesiologists, pathologists, and radiologists don't have to compete for patients. They merely need access to hospitals with reliable patient flows. They don't have to be patient friendly either, so they aren't.

What about insurers? Can't they solve this problem by getting doctors to join their networks? Unfortunately, they can't. Physicians join networks because they need the business that insured patients provide. But the doctors who are responsible for the most surprise bills know that they will have plenty of customers whether they join insurers' networks or not. Consequently, insurers have little leverage over them.

These doctors also know that they'll collect some money from insurers, whether they join insurers' networks or not. Surprise bills are balance bills—they're bills that patients receive after the insurance company has already paid the doctor. Given this, the strategy of staying outside of insurers' networks is more profitable for these physicians. By joining a network, they would limit themselves to the insurance dollars alone. As long as they stay outside, though, they can collect the insurance money plus whatever additional dollars they can extract from patients through surprise bills.

Doctors would be much less likely to play this game if they knew they'd lose patients. The need to compete would temper their zeal to send out surprise bills. But they know that our competition-stifling, government-controlled payment system will direct patients to them regardless, so their enthusiasm for surprise bills is effectively unrestrained.

## How Uniform Is Surprise Billing?

A recent large study of surprise bills makes it clear that the phenomenon is driven by the desire for profit. Out-of-network ER doctors charge far more than in-network physicians do for identical services. They also charge more than six times what Medicare pays.[41]

But the study also found that the frequency with which patients received surprise bills varies widely. Although 22 percent of patients treated at ERs were hit with surprise bills on average, at some hospitals, most or essentially all patients were. "At about 15% of the hospitals, out-of-network rates were over 80 percent."[42]

Much of the variation is explained by the business models of the companies that hospitals engage to manage their ERs. At hospitals that outsourced their ERs to EmCare, one of the two largest outfits in the

United States, both charges for services and the frequency of surprise bills increased. "[W]hen EmCare—which has an average out-of-network billing rate of 62%—takes over the management of emergency services at hospitals with low out-of-network rates, they raise out-of-network rates by over 81 percentage points and [increase] average physician payments by 117%."[43]

Figure 9-4 shows what happened to the rates at which eight hospitals sent out-of-network bills after those hospitals hired EmCare to manage their ERs. At each hospital, the frequency of balance bills increased quickly and markedly, often rising from a low level to 100 percent. One of the authors of the study, which relied on data provided by an insurer, aptly described the change in billing practices as looking "like a light switch was being flipped on."[44]

Why did hospitals allow this to happen to patients treated in their ERs? One obvious reason is that they too made money on the deal.

**Figure 9-4.** Change in Out-of-Network Charges following Changes in Emergency Room Management

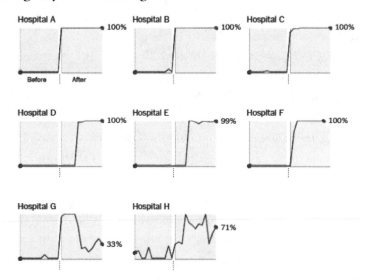

Source: Zack Cooper, Fiona Scott Morton, and Nathan Shekita, "Surprise! Out-of-Network Billing for Emergency Care in the United States," NBER Working Paper no. 23623, July 2017, National Bureau of Economic Research, Figure 3.

After EmCare took over, hospitals' fees increased significantly, owing to more intensive treatments and higher admission rates. In effect, EmCare paid hospitals for the opportunity to balance bill their patients.

When the results just described made nationwide news, how did EmCare respond? It reportedly claimed that hospitals can "treat sicker patients when it takes over, and . . . an increase in such patients explain[s] the higher billing."[45] The Reverse Lake Wobegon Effect strikes again.

### THE EMPIRE STRIKES BACK

We close with a case study that brings together many of the pathologies we discuss in this chapter. In Texas, balance billing has been a particular problem with freestanding emergency departments. These facilities look like urgent care centers, but they are almost never in-network for health insurers. And they bill at rates that are reported to be 10 times those of urgent care centers. When an insurer denies payment of the excess amount, the patient who was treated is on the hook for the balance.

In 2017, researchers associated with Rice University, the Baylor College of Medicine, the University of Texas Health Science Center at Houston, the Michael E. DeBakey VA Medical Center, and Blue Cross and Blue Shield of Texas published a study of ER charges in the *Annals of Emergency Medicine*. They examined more than 16 million insurance claims processed from 2012 to 2015. Their object was "to track the growth in use and prices for freestanding emergency departments relative to hospital-based emergency departments and urgent care centers in Texas."[46] The project was interesting partly because many people think that freestanding ERs and urgent care centers are the same. Both are typically located in neighborhood shopping centers, so how different can they be?

Very different, judging from their bills. The average charge for a freestanding ER visit ($2,199) was about the same as for a hospital-based ER visit ($2,259) but a whopping 13 times the average charge for an urgent care center visit ($168).[47] A patient who visits a freestanding ER expecting an urgent care center charge is in for a nasty surprise.

The prospect of paying substantially more at a freestanding ER seems especially galling when one realizes that these facilities often deliver the same treatments as urgent care centers to patients with the same conditions.

> Fifteen of the 20 most common diagnoses treated at freestanding emergency departments were also in the top 20 for urgent care clinics. However, prices for patients with the same diagnosis were on average almost 10 times higher at freestanding emergency departments relative to urgent care clinics. For example, the most common diagnostic category treated at freestanding emergency departments is "other upper-respiratory infections," which has an average price of $1,351, more than eight times the price of $165 that was paid for the same diagnosis at urgent care clinics.
>
> Thirteen of the most common procedure codes associated with freestanding emergency departments were also among the 20 most common for urgent care clinics. In cases in which the type of procedure overlapped, the total price per visit was 13 times higher in freestanding emergency departments versus urgent care clinics. For example, the price for a therapeutic or intravenous injection at a freestanding emergency department was $203, which was 11.9 times the $17 price at an urgent care clinic.[48]

These staggering price differences could not exist in competitive markets with informed shoppers who were responsible for their bills. Consumers with minor problems would quickly learn that urgent care centers are much better bargains and would stop frequenting freestanding ERs. In fact, however, freestanding ER usage "rose by 236 percent between 2012 and 2015."

These findings provide more evidence that we pay for health care the wrong way. Patients aren't shopping intelligently. They aren't asking about prices or seeking out good values, probably because they're accustomed to relying on their insurers to handle the finances. With time, this may change. As more and more people who visit freestanding ERs get stuck with surprise bills, the focus on costs should intensify and patients who have time to look around will take their business to lower-cost providers. Urgent care centers also have every incentive to advertise the sizable savings they offer by comparison to freestanding ERs.

These findings described above did not sit well with the doctors and business executives who run freestanding ERs. After the study appeared,

Dr. Paul Kivela, president-elect of the American College of Emergency Physicians (ACEP), called Vivian Ho, the lead author. He reportedly "complain[ed] about some numbers in an appendix and implied [that] she could be sued."[49] Then the *Annals of Emergency Medicine* "pulled the study for further review."[50] Although the reason given for taking this step was "'serious concerns over data in the article," the backstory appears to be that the ACEP runs the *Annals* and its member doctors were unhappy that their organization's journal published a study that cast their business model in a bad light. That's Dr. Ho's view, at any rate. She said the ACEP "controls the journal, and they are receiving complaints from emergency physicians, particularly those who could earn a substantial share of their income from the freestanding ER model."[51] She admitted that a minor transcription error occurred in the course of preparing the article for publication, but "said the study findings should stand, once corrected."[52]

The damage inflicted on the reputations of Dr. Ho and her colleagues was partially repaired when the *Annals* reposted the study in late 2017.[53] But the republication was accompanied by a series of letters, policy statements, and other writings in which the researchers' data, findings, and integrity were questioned.[54] The lesson for academics? Study the financial side of health care delivery at your peril because providers whose revenues are at stake may rough you up.

If health care was provided in a competitive market, free-standing ERs would either charge the same prices that urgent care centers do for the same services or they would be out of business. There would be no more need to study freestanding ERs' charges than there is to study the prices charged by Best Buy or Dell. Stated differently, if we want to fix the problem of balance billing, the most direct solution is to reward providers that protect their patients from the risk of receiving surprise bills. And, the best way to do that is to enable cost-conscious consumers to shop for value.

Balance billing is a problem that providers can fix, and would fix, if it were in their interest to do so. But surely the protection of the vulnerable is a job for the government, particularly when people are elderly and dying, right? If you think the government can be relied on to take care of these people, the next chapter will force you to think again.

## CHAPTER 10: MAKING A KILLING ON THE TERMINALLY ILL

### You Have Six Months to Live—Or Do You?

Janet Stubbs was delighted when her elderly Aunt Midge was recommended for transfer from a nursing home to a hospice. One might think Stubbs was happy because terminally ill patients often live longer and enjoy better quality of life when treated in hospices rather than hospitals.[1] Only Aunt Midge wasn't dying. She was old—around 100. But otherwise, she was fine. She was being transferred to hospice care because the doctor who saw her in the nursing home was willing to certify that she was terminally ill when, in fact, she wasn't. The phony certification meant that Aunt Midge would receive better care, including Medicare-paid hospice visits from a nurse and chaplain, plus an extra weekly bath. That's what made Janet Stubbs happy. The offer of free services for Aunt Midge was too good to pass up.[2]

Why was the nursing home doctor willing to falsely certify that Aunt Midge had less than six months to live, the cutoff for being admitted to a hospice? Financial incentives may have had something to do with it. Hospice Care of Kansas (HCK) was holding a "Summer Sizzle" promotion—we are not making this up—during which the company paid its employees bonuses of up to $100 per referral.[3] The nursing home doctor who referred Aunt Midge moonlighted as a medical director at HCK. By sending Aunt Midge to hospice, the doctor made money.

Giving bonuses for referrals wasn't the only way HCK drummed up business from nursing homes. It also gave salespeople $500 a month to buy lunches and other treats for nursing home employees.[4] Other hospices use similar tactics. Some even sponsor trips and family vacations for medical directors they view as good sources of referrals. According to Roger Megli, a former chaplain and marketer for HCK, the company paid nursing home doctors up to $4,000 a month to consult for a day or so per week on patients' conditions and to sign treatment orders. He thought that the practice corrupted doctors' judgment. "If I'm getting $3,000 or $4,000 a month from a hospice to work one day a week," Megli said, "I'm going to refer my patients to hospice, too."[5]

HCK was not alone in adopting aggressive marketing tactics, and these tactics paid off. By 2007, about 1 million Medicare beneficiaries were enrolled in hospices—more than double the enrollment of a decade earlier.[6] By 2015, hospices cared for 1.38 million people, almost half of the Medicare beneficiaries who died that year.[7] Between 2007 and 2015, Medicare spending on hospice services rose 52 percent, from $10.4 billion to $15.8 billion.[8]

The trouble is, there are a lot of Aunt Midges. According to a recent report by the Office of the Inspector General (OIG) for the Department of Health and Human Services, "82 percent of hospice claims for beneficiaries in nursing facilities did not meet Medicare coverage requirements."[9] Why so high? Because the way Medicare pays for hospice care intensifies the incentive to commit fraud.

Most hospice revenue comes from Medicare, which pays a fixed amount per patient per day.[10] This arrangement makes very long stays in hospice profitable for providers.[11] The expensive parts of hospice stays are intake (when patients need to be enrolled and evaluated) and exit (when dying patients require extra care). The time in between is cheap because it requires only routine monitoring and medication. Consequently, hospices benefit when doctors refer patients with long life expectancies, even though this conflicts with Medicare's "six months to live" regulation.

And hospices got what they wanted. In 2000, the average length of stay for hospice patients was 54 days. In 2010, it was 86 days.[12] At HCK's main branch in Wichita, the average length of stay was 109 days.[13]

Nationwide, about 21 percent of hospice patients stayed longer than six months, according to a 2013 report.[14] Recognizing the frequency of abuses, Medicare discouraged hospices from taking healthy patients by reducing payments for care delivered after the 60th day.[15]

### Never Make Forecasts, Especially about the Future

Manipulation of patients' prognoses has led to predictions of imminent death that were amazingly far off the mark. Charles Groomes, who required stiff doses of OxyContin because of painful nerve damage in his feet, was discharged from Horizons Hospice in Pittsburgh after 32 months.[16] When he eventually died, more than five years had elapsed since a doctor first certified that he had less than six months to live. Even then, his illness didn't kill him, exactly. According to his wife, he took his own life by overdosing on pain medication, to which he had become addicted while in hospice care.

Gerald Stout, who spent about a year in hospice care, was still alive more than five years after being discharged.[17] Eight months after being admitted by HCK for Parkinson's disease, he had gained weight, moved about well with a walker, and his doctor determined that he was "not appropriate" for hospice. He was discharged three months later. Medicare paid more than $34,000 for his hospice care.

And remember Aunt Midge? A year after being admitted, she too was deemed "inappropriate for hospice." HCK nonetheless held onto her for another eight months. Throughout her 20-month stay, Medicare paid $3,980 a month and Stubbs added $4,000 to $5,000 more. HCK thus made about $100,000 a year. As for Aunt Midge's predicted encounter with the Grim Reaper, she lived four years after being discharged by HCK and passed away at the ripe old age of 106.

It can be difficult to know when patients will die. We've all heard stories of people who miraculously recovered from illnesses or injuries that seemed certain to be fatal, and of people who succumbed sooner than expected.[18] But the frequency of mistakes is bound to increase when health care providers stand to make money by making wrong predictions. According to Professor Nancy Kane, "The long lengths of stay and high rates of live discharges suggest some hospices are signing up people who don't belong in hospice. Any time there is money to be made, and you have this nebulous, gray area around 'who is terminal,' you get manipulation by some providers."[19] In other words, we rely on providers to assess patients' prospects honestly, but Medicare corrodes their judgment by rewarding dishonesty.

Sometimes hospices scam patients by convincing them they are at death's door—even though they aren't. Misty Wall, a former social worker at a VistaCare hospice unit, explained that her job was to tell patients they were dying so they'd sign up for hospice services. After taking a position as an assistant professor of social work at Boise State University in Idaho, Wall described an incident in which a woman broke down in tears after Wall suggested that, because of renal failure, her father faced imminent death. According to the father's physician, that wasn't true. "I gave her this huge emotional blow, then sat there and soothed her," Wall said. "Of course she signed."[20]

After leaving VistaCare, Wall became a whistleblower. She accused her former employer of admitting patients who were not terminally ill, paying illegal kickbacks to patients and nursing home employees who referred residents, and using friendly doctors to get healthy patients certified for admission. The case was dismissed on a technicality, but many other hospice workers have leveled similar charges at their employers. In 2010, for example, the federal government opened more than 30 new Medicare fraud cases against hospice companies as a result of complaints by whistleblowers. (Of course, whistleblowers have some incentive to exaggerate misconduct, but they get paid only if their charges are proven correct—or the defendant decides to settle.)

In recent years, the federal government has cracked down on hospice fraud by auditing admission practices. Some audits have had stunning results. One, undertaken in connection with a whistleblower complaint, caused the San Diego Hospice (SDH), nominally a nonprofit organization, to drop hundreds of patients "as it target[ed] its services more tightly to only those within the six-month window. The resulting cash crunch forced the business to shed 260 workers and close a 24-bed hospital."[21] The slide didn't end there. After trimming its staff further, the SDH declared bankruptcy and closed its doors in 2013.[22] Fortunately, other local hospice operators took in SDH's patients. In SDH's bankruptcy proceeding, the federal government demanded repayment of $112 million in overpayments allegedly made in response to false claims filed in 2009 and 2010.[23]

DISHONORABLE DISCHARGES

Hospices receive many of their patients from hospitals, which creates another opportunity for gaming the payment rules. Medicare typically pays hospitals a fixed amount, based on patients' discharge diagnoses. The payments, called "DRGs" (for diagnosis-related groups),[24] reflect the expected cost and duration of the hospitalization. Thus, the DRG is a fixed fee that does not vary with the actual number of days that a patient is hospitalized. Previously, Medicare paid for the actual number of hospital days, which caused hospitals to inflate their bills by keeping patients hospitalized for longer than their treatments actually required. The fixed-fee DRG approach has the opposite shortcoming. It encourages hospitals to discharge patients early.

Suppose a DRG required Medicare to pay a hospital $15,000, reflecting the expectation that a patient with a particular diagnosis would need five days of inpatient care at $3,000 per day. By discharging the patient to a hospice in fewer than five days, the hospital would be paid the same $15,000 but would have an empty bed that it could fill with another paying patient. Even if it couldn't fill the bed, the hospital would make a profit by avoiding the incremental costs associated with caring for the patient who was discharged. Minimizing time in-hospital is a profit-maximizing strategy under the fixed-fee DRG approach. When available space in a hospice enables a hospital to discharge a patient quickly, why not?

Would hospitals really send vulnerable patients to hospice just to maximize their profits? Consider the title of another OIG report: *Medicare Could Save Millions by Implementing a Hospital Transfer Payment Policy for Early Discharges to Hospice Care.* The report estimated Medicare could save $602 million by paying hospitals a daily rate (instead of a DRG-based payment) for patients who were discharged to hospice "early," that is, before the end of the period anticipated by the DRG. But, really, it is far from clear such a change would save Medicare money. If Medicare switched to per diem payments for patients who are discharged "early," hospitals would probably adapt by keeping patients just long enough to collect the larger fixed-fee DRG payment. CMS officials who commented on the OIG report said as much.[25] They knew that hospitals would game any set of payment rules Medicare created, so trying to save a paltry $600 million just wasn't worth the trouble.

UPCODING THE TERMINALLY ILL?

Hospices that pay bribes to bring in patients run the risk of doing deals with doctors who are bad actors. For Vitas Health Care Corp. (VHC), the largest hospice company in the United States, that risk became a reality when it "donated" $15,750 to a charity for cancer patients run by the notorious Dr. Farid Fata, the Michigan oncologist we met in Chapter 8. Fata was convicted of giving hundreds of patients false cancer diagnoses so he could make money by giving them chemotherapy and other drugs. A whistleblower filed a complaint alleging that VHC and Fata had a deal. In return for contributing the money, Fata would refer 23 terminally ill patients. VHC paid $200,000 to settle the lawsuit in 2016, while denying that it did anything wrong.[26]

The whistleblower who brought VHC's relationship with Fata to light was Rita Dubois. She knew about VHC's business practices because she once worked as the company's director of marketing development in southeast Michigan. It's common for whistleblowers to be corporate insiders, as we discuss in Chapter 20, because insiders are often the only ones who know what's going on. Companies that defraud the government usually hide what they're doing from public view.

A whistleblower complaint also led to another lawsuit against VHC in 2013. In this suit, which the U.S. Department of Justice (DOJ) joined, the company was accused of admitting patients who weren't terminally ill—the standard charge. But there was also an allegation that VHC inflated its revenues by upcoding, that is, by making terminally ill patients seem to be in worse condition than they actually were. That might not seem possible; but, when you understand how Medicare compensates hospices, you'll see why it would be financially advantageous to do that.

Medicare pays hospices at two different daily rates. In 2015, Medicare paid $156 per day for patients receiving routine palliative care and a much higher rate of $910 per day for patients needing more intensive treatment.[27] Most patients who trigger the higher rate are actively dying, but some are being treated for nonfatal conditions in hope of improving their quality of life during their final days.

The DOJ's complaint accuses VHC of bilking Medicare by listing patients as being in crisis when in fact they were not. According to the government's press release, VHC and its parent company

> set goals for the number of crisis care days that were to be billed to Medicare. The companies also allegedly used aggressive marketing tactics and pressured staff to increase the numbers of crisis care claims submitted to Medicare, without regard to whether the services were appropriate or were actually being provided. For example, the complaint contends that Vitas billed three straight days of crisis care for a patient, even though the patient's medical records do not indicate that the patient required crisis care and, indeed, reflect that the patient was playing bingo part of the time.[28]

One imagines that the patient wasn't the only one shouting "Bingo!" VHC's owners and managers must have thought they were winners too—at least until late 2017, when Chemed Corp., the parent company of VHC, paid $75 million to settle the government's case.[29]

The government's complaint against VHC also revealed, in a surprisingly casual (but candid) manner, one of the main reasons that Medicare fraud can't be policed:

> Because it is not feasible for the Medicare program, or its contractors, to review the patient files for the millions of claims for payments it receives from hospice providers, the Medicare program relies upon the hospice providers to comply with the Medicare requirements, and trusts the providers to submit truthful and accurate claims.[30]

Medicare is ill-equipped to evaluate claims as they come in, so it has no option but to pay providers whatever they demand while trusting them to bill honestly. The government practically invites providers to steal from it by telling them that their claims won't be audited.

Before leaving this case, we cannot resist mentioning its strangest aspect. VHC's founder was Dan Gaetz, who also served as vice chairman of VHC's board of directors during part of the fraud period. When the DOJ filed its complaint, Gaetz was president of the Florida senate. He claimed to have had no active role in VHC's operation when he was vice chairman of the board.[31]

By denying involvement in a long-term health care fraud committed by a company he created, Gaetz joined Florida's governor, Rick Scott, who served as CEO of Columbia/HCA.[32] In 2000, that company agreed to pay $840 million in criminal fines, civil damages, and penalties to settle claims that it defrauded Medicare and Medicaid by billing for tests that were neither needed nor ordered by physicians, using false diagnosis codes to increase reimbursements, and committing other misdeeds. In 2002, Columbia/HCA paid another $881 million in a second settlement involving similar allegations, bringing the total to $1.7 billion. Like Gaetz, Scott claimed to know nothing about the wrongdoing.[33] Florida's governor and senate president were such fantastic managers that they made fortunes running health care businesses, but both somehow remained completely unaware that their businesses were breaking the law.

Hospices also upcode by certifying that patients are in need of something called general inpatient care (GIP). GIP applies when hospice residents need short-term pain control or other symptom management services that must be provided via inpatient facilities, such as hospitals, skilled nursing facilities, or Medicare-certified hospice inpatient units. In 2011, Medicare paid $652.27 per day of GIP, more than four times the rate for routine inpatient hospice care.[34]

Most hospices reserve GIP for cases where it is needed, but some upcode to increase their revenues. In 2014, the DOJ filed a criminal indictment against Seth Gillman, a part-owner of Passages Hospice, LLC, which sends nurses to visit hospice patients in nursing homes and private residences in Illinois. A study of Medicare claims data revealed that Passages' payments for GIP services grew from $4,437 per month in 2006–2008 to $946,743 per month in 2011. A government expert who reviewed the files of several patients treated by Passages concluded that most were not eligible for Medicare hospice benefits for part or all of their admission and that all of the 503 days of GIP submitted for those patients were improper.[35] In hope of covering up the scheme, Gillman allegedly altered patient files that had been requested for auditing.[36] Gillman pled guilty to fraud in early 2016. One month later, Angela Armenta, the director of nursing assistants at Passages, was convicted.[37]

As mentioned above, some hospices have Medicare-certified inpatient units. These hospices can provide GIP in-house instead of referring residents to other facilities—and the ability to profit by doing so has had predictable results. According to a 2013 OIG report, hospices that "owned or leased their own inpatient units provided that care to 35% of their Medicare patients," while those "that had to send their inpatients to other companies' hospitals or skilled-nursing facilities did so for only 12% of their Medicare beneficiaries."[38] Finally, when hospices had their own facilities, GIP stays were 50 percent longer than when residents were sent to hospitals for treatment. The odor of excessive use of medical treatments is hard to miss.

## Garden-Variety Hospice Fraud

Most hospices are run by trained professionals who care deeply about their patients and treat them well. But fraud permeates every part of our government-controlled, third-party payer health care system, hospices included. The case of Matthew Kolodesh, the owner of Home Care Hospice, Inc. (HCH), shows how rotten a hospice operation can be.

In 2011, the federal government filed a criminal complaint in which it accused HCH of submitting false claims to the tune of roughly $14.3 million. Thirty percent of the patients treated at HCH were said to be ineligible for hospice care, and 90 percent of HCH's charges for more expensive and intensive continuous care were deemed wholly fraudulent. The services were never delivered. The complaint also charged

Kolodesh with paying doctors and other health care professionals to refer patients and provide false eligibility certifications and accused him of disguising the payments by hiring the recipients as medical directors, hospice physicians, and advisers. A jury convicted Kolodesh in late 2013. He was sentenced to spend more than 14 years in prison and ordered to pay over $16 million in restitution.

Kolodesh hid HCH's malfeasance by altering patients' records or creating phony ones. To make HCH's patients seem sicker, he ordered employees to alter charts, falsify nursing notes, change diagnoses, and invent instances of weight loss, fever, and infection. To disguise billings for services that were never delivered, he had his nurse concoct phony schedules of continuous care visits. Often, the schedules used real events, such as death dates or hospitalizations, as anchors, falsely showing that services were delivered in the days immediately before the events occurred. To secure staff members' cooperation, Kolodesh reportedly paid nurses $20–$25 per hour for every hour they falsely certified as having been devoted to a patient. Home health care aides allegedly received $11 per hour for participating in the scam.

Kolodesh is reported to have diverted $9.4 million of these fraudulent billings to his family, of which $5.3 million went in the form of salary and bonuses for his wife (who held a nominal position in HCH); $3.6 million went to other businesses Kolodesh owned; and $500,000 went to vendors who supposedly paid kickbacks to Kolodesh. He is even said to have committed tax fraud by conspiring with his synagogue to inflate his charitable contributions. According to the feds, Kolodesh gave his synagogue almost $150,000 written on HCH checks and the synagogue handed him back $55,700 in cash. He thus took a $150,000 charitable deduction while actually donating $55,700 less, and also avoided paying income taxes on the latter amount.[39]


## MAKING MONEY MEDICATING SENIORS

Hospice companies, which are paid by Medicare, often operate nursing homes too. They frequently bill Medicaid for the services that the latter operations provide. Many patients, called "dual eligibles," reside in nursing homes and receive hospice care at the same time. The prospect of collecting from both payers gives hospices that are affiliated with nursing homes an obvious temptation to double dip.

This temptation appears to have been more than the managers of Voyager HospiceCare, Inc., could resist. At a time when about one-third of hospice patients resided in nursing homes, more than half of Voyager's patients did.[40] According to Larry Anderson, a former president of the Kansas Medical Society, Voyager used its network of nursing home doctors to provide a ready supply of hospice patients. He called this arrangement "a win-win for everybody but the taxpayer."[41] Anderson also observed that, after he declined to approve several patients for hospice care because they were not terminally ill, a nursing-home doctor made the certification. The rate at which nursing homes falsely certify residents as hospice ready is unknown, but many fraud cases make this allegation.

Nursing homes also commit abuses on their own. A particular concern has been their tendency to render the vulnerable seniors who are left in their care more docile by dosing them with anti-psychotic drugs, like Risperdal, Haldol, and Seroquel. In 2010, for example, about 185,000 nursing home residents received drugs of this type, against the recommendations of federal nursing home regulators.[42] Use of anti-psychotics for this purpose, known as "chemical restraint," is usually off-label. "In 2011, a government study found that 88 percent of Medicare claims for antipsychotics prescribed in nursing homes were for treating symptoms of dementia, even though the drugs aren't approved for that."[43] The federal government has campaigned against this practice, but chemical restraints are still common. Across the country, 19 percent of long-stay residents in nursing homes have received anti-psychotics, ranging from a high of over 25 percent in Texas to a low of only 9 percent in Hawaii.[44]

When asked, nursing home operators often say that chemical restraints are needed because residents would otherwise have to be restrained physically. Sometimes, that is true. But many experts believe that nursing homes administer anti-psychotics far too freely, and that financial incentives play a role in this. Citing Charlene Harrington, professor of nursing and sociology at the University of California,

San Francisco, the *AARP Bulletin* reported that "as many as 1 in 5 patients in the nation's 15,500 nursing homes are given antipsychotic drugs that are not only unnecessary, but also extremely dangerous for older patients" and that "an aggressive push by pharmaceutical companies to market their products" is one reason why.[45]

But it is not just pharma companies that push anti-psychotics. In the scam we are about to describe, a pharmacy company, two drug companies, and two nursing home chains all worked together to load up residents with expensive prescription drugs.

Omnicare operates pharmacies that provide prescription medications for more than one million people who reside in nursing homes and other long-term care facilities. As a pharmacy company, it doesn't directly control the quantity of medications it delivers: it fills prescriptions written by physicians. Its revenues therefore depend on the frequency with which doctors order drugs and the cost of the drugs they prescribe.

Recognizing this, Omnicare set about convincing doctors to use their prescription pads more often. Its pharmacists had good working relationships with doctors employed at long-term care facilities, so Omnicare implemented a policy of having its pharmacists prompt nursing home physicians to write prescriptions. The policy worked. According to the DOJ, which eventually sued Omnicare, physicians employed by nursing homes accepted the recommendations of Omnicare's pharmacists more than 80 percent of the time.[46]

Omnicare also had cozy relationships with two companies that operate nursing homes.[47] One was Mariner, which ran more than 250 facilities. The other was Sava, a Mariner spinoff that operated 190 skilled nursing and assisted living facilities in nearly 20 states.[48] According to the federal government's complaint, Omnicare paid Mariner and Sava $50 million in exchange for the exclusive right to provide pharmacy services to their nursing homes. The parties disguised the $50 million kickback by making it part of a transaction in which Omnicare acquired a small Mariner business unit.

The right to be the sole pharmacy supplying Mariner's and Sava's facilities gave Omnicare significant power to influence the selection of drugs for large numbers of residents. Omnicare's pharmacists could push certain drugs by advising doctors to prescribe them. They could also steer doctors away from other drugs by recommending alternatives.

Recognizing that pharmaceutical companies might pay handsomely to have this power exercised in their favor, Omnicare went hunting for treasure. According to the government, Omnicare solicited a drug company known as IVAX, which paid $8 million in kickbacks in exchange for Omnicare's agreement to purchase $50 million worth of IVAX drugs.[49]

Omnicare also approached Johnson & Johnson (J&J), with which it had a longstanding business relationship. The relationship was so close that J&J effectively used Omnicare's pharmacists as an "[e]xtension of [the J&J] sales force."[50] Again, the kickback was disguised. Formally, J&J paid Omnicare tens of millions of dollars and gave Omnicare millions of dollars in interest-free loans to create "incentives" for pharmacists "to advocate appropriate use of J&J products."[51] No such incentive was needed, of course. Pharmacists are paid salaries to do precisely that job. The objective was to influence the professional judgment of Omnicare's pharmacists, so they would recommend J&J's products more often.

The plan worked. Omnicare's purchases of Risperdal, an anti–psychotic drug produced by J&J, nearly tripled. J&J's Levaquin, an antibiotic, rose from its initial 19.2 percent share of Omnicare's deliveries to 66.4 percent, while deliveries of Cipro, an antibiotic manufactured by a competitor, declined from 80 percent to 20 percent.[52] In 2001, Omnicare's senior vice president of professional services and purchasing wrote a letter to J&J exclaiming, "WE ARE SELLING MORE HIGH PRICED DRUGS FOR THE PHARMACEUTICAL INDUSTRY!!"[53]

As we said above, the scheme was complex. The key to understanding it is that all of the companies involved stood to gain by pumping drugs into nursing home residents and by substituting more expensive drugs for cheaper ones. Omnicare benefited because its sales increased. It shared part of its gain with Mariner and Sava to ensure their cooperation and obtained in return the exclusive right to deliver drugs to their residents. Then, it used its control of the nursing home market to obtain payments from IVAX and J&J, both of which gained by having Omnicare deliver their drugs.

In view of the money to be made and the vulnerability of many nursing home residents, it is easy to see why anti-psychotics are over-prescribed. In 2011, the U.S. Senate Select Committee on Aging held a hearing on the overuse of anti-psychotics in nursing homes at which Daniel R. Levinson, the inspector general for the U.S. Department of Health and Human Services, testified.[54] According to his written sub-mission, the OIG "hired psychiatrists expert in treating elderly patients to review a sample of medical records. Their review found the following:

- "14% of nursing home residents, or nearly 305,000 patients, had Medicare claims for atypical antipsychotic drugs.
- "Half of these drug claims should not have been paid for by Medicare because the drugs were not used for medically accepted indications.
- "For one in five drug claims, nursing homes dispensed these drugs in a way that violated the Government's standards for their use. For example, the prescribed dose was too high, or residents were on the medications for too long.
- "Part D prescription drug plan . . . sponsors lack access to the information necessary to ensure appropriate reimbursement of Part D drugs, including antipsychotics."[55]

Inspector Levinson also testified that off-label prescribing of anti-psychotics for unapproved uses was common and that "the large major-ity of claims for atypical antipsychotics were for elderly patients with dementia. These findings are . . . troubling given that there is ample evidence that some drug manufacturers have illegally marketed these drugs for off-label use."[56]

The danger that elderly nursing home residents will be overmedicated and mistreated in other ways has been known about for decades. In 1986, the Institute of Medicine issued a report finding that nursing home res-idents were often abused, neglected, and cared for inadequately.[57] As a result, Congress enacted the Nursing Home Reform Act, a law that, among other things, requires nursing homes to protect residents from chemical restraints imposed for purposes of discipline or convenience rather than to treat medical conditions. Regulations also require consulting pharmacists to review residents' records every month, so the pharmacists can monitor the use of anti-psychotics and discourage doctors from misusing them.

Omnicare's kickback arrangement with J&J stood the practice of pharmacist review on its head. Instead of *discouraging* doctors from overusing Risperdal, Omnicare's pharmacists *en*couraged them to do so because their objective was to move the largest possible volume of J&J products. The predictable result was overmedication.

When the federal government finally caught on to the scam, each of the conspirators paid millions to settle the resulting fraud claims. In 2009, Omnicare paid $98 million and IVAX paid $14 million.[58] In 2010, the nursing homes paid $14 million.[59] Finally, J&J paid $2.2 billion in 2013 to settle multiple fraud claims, with $149 million attributable to its pact with Omnicare.[60] Of course, the human cost of overmedicating vulnerable seniors is incalculable.

## THE DEVIL WENT DOWN TO GEORGIA

As the federal government admitted when suing Vitas Healthcare, Medicare and Medicaid, which pay for about 75 percent of all nursing home services, work on the honor system. The government expects providers to be honest and doesn't do nearly enough to monitor them. This is true for the quality of the services that providers deliver, as well as for the accuracy of their bills. There are far too many providers for Medicare and Medicaid to police them.[61]

What happens when nursing home providers deliver services of such low quality as to be worthless? Ordinarily, they get paid, just as they would if they were treating residents exceptionally well. The government assumes that the beneficiaries of its programs are receiving appropriate treatment when, in fact, they may be suffering severely.

Consider the case of George D. Houser, for whom we hope a special place in hell has been reserved. Houser ran three nursing homes in Georgia. Over a four-year period (2004–2007), Medicare and Medicaid paid almost $33 million for services they delivered.[62] But Houser wasn't using the money to take care of the residents. At a trial that occurred years later, the evidence showed "a long-term pattern and practice of conditions . . . that were so poor, including food shortages bordering on starvation, leaking roofs, virtually no nursing or housekeeping supplies, poor sanitary conditions, major staff shortages and safety concerns that, in essence, any services actually provided were of no value to the residents."[63] A state official who inspected Houser's operation in Rome, Georgia, testified that "the heat, flies, filth, and stench created an environment that was 'appalling' and 'horrendous.'"[64] The facilities were repeatedly cited for violations, and in 2007, the state of Georgia terminated the Medicaid provider agreements and ordered the closure of all three nursing homes.[65]

The conditions were so egregious that Houser was charged with criminal health care fraud. Houser is one of the few persons ever tried for defrauding the government on the basis of providing services that were of such poor quality as to be worthless. He was sentenced to 20 years in prison and ordered to repay $6.7 million in restitution to Medicare and Medicaid. At sentencing, the trial judge noted that, if these nursing homes had been prisons, he would have ordered them closed for violating the Eighth Amendment's prohibition of cruel and unusual punishment.[66]

Of course, Houser treated himself much better than the vulnerable seniors in his charge. Evidence presented in the criminal case showed that he diverted $8 million of federal money to himself. He is said to have used the money to buy real estate worth $4.2 million upon which he planned to develop hotels, a $1.4 million house in Atlanta for his ex-wife, two Mercedes-Benzes, furniture, and vacations. The government also accused Houser of writing bad checks to employees, failing to pay vendors for such essentials as utilities and garbage pickup, and failing to repair leaking roofs and broken air-conditioning units. Commenting on the fraud verdict, U.S. Attorney and Georgia native Sally Quillian Yates—who went on to be President Donald Trump's acting attorney general for all of 10 days—stated, "It almost defies the imagination to believe that someone would use millions of dollars in Medicare and Medicaid money to buy real estate for hotels and a house while his elderly and defenseless nursing home residents went hungry and lived in filth and mold."[67] No, it doesn't—and that degree of willful blindness is unhelpful if you want to understand and fix America's health care system.

Our politicized third-party payment system creates bad incentives that attract the already corrupt, and also corrupt the virtuous. Although many angels work in the health care sector, the easy money to be made by committing fraud attracts many devils as well. When left unsupervised and put in charge of vulnerable patients, the devils will exploit those patients for personal gain. They'll pump them full of drugs they don't need; subject them to treatments that do not work; lie to them about how long they have to live; move them like cattle between nursing homes, hospitals, and hospices; and leave them to rot in filth and be harassed by flies. The puzzle is not that such people exist. The puzzle is why Congress creates and defends government programs that allow and even encourage the devils to operate in this fashion.

## SHELTER FROM THE STORM

In 2017, Hurricane Irma inflicted considerable damage in the United States. When it made its way up Florida's peninsula, it knocked out power for millions of people and caused more than 30 deaths. Fourteen of the victims were nursing home residents who lived at the Rehabilitation Center at Hollywood Hills (RCHH). Irma didn't kill them directly. It didn't knock down a wall, blow off the roof, or flood the building. The residents died during the heat wave that followed the gale. When the power went out, RCHH's air-conditioning system stopped working and the temperature inside the facility soared. Some of those who perished reportedly had body temperatures as high as 109.9 degrees.[68] A cooling tower and stand-by generator had both been installed defectively and without required permits. When Irma struck, the equipment failed.[69]

When they chose to reside at RCHH, neither the residents who died nor those who survived likely had any inkling that they were entrusting their lives to someone with a history of committing health care fraud.[70] According to a federal complaint filed in 2004, Dr. Jack Michel, who purchased RCHH in 2015, conspired with other doctors and facility operators—including Morris and Philip Esformes, a father/son duo we discuss further in Chapter 12—to generate phony bills by sending patients to the Larkin Community Hospital of Miami (LCH) for treatments they didn't need.[71]

In one scam, dubbed "The 1997 Scheme" in the complaint, Jack Michel and his brother, Dr. George Michel, engaged in seven types of kickback arrangements with LCH. For example, they referred patients to LCH and received $70,000 per month in return. "Many of the patients . . . were residents of Oceanside, a skilled nursing facility located in North Miami Beach" where Jack Michel served as medical director. "Oceanside residents were transported to Larkin where the[y] were provided with medically unnecessary services with the knowledge of Oceanside's ownership, Morris Esformes and Philip Esformes."[72] Altogether, these referrals were said to have generated over $5 million in payments from Medicare and Medicaid for LCH. The government also accused LCH of disguising kickbacks to Michel as fees for running its emergency room, staffing its radiology department, and operating his house call program, and as payments to a pharmacy Michel owned.

In The 1997 Scheme, LCH also paid kickbacks to other physicians who referred patients. The involvement of other doctors allegedly ended in 1998, when Michel purchased LCH and started the second scam, labeled "The 1998–1999 Scheme" in the government's complaint. The 1998–1999 Scheme was described as a cozier arrangement that involved just the Michel brothers, the Esformes, and the assisted living facilities, skilled nursing facilities, and similar operations that they owned, controlled, or planned to buy. The scam was simple. The facilities sent residents to LCH for unnecessary treatments, LCH billed Medicare and Medicaid, and the conspirators split the cash. An examination of the files of patients "admitted to [LCH] in 1998 and 1999 demonstrated that a minimum of 50 percent of the services [they received] . . . were medically unnecessary."[73]

In 2006, Michel and the other defendants paid $15.4 million to settle with the government.[74] In the press release announcing the settlement, Peter D. Keisler, assistant attorney general for the Justice Department's

Civil Division, stated, "We will not tolerate health care providers who pay kickbacks or perform medically unnecessary treatments on elderly beneficiaries in order to generate Medicare and Medicaid payments."[75]

But tolerate Dr. Jack Michel is exactly what the government did. It let him retain his medical license and also let him keep on billing Medicare and Medicaid. After the case settled, Michel continued to operate nursing homes and LCH, as before. And the government kept cutting him checks like clockwork, each and every month.

Michel even expanded the network of nursing homes he owned. In 2015, he purchased RCHH, which was on the auction block because its former operator had committed health care fraud and was on her way to jail. "The nursing home's previous CEO, Karen Kallen-Zury, was sentenced to 25 years in federal prison" for her role "in a $67 million Medicare fraud scheme, a case [that] federal prosecutors described as a 'massive criminal fraud conspiracy involving fake documents . . . fake patients, fake services, and bribes.'"[76] (It was during Kallen-Zury's watch that the standby generator and cooling tower were installed improperly and illegally.) Three other executives were also sent to prison and ordered to pay millions in restitution.

The prospect that one fraudster would succeed another did not sit well with the folks at Florida's Agency for Health Care Administration (AHCA), the state's nursing home regulator, so they "moved to block" Michel's attempt to purchase RCHH.[77] "But months later, after Michel retained a lobbyist confidant of Gov. Rick Scott—Fort Lauderdale's William 'Billy' Rubin—the [AHCA] reversed course" and "approved a pair of license transfers that Michel and [LCH] needed to buy and operate [RCHH] and an adjacent mental health hospital."[78] As noted above, Governor Scott is the former CEO of Columbia/HCA, which paid $1.7 billion to resolve fraud claims in 2000 and 2002.[79] "What role Scott and Rubin may have played in the process, or what impact their relationship may have had on AHCA's ultimate decision, isn't known," according to Florida Bulldog, an independent watchdog group. What is known is that "Rubin's firm, The Rubin Group, [received] between $50,000 and $80,000 for lobbying the executive branch" on behalf of Hollywood Property Investments LLC, the vehicle Michel used to

purchase RCHH.[80] Other entities associated with Michel had sizable
dealings with the state, including a $23 million contract to train physi-
cians and a $48 million contract to treat state prisoners.[81] The full story
of the relationship between Scott, Rubin, and Michel remains to be
written, but the decision to allow Michel to acquire and operate RCHH
was, at least in retrospect, clearly a mistake.

The deaths at RCHH outraged the public. Seeing an opportunity
to play to the crowd, Florida officials initiated criminal and legislative investigations and condemned everyone responsible for the loss.
After learning of Michel's history of fraud charges, state senator Gary
Farmer said that Florida's "skilled nursing facilities have really become
death warehouses," adding, "Our elderly patients are being treated as
cash crops." He denounced the practice of allowing providers who settle
fraud cases to go into business again and promised to sponsor legislation
that would permanently ban them from running nursing homes.[82]

The best guess, unfortunately, is that these promises are hollow.
The government has neither the means nor the motivation to bring
providers to heel. The threat to exclude providers that settle false claims
cases from the Medicare and Medicaid programs is empty too. To see
that, one need only ask why such persons are not excluded already.
Medicare and Medicaid have existed since the mid–1960s, but 50 years
later they are still allowing known fraudsters like the Michels and the
Esformes to bill. Unscrupulous nursing home operators treat America's
elderly citizens as "cash crops" because, as far as both the providers and
the government are concerned, that is what they are. For providers,
senior citizens are opportunities to submit bills and get paid. For the
government, senior citizens are opportunities to cut checks in exchange
for political support. In a health care payment system whose chief purpose is to move money, elderly nursing home residents are simply means
to an end.

# CHAPTER 11: MY DOCTOR, MY DRUG DEALER

## GETTING YOUR FIX AT STARBUCKS

Doctors can be inaccessible. They work limited hours at inconvenient locations and are often booked weeks in advance. Physician Alvin Yee was more customer friendly.[1] He'd see a dozen or more patients a night, at eateries like Carl's Jr. and Denny's and at coffee shops like Starbucks. He once met a patient at an auto dealership. Wherever he was, Dr. Yee would take out his stethoscope, listen to patients' hearts and lungs, and evaluate their vital signs. Sometimes, he performed neurological exams.

Yee's unusual practice style appealed to Millennials. One-third of his patients were in their 20s. Remarkably, many of these young people needed help with pain. Yee gave them prescriptions for OxyContin, Xanax, Roxicodone, and Vicodin. Some patients had trouble concentrating. He wrote them scripts for Adderall, an amphetamine. Despite his low overhead, Yee wasn't cheap. Initial visits cost $600; follow-ups were $300. Convenience came at a price.

Yee stopped seeing patients after two of his patients died and the feds arrested him for prescription drug fraud. A few of the folks who visited him before he shuttered his practice were U.S. Drug Enforcement Administration agents. Yee gave them prescriptions for controlled substances too. He wrote prescriptions for one agent after being told that the medicine was for a friend who was unable to keep her appointment.

Another undercover agent said he was a former heroin addict who'd been borrowing painkillers from others. Yee gave that agent a prescription too, telling him, "You won't be having to bum off of your friends anymore."[2] Yee was so quick on the draw that he once reportedly pulled out his prescription pad while gambling at a Las Vegas casino.[3] After being indicted on 56 counts of illegally distributing controlled substances, Yee pled guilty and agreed to a minimum punishment of eight years in prison. The judge gave him 11 years.[4]

Some of Yee's patients wanted drugs for themselves. The two who died from overdoses obviously fell into this category. Others sold the drugs they obtained on the black market. Yee was practicing in Orange County, California, but investigators seized large quantities of the drugs he prescribed during busts in Seattle, Phoenix, and Detroit. But Yee didn't see himself as a criminal. In a televised interview, he accepted "responsibility for . . . lapses in judgment," but he seems to have thought he was mostly helping people.[5] Yee's attitude is not unusual. A study of physicians who were imprisoned for Medicaid fraud found that none thought they had done anything wrong. They "saw themselves as sacrificial lambs hung out to dry because of incompetent or backstabbing employees, stupid laws, bureaucratic nonsense, and a host of similar reasons."[6]

## The Drug Warriors Lost, the Drug Market Won

The prevalence of prescription drug fraud has a lot to do with the War on Drugs. Policies that criminalize access to controlled substances create lucrative black market opportunities for people willing to sell them illegally. Consider OxyContin. Its street value is about ten times the price at a pharmacy.[7] Arbitrageurs (i.e., middlemen) can make an enormous amount of money on the spread, and the harder law enforcement officers crack down on illegal sales, the higher street prices rise, automatically rewarding dealers for running greater risks. When Florida clamped down on illegal sales of oxycodone (the drug that is the active ingredient in OxyContin) in 2011, the street price went from $8 a pill to $15.[8] The incentive to run the risk of arrest and imprisonment was preserved and will last as long as the War on Drugs continues.

The black market in prescription drugs is good at meeting customers' demands too. After the U.S. Food and Drug Administration approved a generic version of OxyContin, the generic pills showed up on the street in some parts of the country before they were available in local pharmacies.[9] Undercover agents who bought the pills didn't even know what they were. Today, dealers are distributing new opioids so quickly that forensic labs are having trouble figuring out what's being sold, and first responders have no idea how to help people who overdose.[10]

If the War on Drugs were to end tomorrow, the street price of controlled substances would drop and a good deal of prescription drug fraud would vanish overnight. But illegal behavior would not disappear entirely. Prescription drug fraud that rips off Medicaid, Medicare, and private insurers will persist as long as patients rely on third-party payers to cover the cost of their medicines. Indeed, these other types of fraud are likely to become more of a problem as criminals who formerly sold drugs on the black market look for new ways to make money.

Perhaps the most surprising unintended consequence of the War on Drugs is that it turned urine into liquid gold. Monitoring the use of controlled substances, including both those that are prescribed and those that are acquired illegally, requires doctors and independent laboratories to test millions of urine samples, for which payers dole out billions of dollars. In just one year, Medicare alone paid for about 19 million urine screens. All together, "[t]he federal government paid providers more to conduct urine drug tests in 2014 than it spent on the four most recommended cancer screenings combined."[11] It is hard to imagine better evidence that our priorities are reversed.


## GETTING HIGH AT THIRD-PARTY PAYERS' EXPENSE

In 2013, twin brothers Robert and William Carlucci, both 70-year-old pharmacists in New Jersey, pled guilty to charges of submitting fraudulent bills to health care payers, including Medicare and Medicaid.[12] Their schemes covered the waterfront: underfilling prescriptions while billing for the full amount; charging for name brand drugs while substituting generics; billing insurers for refills without patients' knowledge; and buying drugs from nonlicensed wholesalers at substantial discounts while charging insurers their normal cost. The Carlucci brothers were comparatively small fry: they took insurers for only $1.5 million.

In October of 2011, a much larger criminal conspiracy came to light when the federal government indicted 24 defendants in South Florida for trafficking in oxycodone and other synthetic painkillers to the tune of $40 million.[13] The defendants included a doctor, two pain clinic operators, the owner of four Robert's Pharmacies, recruiters, and several professional patients.

The scheme worked this way. Recruiters paid people $600 to visit pain clinics in South Florida. Physicians at the pain clinics wrote prescriptions for controlled substances, even though the patients did not need them. The patients filled the prescriptions at Robert's Pharmacies and gave the drugs to the recruiters, who sold them on the black market. Finally, the pain clinics and pharmacies billed Medicare, Medicaid, and private insurers for the services and drugs they had provided. Everyone made money, and Robert's Pharmacies became one of the largest purchasers of oxycodone in South Florida.

This case is typical. South Florida has long been a hot spot of pharmaceutical fraud in all of its many varieties. In 2017, the Department of Justice charged the owner of a drug-treatment center in Delray Beach, Florida. He allegedly "recruited addicts to aid him in his schemes, attending Alcoholics Anonymous meetings and visiting 'crack motels' to persuade people to move to South Florida to help him. He offered kickbacks in the form of gift cards, plane tickets, trips to casinos and strip clubs as well as drugs."[14] In 2011, the *New York Times* observed that "pill mills" were everywhere in Florida; "so many out-of-staters flocked to Florida to buy drugs at more than 1,000 pain clinics that the state earned the nickname 'Oxy Express.'"[15] Substantially more people were dying each year from prescription drug overdoses than from illegal drugs. Florida subsequently cracked down on illegal prescribing by prohibiting physicians from dispensing narcotics themselves and by creating a statewide prescription drug monitoring system. Roughly half of the pain clinics shut down immediately.

But Floridians who want painkillers and can't find them locally don't have to travel far. Doctors in southern states are happy to get out their pads. When the U.S. Centers for Disease Control (CDC) tracked the number of opioid-based painkiller prescriptions per 100 residents, states in the South and the Midwest stood out like sore thumbs. Alabama, Arkansas,

Indiana, Kentucky, Louisiana, Michigan, Mississippi, Ohio, Oklahoma, South Carolina, Tennessee, and West Virginia all had at least one prescription for every man, woman, and child in the state. Some southern states had 1.25 prescriptions. In Alabama, Tennessee, and West Virginia, the figure was 1.4 prescriptions per resident. All other states had less than one prescription per resident. California, Hawaii, Minnesota, New Jersey, and New York all had between 0.52 and 0.63 prescriptions per resident.[16]

In fairness, the South doesn't have a monopoly on opioid fraud. A New York clinic was charged with fraudulently issuing prescriptions for more than five million oxycodone tablets, which reportedly fetched from $30 to $90 apiece on the street.[17] That said, the number of pills needed to fill the prescriptions written in southern states boggles the mind. Consider West Virginia. Studying sales records provided by the Drug Enforcement Administration, journalists learned that "drug wholesalers shipped 780 million prescription painkillers to West Virginia over a six-year period."[18] Nearly nine million hydrocodone pills went to a pharmacy in the tiny town of Kermit, home to 392 people. If you divide the sales volume by West Virginia's population, the shipments totaled "433 pain pills for every man, woman and child" in the state.[19]

Not surprisingly, the opioid crisis that has gripped the nation in recent years has hit West Virginia especially hard. When the CDC studied trends in drug overdose mortality per capita, it found that West Virginia had moved from the bottom quartile of the states in 1999 to the very top of the list in 2015. In comparison with the national average of 16.3 deaths per 100,000 people, West Virginia's rate of 41.5 was almost off the charts. This wasn't a one-time blip. In 2016, West Virginia again led the nation in drug overdose deaths per capita, with 35.5 per 100,000.[20] Things are so bad in West Virginia that in August 2016, 28 people overdosed in a four-hour span in Huntington, a town of 50,000 residents.[21] The spike in deaths even overwhelmed a state program providing burial assistance to indigent families.[22]

Of course, these problems aren't limited to West Virginia. Drug overdoses have increased the death rate of young white Americans to levels not seen since the height of the AIDS epidemic. Nationwide, drug overdoses account for 28 percent of deaths among white males aged 15–34, and 8 percent of all fatalities among white males age 35–64.[23]

Problems caused by opioid abuse affect people who aren't users too, as U.S. District Court Judge Joseph Goodwin explained in a thoughtful opinion providing a detailed description of the nationwide opioid crisis and West Virginia's particular situation:

> West Virginia leads the nation in the incidence of babies born exposed to drugs and has the highest rate of babies born dependent on opioids. In Huntington, for example, one in ten babies born at the hospital suffers withdrawal from substances such as heroin, opiates, cocaine, or alcohol. That is about fifteen times the national average.[24]

If there is one bright note in this sea of bad news, it is that West Virginia Governor Jim Justice (R) signed a law in 2017 that will make medical marijuana available in the state starting in mid-2019.[25] A 2017 study by researchers at the University of California San Diego found that in states that legalized medical marijuana, the number of hospitalizations for abuse and addiction to painkillers fell by 23 percent from 1997 to 2014, and hospitalizations for opioid overdoses declined by 13 percent.[26] These declines occurred at the same time that opioid-related deaths and hospitalizations in other states were skyrocketing. These findings suggest that people wanting to experience pain relief or drug-induced euphoria will use safer substances when they are available. Addicts may be addicts, but they're not suicidal. If we're right about that, West Virginia's opioid crisis might be nearing its end—even though the law was intended to help cancer victims and other people with terminal illnesses who need help managing pain.

### DOCTORS WHO DEAL—OR "JUST" OVERPRESCRIBE

Writing prescriptions for millions of pills requires a terrific work ethic, which Dr. Michael R. Brown certainly had. Known as "Dr. Feel-Good" by his clients, Brown was responsible for almost one-third of the Oxy-Contin prescriptions filled at Massachusetts pharmacies in 2004—an astonishing 288,859 prescriptions out of a statewide total of 922,985. To sustain that rate, Brown would have had to write 33 prescriptions an hour, 24 hours a day, 7 days a week, every week of the year. He was convicted of dealing drugs and committing Medicaid fraud in 2007. When the state medical board finally stripped him of his license, its investigator reported that Brown had been "dealing OxyContin to the entire South Shore."[27]

Prescription drug fraud isn't limited to narcotics either. For years, Dr. Huberto Merayo wrote hundreds of prescriptions for powerful and expensive anti-psychotic drugs at his office in Coral Gables, Florida. In 2009 alone, these prescriptions cost Florida's Medicaid program nearly $2 million. But, by comparison to Dr. Fernando Mendez-Villamil, Merayo was a rank amateur. Mendez-Villamil wrote more than 96,000 Medicaid prescriptions for mental health drugs from July 2007 to March 2009. In 2009 alone, his prescriptions for anti-psychotics cost the state's Medicaid program $4.7 million. Eventually, the state caught up with both Merayo and Mendez-Villamil, but it took years for it to do so.[28] Both doctors eventually pled guilty to health care fraud.[29]

## DRUG FRAUDS COST BILLIONS

Egregious overprescribing of the sort just described is easy to detect. Just look for extreme outliers. "Pill mill" doctors get away with their frauds for so long because no one is paying attention. But even if someone were looking for outliers, lower-volume frauds would fly under the radar. Unlike consumers, law enforcement officers cannot be present every time a prescription is written. They have to rely on physicians' honesty and records. But honesty cannot always be assumed. Records may be phony. Barring extreme facts, regulators are inevitably left guessing much of the time—and they will understandably tend to give physicians the benefit of the doubt. Meanwhile, in 2010, Medicaid spent more than $27 billion nationwide on prescription drugs. We don't know exactly how much of that was wasted, but we can be sure that billions were.

How do we know that? The government has studied prescription drug fraud in public programs repeatedly, and each time it has concluded that fraud is rampant. A 2009 GAO report on the Medicaid programs in five large states (California, Illinois, New York, North Carolina, and Texas) opened with the observation that investigators "found tens of thousands of Medicaid beneficiaries and providers involved in potential[ly] fraudulent purchases of controlled substances, abusive purchases of controlled substances, or both."[30] Sixty-five thousand beneficiaries had engaged in "doctor shopping," by acquiring prescriptions for the same type of controlled substances from six or more different medical practitioners during fiscal years 2006 and 2007. Four hundred of them got prescriptions for controlled substances from 21 to 112 medical practitioners and visited up to 46 different pharmacies to have them filled.[31]

Some of the specific findings were macabre. An Ohio physician who specialized in pain management was convicted of filing $60 million worth of fraudulent Medicaid, Medicare, and insurance claims. The doctor got patients hooked on controlled substances "so that he could profit from their habit[s] and increase the income he received from their medical claims. Two patients who regularly saw him died under his care, one from a multiple-drug overdose in the physician's office and one from an overdose of OxyContin taken on the same day that the prescription was written."[32]

Other findings remind us that the government often misses even patently fraudulent claims. Medicaid paid pharmacists for dispensing controlled substances to over 1,800 dead beneficiaries and for filling prescriptions for controlled substances written by more than 1,200 dead physicians. No wonder the GAO concluded that the five states it examined "did not have a comprehensive fraud prevention framework" for dealing with controlled substances.[33]

### MEDICARE PART D: THE ALWAYS-POURING PITCHER OF DRUG FRAUD

Similar problems beset Medicare Part D, which was enacted during President George W. Bush's administration and now pays for one out of every four prescriptions filled nationwide. A 2011 GAO report found that doctor shopping was widespread, with more than 170,000 Medicare beneficiaries receiving prescriptions for controlled substances from five or more medical practitioners in 2008. Six hundred Medicare beneficiaries obtained prescriptions from 21 to 87 medical practitioners in a single year.[34]

These examples are part of a much larger phenomenon. In 2014, researchers at Harvard Medical School released the results of a study of more than 1.2 million medical records of Medicare patients who took opioids like hydrocodone, fentanyl, morphine, and oxycodone. Nearly

35 percent had prescriptions from more than one doctor. One-third of this group got their prescriptions from four or more doctors.[35] In 2016, half a million Medicare beneficiaries (excluding those with cancer or in hospice) were prescribed "excessive" amounts of opioids (relative to standards set by the CDC), including 70,000 who received "extreme" amounts of narcotics (i.e., more than 240 mg of morphine every day for the entire year), and 22,000 who appeared to be "doctor shopping" (i.e., going to multiple physicians to obtain multiple prescriptions for opioids).[36]

*ProPublica*, a leading source of investigative journalism, has also documented fraud problems under Medicare Part D. After analyzing Medicare records it obtained via the Freedom of Information Act, it reported a host of abuses:

- Medicare allows doctors to write prescriptions for seniors even though the doctors have been barred from state Medicaid programs for questionable prescribing practices—or even criminal charges.
- "About 70 providers each wrote more than 50,000 prescriptions and refills in 2010, averaging at least 137 a day."
- A single Chicago psychiatrist who worked at a string of nursing homes for the mentally ill prescribed more of a potent schizophrenia drug (clozapine) than all the physicians in Texas combined. "He wrote an average of 20,000 Medicare prescriptions annually for clozapine and a brand-name version, FazaClo, with most going to disabled patients younger than 65."
- In 2010, "half of Medicare's top 20 prescribers of OxyContin had been criminally charged, convicted, or settled fraud claims, or had been disciplined by their state medical boards. . . . Similarly, eight of the top 20 prescribers of 30-milligram oxycodone pills— the strongest dose—have been charged, convicted, or barred from prescribing controlled substances, or faced discipline by licensing boards. Yet as of [May of 2013], only one of those doctors had been barred from Medicare, and that wasn't until nearly a year after his conviction for drug trafficking and health-care fraud."
- In 2007, Medicare Part D paid $1.2 billion for drugs prescribed by providers whose identities were unknown, because they provided invalid prescriber identifiers.[37]

The underlying scams take many forms, but one common strategy involves identity theft. Dr. Ernest Bagner III worked at a clinic in a strip mall in Hollywood, California, and saw a small number of patients with psychiatric problems. Then someone began forging his name on prescriptions for expensive medications for a wide array of nonpsychiatric problems. Medicare paid $3.8 million for phony prescriptions supposedly written by Bagner in 2010, and another $2.6 million in 2011. Even though Bagner repeatedly informed fraud control personnel that he had not written the prescriptions in question, Medicare took no action to prevent payment on newly submitted prescriptions.[38] Instead, the U.S. Centers for Medicare and Medicaid Services (CMS) kept shoveling money out the door.

Bagner's case is not an isolated event. According to a 2012 article in the *Journal of the American Medical Association*, there were more than 12,000 cases of identity theft involving physicians between 2007 and 2009. In 32 percent of these cases, the thefts went undiscovered for more than a year, meaning that the criminals had many months in which to submit fraudulent bills in the names of the doctors whose identities they purloined.[39]

A much more elaborate phony prescription operation involved Babubhai Patel, the owner of several Detroit-area pharmacies. Patel "had a stable of doctors willing to write Part D prescriptions for any drug he wanted, any time he wanted. In return, the doctors got cash, a flock of new patients and, in at least one case, a down payment for an office building."[40] Patel got paid by Medicare and other insurers for filling the bogus prescriptions and then made even more money by reselling the drugs. Thirty-nine people were indicted in August 2011 for participating in Patel's scheme, including 8 doctors, a podiatrist, 15 pharmacists, 3 home health agency owners, an accountant, and a psychologist. Most pled guilty. Patel was convicted in 2012 and is serving 17 years in prison.[41]

One of the physicians who went down with Patel was Dr. Mark Greenbain. Patel paid him $500 a week for prescribing expensive antipsychotics in 2011, the year Greenbain was indicted. Within a month, Medicaid suspended Greenbain from further billing. But Medicare kept him on and paid $862,000 for prescriptions he had written in 2012, even though Greenbain was under indictment for health care fraud. Even after Greenbain pled guilty in 2013, Medicare took several months to revoke his billing authorization.[42]

Scams like Patel's succeed for many reasons. First, to external appearances nothing was amiss, apart from the total volume of drugs being prescribed. Physicians were writing prescriptions for patients, and patients were having those prescriptions filled at pharmacies. To a bureaucracy, paperwork is reality, and all the paperwork was in order. One key to a successful scam is for everything to look normal. Second, Medicare's structure makes it easy for fraudsters. Medicare Part D gives the private insurance companies that administer the program only 14 days to pay for prescriptions. And once the money goes out the door, there's little hope of recovering it. Third, the insurers can't block suspect doctors' prescriptions or review patients' medical records to confirm that the patient actually saw the doctor who wrote the script. Fourth, the frauds often involve multiple insurers, each of which sees only part of the picture.

Finally, many patients in whose names bogus prescriptions are written either cannot detect the frauds or do not care because the frauds cost them no money. A scam that used identities stolen from nursing home patients came to light only because Denise Heap happened to check a form Medicare sent about her mother, a victim of Alzheimer's disease. Upon learning that her mother was being given all sorts of unnecessary and expensive medications, Heap complained to Medicare. Predictably enough, Medicare wasn't interested. But Heap persisted and contacted local law enforcement officials. Her call "launched an investigation that uncovered a large Part D scheme allegedly connecting the owners of the nursing home to a North Hollywood pharmacy operation, including evidence that other residents' identities were used." Reporters who interviewed Sergeant Steve Opferman, head of the local anti-drug task force, wrote that "investigators might never have known of the scheme without Heap's tip."[43]

In 2014, the federal government finally adopted a rule allowing officials to exclude overprescribing doctors from Medicare. But the rule isn't self-enforcing, and there are good reasons to be skeptical of the ability and willingness of CMS to use their newly granted powers to crack down on problem overprescribers. After all, CMS swung into action only because the media exposed its ineptness, not from a deep-seated desire to protect taxpayers' money. Even as the new rule was being announced, Medicare officials were reassuring providers that they intended to use it only in "very limited and exceptional circumstances."[44]

For this reason, we weren't surprised when, in a follow-up article published in 2015, *ProPublica* reported, "Fraud and abuse continue to dog Medicare's popular prescription drug program despite a bevy of initiatives launched to prevent them." Examples included the following:

- In 2014, "more than 1,400 pharmacies had questionable billing practices," meaning that they filled unusually high numbers of prescriptions per patient or billed for prescriptions for controlled substances unusually often.
- Prescriptions for opioids continued to rise, despite efforts to rein them in.
- New York and Los Angeles continued to be "hotbeds for questionable prescribing, with far higher use of expensive drugs associated with fraud than other parts of the country."
- CMS twice delayed implementation of measures designed to prevent fraud by requiring all doctors who wrote covered prescriptions to register with CMS.[45]

Oscar Wilde famously said, "Second marriage is the triumph of hope over experience." The same is true of anti-fraud measures like those adopted in 2014. They may save a billion dollars here or there, but that's no reason to celebrate when criminals are carting off an order of magnitude more. Sterner measures are required, but Congress will never embrace them. They'd be of limited effectiveness anyway because anything that restricts the flow of illegal prescription drugs will only strengthen the incentive to violate the law by causing their price to rise. Like the police officers who carry out the War on Drugs, the administrators responsible for preventing fraud in the Medicare and Medicaid prescription drug programs are playing an unwinnable game of Whac-a-Mole. The next chapter explains why this metaphor is apt.

# CHAPTER 12: WHAC-A-MOLE

## WITH THIRD-PARTY PAYMENT, THE MOLES WIN BIG

Whac-a-Mole is the arcade game in which players try to clobber as many moles with a mallet as they can before time runs out. Even the fastest player can't exhaust the supply of moles, though. Every time one gets bopped on the head, a new one pops up in a different place. Not knowing where the next mole will appear is part of the fun.

Policing health care fraud in America's politically controlled, third-party payer system is like playing an endless game of Whac-a-Mole. The main differences are that the game involves billions of dollars and the moles always win. Of course, some criminals do get clobbered. But third-party payment makes fraud so easy and lucrative—particularly when the government is the payer—that the supply of fraudsters is endless. No matter how fast prosecutors put them in jail, more get busy. And these moles are stealthy. Instead of signaling their locations by sticking their heads out, they hide their phony claims by making them look just like real ones. Before it can whack these moles, the government has to find them. Worse, by the time it figures out their locations, they've often shut down their criminal operations and started new ones in new places. For the government, looking for fraudsters and putting them away is a never-ending, full-time job.

As we said, the moles that the government misses cost taxpayers real money, not meaningless points in an amusing game. How much? By its nature, fraud is hidden, so no one knows for sure. The government says that fraud accounts for 10 percent of the dollars it pays out to health care providers.[1] This implies that criminals steal more than $100 billion a year from Medicare and Medicaid alone.

Some experts believe that the toll is far higher. Malcolm K. Sparrow, a professor at the Kennedy School of Government at Harvard University whose book *License to Steal* is a classic in the field, thinks that Medicare's fraud-related losses may run "as high as 30 to 35 percent" of its budget.[2] If Sparrow is right, criminals steal a staggering $185 billion to $216 billion from Medicare alone. And they steal tens or hundreds of billions more from Medicaid, other federal programs, and private insurers.

In the arcade game, it's tough being a mole. You keep getting bashed on the head. In real life, being a mole can be sweet. Fraudsters amass fortunes while running little risk of being caught. In some of the stories we discuss below, they literally needed help carrying away bags filled with money. You may think that you pay taxes to provide medical services for the elderly and the poor, but you're often just helping some scam artist enjoy a fancier lifestyle than you can afford.


### THE COPS ARE OUTNUMBERED

It may seem hard to understand why the government lets criminals rob it blind year after year, often by using the same scams. But it's really fairly easy. One must see, first, that opportunities to commit fraud are everywhere. Every filed claim has the potential to be fraudulent in numerous ways. A doctor may have rendered a service that was unnecessary or inappropriate, delivered a less-expensive service than claimed, performed a service poorly, supplied no service at all, or paid a kickback to a patient in return for an insurance number. A hospital's bill could include inflated charges, result from an illegal referral arrangement with a physician, seek compensation for medical conditions a patient did not have, or be wholly fictitious. A pharmacist may have filled a prescription with a generic while billing for a name brand, be part of a ring that supplies drugs to the street by filling phony prescriptions written by corrupt doctors for phantom patients, or have created additional doses by diluting drugs. In theory, every claim that a payer receives can be tainted by fraud.

The second thing one must know is that the number of claims is extraordinary. In 2015, the outside contractors that handle bills for Medicare processed 1,222,500,000 claims. That's almost 3.4 million claims per day.[3] And that was just for Medicare Part A and Medicare Part B, which cover treatments delivered by hospitals and physicians, respectively. Medicare Part D, the prescription drug program, generated hundreds of millions of additional claims.[4]

Medicaid must be considered too. Because each state runs its own system, comprehensive statistics for this program are not available. But Medicaid is now almost as large as Medicare in terms of the total number of dollars that are paid out. So the flow of claims relating to that program is presumably at least as great.

All things considered, Medicare and Medicaid receive something like three billion claims a year. For a human being to spend five minutes reviewing each claim would require 125,000 people each working 2,000 hours a year. That's not enough time to find and flag a fraud, much less to investigate one. More searching assessments are out of the question. So most claims are submitted and processed electronically without any substantive review. Computer programs check to see if all of the fields in a bill have been completed as the relevant regulations require and, if they have, the bill is paid. Only a tiny fraction of the bills submitted to CMS are individually screened.

The result is predictable. Scammers hide millions of fraud-tainted bills in the stream by making them look ordinary. They fill in the blanks the same way honest providers do, so the bill-processing computers approve their claims. The hard part for the scammers is acquiring the necessary billing numbers for providers and patients. They use many schemes to get them, some of which we describe below.

The ratio of bad guys to good guys is a big part of the problem too. There are far more people trying to defraud the government than there are cops on the beat trying to protect it. In 1991, the Office of the

Inspector General (OIG) of the U.S. Department of Health and Human Services (HHS) had a grand total of 1,150 employees who were collectively responsible for preventing fraud and abuse in a combined HHS budget of $485 billion. In 2013, even though HHS's budget had more than doubled (to $1.01 trillion), the OIG's headcount had risen only to 1,700 employees, or a 48 percent increase. Stated differently, in 1991, each OIG employee was responsible for preventing fraud in roughly $425 million in annual federal spending; in 2013, the number was $595 million. The states, which run Medicaid programs, are also outgunned. In 2014, "New York ha[d] a Medicaid investigations division of 110 souls (including support staff) to scrutinise [sic] $55 billion of annual payments and 137,000 providers."[5] That works out to $500 million and 1,245 providers per person. Even working every day of the year, no one could police that many claims or keep that many providers honest.

The police forces are small because preventing fraud is a low priority. Total federal spending on health care fraud and abuse is about $1.25 billion.[6] That's way too little, as the government's own statistics show. Government sources often boast that every dollar spent on health care–related fraud and abuse investigations generates $7–$8 dollars in recoveries.[7] If we assume that this is the marginal rate of return, the government should be spending much more. Instead, it is dropping investigations because it hasn't the manpower or the money to pursue them.[8]

How ineffectual are the fraud police? A 2011 article provides one indication. Its title was "How to Commit Medicare Fraud in Six Easy Steps."[9] The ratio of dollars lost to fraud to dollars recovered provides another. In 2016—a banner year—the federal government collected about $4.7 billion in fraud recoveries.[10] According to the government's low-end estimate, criminals stole more than $100 billion from taxpayers that year. The fraud police recovered less than five cents on the dollar.

## Fraud-Laced Industries: Home Health Care

The size of some conspiracies, the amounts stolen, and the number of years they persist all highlight the inadequacies of the fraud police. The home health care industry provides a raft of examples, many of which follow a pattern. Working with corrupt physicians, home health care agencies (HHAs) defraud Medicare by delivering or claiming to have delivered services to people who don't qualify for them. The doctors falsely certify that the patients need the visits, then the HHAs bill Medicare and share the proceeds with the doctors and, often, the patients. For the conspirators, the arrangement is win-win-win. For taxpayers, of course, it's a different story.

In 2012, a single Texas physician, Dr. Jacques Roy, was arrested for helping 500 different HHAs bilk Medicare and Medicaid out of almost $375 million. Over the preceding six years, Roy had signed more than 11,000 eligibility certifications, more than any other medical practice in the United States.[11] It should have been easy for Medicare to spot Roy. In 2010, 99 percent of the physicians who evaluated patients for home health services certified fewer than 104 patients. Roy certified about 5,000 patients that year, almost 50 times as many. For years, Medicare simply failed to notice that Roy was running a certification mill even though it bragged in the press release announcing his arrest that, "thanks to our new fraud detection tools, we have greater abilities to identify the kind of sophisticated fraud scheme that previously could have escaped scrutiny." What about this scam was "sophisticated"?

The story didn't end there. Prior to his arrest, Medicare had suspended Roy in June 2011 because of suspicions about his billing practices. In response, Roy continued certifying patients and billing, this time under someone else's name and provider number. Medicare blithely paid the bills. Roy didn't limit himself to home health care certification fraud either. At his trial, evidence was presented that he had gotten two patients hooked on prescription drugs so he could have sex with them.[12] A jury convicted Roy in 2016, and he was sentenced to 35 years in prison.[13]

Roy didn't even hold the record for most HHA certifications. Between 2006 and 2011, Dr. Joseph Megwa of Arlington, Texas, signed 33,000 phony prescriptions for home health services. According to Attorney General Eric Holder, Megwa was responsible for more than $100 million in false claims, attributable to more than 230 Dallas area HHAs.[14] Similar home health frauds were perpetrated in Florida,[15] Illinois,

Maryland, Michigan,[16] and other states. Many of these scams ran for years before they were finally detected and shut down.

HHA fraudsters are adaptive, too, and often circumvent the controls that CMS imposes. Consider the case of Florence Bikundi, who was suspended from participating in all federal health care programs in 2000. In 2009, she got married, changed her name, opened three HHAs, and secured new Medicaid provider numbers for each. Over the next five years, Medicaid paid Bikundi almost $80 million.[17] Another successful con.

Bad behavior is not limited to fly-by-night marginal players in home health care, either. In 2014, Amedisys, the largest home health care provider in the United States, paid $150 million to resolve a host of fraud claims, including the charge that it gamed the payment system by rigging the number of visits that patients received. From 2000 to 2007, Medicare paid a flat rate of $2,200 for the first nine home care visits, plus a second $2,200 for 10 visits or more. According to a 2010 *Wall Street Journal* article, "Amedisys provided many of its patients just enough therapy visits to trigger the extra $2,200 payment. In 2005, 2006 and 2007, very few Amedisys patients received nine therapy visits while a much higher percentage got 10 visits or more. In 2007, for instance, only 2.88 percent of patients got nine visits, while 9.53% of patients got 10 visits." A nurse who worked for Amedisys in Tennessee reported that her supervisors had her comb through patients' files and identify those who were just shy of the 10-visit mark. She would then call the patients' therapists and have them set up the tenth visit, triggering the second payment.[18]

When challenged, Amedisys defended itself by saying that its practices were "in line with the industry trends." That was true. The company's competitors were gaming Medicare's fee structure too. The full extent of their strategizing was revealed in 2008, when Medicare scrapped the old approach and adopted a new one that paid an extra fee of several hundred dollars at the 6-visit, 14-visit, and 20-visit levels. After the switch, the industry-wide percentage of therapy visits in the 10-to-13 range dropped by about a third, and new clusters formed around the new break points.[19] Of course, this behavior is not unique to this setting. Whenever people can adapt to a payment system in ways that serve their interests, they will attempt to do so.

The history of fraud in the home health care sector is so lengthy that one would expect the police to have gained a handle on it long ago. One wouldn't think that they'd have allowed a known bad guy to run the largest such fraud in history right under their noses—and of all places in Florida, the hotbed of fraud.

But that is exactly what they did. In 2016, the feds charged Philip Esformes and two accomplices with running a scam that lasted at least seven years. The scam involved a network of corrupt doctors, hospitals, skilled nursing homes, assisted living facilities, community mental health centers, and HHAs that filed false claims for treatments they claimed to have delivered to 14,000 patients. All told, the scam took Medicare and Medicaid for more than $1 *billion*. In 2006, the very same person (Philip Esformes) had paid $15.4 million "to resolve civil federal health care fraud claims for essentially identical conduct." And, as we describe in Chapter 10, in 2013, he and his father had shelled out $5 million to settle a whistleblower case that accused them of having an illegal kickback arrangement with Omnicare, which was said to have paid them millions of dollars in return for the right to deliver pharmacy services at certain nursing homes. According to the press release that announced his indictment, Esformes continued his criminal ways after the 2006 settlement, and he and his accomplices used "sophisticated money laundering techniques in order to hide the scheme and Esformes' identify from investigators."[20]

That's not all they did. According to the revised indictment and news reports, Esformes allegedly paid a state employee thousands of dollars in return for information about upcoming inspections; allowed patients at his company's facilities to be "used as guinea pigs for the sole purpose of billing medically unnecessary procedures to Medicare and Medicaid"; plied elderly patients with opioids to render them dependent on the drugs and on their facilities to supply more; and plotted to help one of his collaborators flee the country to avoid prosecution.[21] Esformes denies the accusations, but two federal judges deemed him to be a flight risk and denied his repeated requests for bail. Because Esformes owned his own jet, that seems an accurate assessment. His trial is scheduled for 2018.

Assuming that the charges against Esformes are true, U.S. Attorney Wifredo Ferrer wasn't exaggerating when he said, "The magnitude of

[the] alleged false claims in this scheme is staggering and outrageous, even by South Florida health care fraud standards. This case illustrates once again that Medicare fraud has infected every aspect of the health care system."[22] He might have added that the fraud police can do little to put the bad guys out of business. Esformes may be behind bars, but there are lots of other moles where he came from.

### FRAUD-LACED INDUSTRIES: MENTAL HEALTH SERVICES

The impotence of the fraud police is also indicated by the brazenness with which some frauds are committed. In 2010, the U.S. Department of Justice (DOJ) announced that it was prosecuting American Therapeutic Corp. (ATC) for attempting to defraud the government out of $205 million as part of a partial hospitalization program (PHP) scam. ATC was the nation's largest community mental health center chain, with seven clinics stretching from Miami to Ft. Lauderdale to Orlando. It grew so large partly because its owners, Marianella Valera, Lawrence Duran, and Judith Negron paid illegal kickbacks to assisted living facilities and halfway houses for sending over patients who suffered from dementia, Alzheimer's disease, and addictions. Valera, Duran, and Negron paid patients kickbacks too. Altogether, ATC filed 866,000 payment claims between 2002 and 2010 and took the federal government for $87.5 million. In a plea agreement, Valera admitted that *all* of the bills were dishonest. She was sentenced to 35 years behind bars while Duran, her boyfriend and collaborator, got 50 years, reportedly the longest prison term ever imposed for health care fraud. A jury convicted Judith Negron on 24 felony counts in August of 2011, and she was subsequently sentenced to 35 years in prison.[23]

The ATC fraud lasted eight years before federal prosecutors finally brought the hammer down. The duration of the fraud is remarkable given the patently fraudulent nature of some of ATC's bills. At Negron's trial, prosecutors showed that she claimed to have treated patients in Boca Raton and Homestead—cities in Florida that are 80 miles apart—at the exact same time. "In one particularly troubling case, prosecutors claimed that Negron charged for group psychotherapy provided to a patient who was in a neuro-vegetative state, who could not lift her head or respond." ATC also threw "charting parties" where employees altered patients' records. Its bills were wholly fictitious, but it took years for federal auditors to figure things out.[24]

Valera, Duran, and Negron also built a network of cooperating providers, all of whom were in on the fraud.[25] For example, they paid Dr. Alan Gumer, a psychiatrist, to certify that patients needed group therapy services, to prescribe psychiatric medications, and to refer hundreds of ATC patients to a related company, the American Sleep Institute, for unnecessary diagnostic sleep disorder testing. Altogether, the feds indicted about 40 people, including ATC employees, psychiatrists, counselors, nurses, marketers, patient recruiters, and others who supplied Medicare beneficiaries in exchange for kickbacks.[26]

Most criminals keep a low profile to evade detection, but Duran enjoyed rubbing elbows with the elite. He created and served on the board of the National Association for Behavioral Health (NABH), a Washington, D.C., lobbying group that encouraged Congress to provide greater financial support for community mental health centers. NABH, which spent more than $750,000 on lobbying, threw fundraisers for Rep. Kendrick Meek (D) from Florida and Sen. Mary Landrieu (D) from Louisiana.

According to the DOJ, Duran used NABH to "franchise his fraud to others."[27] In view of this, it isn't all that surprising that there were multiple PHP facilities scamming the government. In 2014, federal agents arrested 42 suspects who lured out-of-state Medicare patients to South Florida with the promise of providing shelter.[28] Once the patients arrived, they were placed in assisted living facilities and steered to PHP mental health programs. If they dropped out of the group therapy sessions, they were dumped on the street. The network of corrupt providers included the owners of the Biscayne Milieu Health Center in Miami, physicians, patient recruiters, owners of assisted living facilities, and operators of home health care agencies, HIV-therapy clinics, and medical equipment businesses. Collectively, the defendants were accused of submitting $160 million in false claims on which Medicare paid out more than $90 million. The prosecution produced eight criminal convictions and a host of guilty pleas.[29]

PHP scams were also being perpetrated in other states. In 2011, the feds arrested the owners of Spectrum Care P.A., located in Houston, Texas, and accused them of attempting to bilk the government out of $97 million. "The indictment allege[d] that Spectrum billed Medicare for mental health services when patients were actually watching movies, playing bingo or engaging in other activities." Spectrum's owners allegedly paid the owners of assisted living facilities for referring Medicare patients. Sometimes, they paid kickbacks to Medicare patients as well.[30]

A year later, the DOJ filed criminal charges against 10 people running a PHP scam out of Riverside General Hospital (RGH), another Houston establishment.[31] Assisted living facilities and group care homes allegedly received kickbacks to refer Medicare beneficiaries for treatment at RGH. Patients got cigarettes, food, and coupons redeemable for items available at RGH's "country stores" in exchange for their participation. Everybody won, except the taxpayers, who had to deal with fraudulent bills totaling $158 million, on which at least $45 million was paid. When Medicare finally responded to the fraud by cutting off all payments to RGH, Texas Rep. Sheila Jackson Lee (D) lodged a protest in which she claimed that CMS was jeopardizing access to care for vulnerable Medicare patients. CMS responded two months later by restoring 70 percent of the payments.[32]

## FRAUD-LACED INDUSTRIES: DURABLE MEDICAL EQUIPMENT

Durable medical equipment (DME) includes things like oxygen supplies, mail-order diabetic supplies, power wheelchairs and scooters, knee braces, prosthetic limbs, and surgical dressings. From 2009 to 2012, Medicare paid a total of $43 billion for DME. According to some reports, more than 60 percent of that amount—$25 billion plus—may have been paid out improperly.[33] Unsurprisingly, DME suppliers lead the list of entities investigated for criminal health care fraud violations.[34] But the federal government has recovered only about 3 percent of overpayments.[35] Criminals are all about stealing money. They're not inclined to give it back.

The largest known DME fraud involved Abner and Mabel Diaz, of Miami Lakes, Florida, who pled guilty in 2008. They ran All-Med Billing Corp. (All-Med), a Miami medical billing company that submitted claims to Medicare on behalf of DME suppliers. All-Med submitted almost $420 million in fraudulent claims for 85 separate DME suppliers. The equipment had not been ordered by physicians or delivered to the beneficiaries. Medicare paid the suppliers almost $149 million on these fraudulent claims.[36]

Most DME frauds are smaller. Some involve hundreds of thousands of dollars or even less. But corrupt DME sellers make up in volume what they lack in size. In July of 2010, the federal government announced that it had indicted an astonishing 94 doctors, health care company owners, and others for participating in DME scams across the United States. These scams collectively generated more than $251 million in false billings. The variety of scams and scammers is also incredible. One scheme involved a pastor who ran a corrupt DME business on the side.[37] Another involved a husband and wife team of co-pastors who defrauded Medicare with help from members of their church.[38] In a third, Medicare was billed for leg braces that were sent to a customer whose legs had been amputated.[39]

Frauds involving power wheelchairs and scooters could fill an entire book. To give just one example, in 2013, FBI agents raided the headquarters of the Scooter Store in New Braunfels, Texas, after a federal audit found the company had overbilled Medicare by as much as $87 million from 2009 to 2011. The Scooter Store advertised widely, telling Medicare recipients: "You may qualify for a power chair or scooter at little or no cost to you."[40] Who wouldn't want one? DME suppliers even exploited Medicare's generosity after hurricanes Katrina and Rita by falsifying applications for new power wheelchairs that were intended to replace ones that were destroyed by the storms.[41]

DME fraudsters adapt quickly and are willing to change tactics, making them hard to stamp out. In 2011, the HHS inspector general testified that "investigations have found that criminals set up sham DME storefronts to create the appearance that they are bona fide providers; fraudulently bill Medicare for millions of dollars; and then close up shop, only to reopen in a new location under a new name and continue the fraud."[42] A year earlier, testimony by the chief counsel to the OIG included almost exactly the same language, plus the observation that fraud is viral, in that it replicates rapidly within geographic and ethnic communities. Indeed, he noted that health care fraud "migrates: as law enforcement cracks down on a particular scheme, the criminals may shift the scheme (e.g., suppliers fraudulently billing for DME have shifted to fraudulent billing for home health services) or relocate to a new geographic area."[43]

## TAKING TAXPAYERS FOR AN AMBULANCE RIDE

People receive health care in hospitals, emergency rooms, dialysis clinics, therapy centers, and other locations. To receive care in these settings, some need to get there by ambulance. Ambulance companies are supposed to obtain a physician's certification that a patient needs special treatment, but they can obtain payments without submitting them. Once again, Medicare trusts providers to do the right thing. Want to guess how that has worked out?

Ambulance rides have been a cesspool of corruption. Consider Houston, Texas, where problems with ambulance transportation fraud emerged in the early 2000s, then ballooned. By 2009, Medicare was paying $62 million for ambulance rides in Houston, compared to a mere $7 million for New York.[44] And 2009 was not an especially expensive year. During 2005–2010, Medicare paid a total of $488 million, or about $81 million per year, for ambulance trips in Houston. Medicare's billing contractor for Texas identified nonemergency transports as its number one problem.[45]

The array of fraud was breathtaking in its variety and simplicity. Ambulances were used to transport patients to routine appointments for medical services of dubious value, even though the patients could have traveled safely, and much less expensively, by ordinary means. When interviewed after being dropped off by an emergency medical services (EMS) company at home, 23-year-old Daniel McCall said he had just returned from "a place where 'they just fed us junk food . . . we watch TV and stuff.'"[46] McCall, who was neither bedridden nor physically disabled, didn't know why he went to therapy, why he rode in an ambulance, or who paid for it. He did know that he took a 25-mile ambulance ride to the Cadwalder Behavioral Clinic (CBC)—a three-bedroom house with portable toilets in its driveway—six days a week. EMS companies transported many other patients to CBC too. Investigative reporters who visited CBC "found a steady stream of EMS vehicles picking up and dropping off dozens of people."[47]

McCall's trip wasn't nearly the longest, either. The *Houston Chronicle*'s reporters watched as three vehicles operated by Promise EMS pulled into the driveway at Desire to Live, an unlicensed and illegal assisted living facility in Alvin, Texas. Each vehicle dropped off an elderly female patient who, like McCall, had received therapy at CBC. For these women, the round-trip ride, which they too made almost every day, covered 135 miles. The cost? More than $1,000 per trip.

Houston may once have been ground zero for ambulance fraud, but the problem has now spread. Thousands of ambulance companies have been investigated, in locations as far-flung as upstate New York,[48] Pennsylvania,[49] South Carolina,[50] Tennessee,[51] and Virginia.[52] But the prize for sheer chutzpah goes to three services that operated in New York City. After Medicare demanded millions of dollars back from them for ambulance rides that were unnecessary or lacked supporting documentation, the companies appealed. Then they forged and submitted hundreds of documents attesting that the rides at issue were necessary and appropriate.[53] When accused of fraud, these companies committed more fraud.

## ORGANIZED CRIME

Organized crime has long recognized the benefits of stealing from government health care programs. In 1995, Louis Freeh, then the director of the FBI, observed that, "in South Florida and Southern California, we have seen cocaine distributors switch from drug dealing to health-care fraud schemes. The reason: The risks of being caught and imprisoned are less."[54] Seven years later, a representative of the OIG noted that "drug dealers are switching from trafficking in narcotics to health care fraud, having discovered that defrauding Medicare is safer and more lucrative and carries a lower risk of detection and prosecution. . . . In several major cities, including Miami, Los Angles, and Houston, organized crime is a driving force behind the growing problem."[55]

A few examples help make the point more concrete. In 2010, the DOJ indicted 73 individuals, many of whom belonged to an Armenian-American organized crime syndicate known as Mirzoyan-Terdjanian, for $163 million in fraudulent billing.[56] The defendants stole the identities of doctors and thousands of Medicare beneficiaries and operated at least 118 different phony clinics in 25 states. When the arrests and indictments were announced, the acting deputy attorney general observed, "The emergence of international organized crime in domestic health care fraud schemes signals a dangerous expansion that poses a serious threat to consumers as these syndicates are willing to exploit almost any program, business or individual to earn an illegal profit." Mirzoyan-Terdjanian is named for its principal leaders, Davit Mirzoyan and Robert Terdjanian, who are thought to oversee the gang's U.S. and international activities from Los Angeles and New York. Mirzoyan pled guilty in 2012, and Terdjanian, whose rap sheet included burglary and weapons convictions, was sentenced to 10 years of prison time in 2013.[57]

Fast-forward four more years. Special Agent Brian Martens testi-fied before the Senate Special Committee on Aging in 2014 that federal agents assigned to Medicare fraud investigations "regularly encounter stockpiles of weapons when we execute arrests and enforcement oper-ations."[58] One news report said that he compared anti-fraud efforts to a game of Whac-a-Mole, noting that, "as enforcement efforts target certain [schemes], others pop up. [Criminal gangs] switch between different parts of the Medicare program, they move from area to area, and they often rely on the muscle of organized crime."[59] Martens also admitted, "we don't have the staff that we need with the amount of fraud that goes on."

### THE COMPLETE IDIOT'S GUIDE TO HEALTH CARE FRAUD

Perhaps you're thinking that the wrongdoers who rip off the health care system are criminal masterminds. They aren't. Health care fraud is so simple that even high school dropouts have stolen millions of dollars. Aghaegbuna "Ike" Odelugo, a Nigerian immigrant, took Medicare for almost $10 million. After being convicted, he told the Subcommittee on Oversight of the House Ways and Means Committee that "DME fraud is incredibly easy to commit. The primary skill required to do it successfully is knowledge of basic data entry on a computer."[60] Odelugo's billing scheme involved 14 DME suppliers located in 10 different states.

Angel Castillo Jr., of West Miami-Dade, Florida, made an even bigger dent in the Treasury. He was a small-time drug dealer who discovered that his 9th-grade education was more than sufficient to commit Medicare fraud. After serving a couple of years in prison for trafficking in cocaine, he became an electrician and used his newfound skills to build marijuana grow-houses. Then his best friend told him there was money to be made in Medicare fraud, so he concentrated his energies on that. Before he went to jail again in 2008, Castillo controlled about a dozen phony medical equipment companies, all incorporated in the names of Cuban straw owners, that sent fraudulent bills to Medicare for mattresses, knee braces, artificial limbs, and other items that were never delivered. Altogether, these companies submitted almost $50 million in phony bills. So much money poured into his account that "Castillo bribed bank tellers to let his associates pick up bags of cash totaling as much as $100,000 from Bank of America, Union Planters, and Washington Mutual."[61]

The government has such difficulty detecting fraudulent providers that even recent immigrants and career criminals can rob it blind. In 2012, the *Miami Herald* reported, "Dozens of Cuban immigrants charged in South Florida with trying to bilk [Medicare] have fled to the island nation, which historically has turned a blind eye and doesn't return the fugitives to the United States."[62] The occasion for this observation was provided by the arrest of Armando "Manny" Gonzalez on charges of attempting to steal $63 million from the federal government. Gonzalez was "a convicted cocaine trafficker who joined the Medicare rackets in the mid-2000 era when he opened a pair of mental health clinics in the Kendall and Cutler Bay areas."

Gonzalez's clinics were highly successful. Over the seven-year period extending from 2004 to 2011, they reportedly collected $28 million from

the Medicare program. What services did they provide? According to the
DOJ, Gonzalez used the same approach that Duran employed at ATC.
While purporting to offer group therapy treatments, his clinics actually
entertained patients with TV shows and movies. Gonzalez even joined
Duran's NABH and helped lobby congressional leaders to provide more
Medicare dollars for psychotherapy treatments at community clinics.

And like Duran, Gonzalez lived extremely well. The assets of his
that the feds tried to seize included a $750,000 house in Henderson-
ville, North Carolina, and 17 vehicles, including two Cadillac Esca-
lades, a BMW, and a Mercedes-Benz, all paid for with taxpayers' money.
Because the "vast majority" of the money Gonzalez's clinics took in was
"laundered through shell corporations," there was no hope of recovering
it. "Pay and chase" failed again.

But the record, so far as we can tell, goes to Alexis C. Norman,
who was sentenced to eight years in prison for defrauding Medicaid by
submitting bills for counseling services that were never provided. While
awaiting sentencing for this crime, Norman set up two companies to
continue the fraud under different provider names. She started submitting bills immediately, including the day before her sentencing hearing.
And she kept her counseling scam 2.0 going while she was incarcerated,
billing the Medicaid program an additional $800,000, on top of the
$5.5 million that counseling scam 1.0 billed. The "good" news is that
the Medicaid program paid her only $2.5 million on counseling scams
1.0 and 2.0 before they caught on.

### When Patients Are the Problem

Patients also help bleed the treasury. The most famous recent example
involves the five dozen Russian diplomats and spouses who got New
York's Medicaid program to cover the medical costs associated with
pregnancies and deliveries.[63] From 2004 to 2013, they cheated the system the old-fashioned way: by lying about their income.

Patients can rip off the system in multiple ways. We've already discussed doctor-shoppers, who accumulate pills to sell on the black market. There are also patients who knowingly allow providers to upcode or

provide them unnecessary products and services. And, of course, there are patients who receive cash payments for allowing fraudulent providers use of their Medicare or Medicaid numbers.

Perhaps the most stomach-turning examples are "rent-a-patient" scams, in which bribed patients allow corrupt doctors to perform unnecessary surgeries on them. According to one of the willing victims, during a five-month period, he underwent a circumcision, removal of his sweat glands, a nose operation, a colonoscopy, and an endoscopy at a surgery center in Orange County, California, even though he was "healthy as a horse." For each procedure, he was paid $800, and the surgery center billed the victim's insurer for tens of thousands of dollars for the unnecessary surgery.[64] The scam came to light only after the insurer sent the check to the patient, who cashed it, rather than sign it over to the surgery center.[65] The surgery center sued its former patient to collect its ill-gotten gains, along with another 11 former patients who had also had unnecessary surgeries, and received checks from their insurers. The rent-a-patient scam triggered an FBI investigation of roughly 100 surgery centers and a lawsuit brought by 12 major insurers against 16 clinics or management companies and 34 individuals, seeking $30 million in damages.[66]

Patient complicity is so common as to stagger the imagination. Most stories simply report that patients were recruited and omit the details. For example, Dora Binimelis, the owner of Blessed Medical Clinic, took Medicare for $2.4 million by bribing senior citizens to sit through unnecessary tests.[67] The payments aren't always in cash, though. In 2014, Drs. Hoi Yat Kam and Chang Ho Lee pled guilty to fraudulently billing Medicare for more than $13 million.[68] Their clinics offered seniors free massages, facials, meals, prizes, and social events in return for their Medicare numbers, which were used to bill for medical services that were never provided.

When details do come to light, they can be interesting. Did you know that thousands of patients are enthusiastic co-conspirators in the commission of health care fraud? Prosecutors focus on fraudulent providers, not patients. Consequently, corrupt patients "remain free to move from clinic to clinic, scam to scam, from durable medical equipment and

HIV infusion therapy to home health care. Another year, another disease."[69] In the words of Peggy Sposato, a former emergency room nurse who joined the DOJ as an investigator, "To look at health care fraud and not [see] that the beneficiaries are somehow involved is to be blind to the problem. We've got people out there who brag about the fact that they are making large amounts of money abusing Medicare."[70]

One professional patient was Alexander McCray, a crack addict who needed money to support his habit. According to a news report, McCray received kickbacks of $150 to $300 each time he visited a private clinic, which he did as often as three times a day, three days a week over seven years. Using McCray's name and Medicare number, clinic operators filed more than $1.1 million in false claims for fabricated HIV-infusion treatments billed in his name. Some 90 doctors signed off on phony prescriptions for drugs that were supposedly given to McCray.[71]

McCray isn't an exception. According to the *Miami Herald*, which has a series of investigative articles devoted to Medicare fraud, there are "thousands of con artists" like McCray in South Florida alone.[72] South Florida isn't exceptional either. Patient recruiters do a thriving business in many cities. Often, they focus their efforts on locations where homeless people and drug addicts gather.

### THE SONG REMAINS THE SAME

Although federal prosecutors are putting away bad guys as fast as they can, fraud is still rampant. High profile sweeps conducted by the Medicare Fraud Strike Force (MFSF) in back-to-back years make both points. In 2014, the MFSF sweep netted 90 people, including 27 doctors, nurses, and other medical professionals who collectively submitted about $260 million in false bills. The 2015 haul was even bigger, resulting in charges against "243 individuals, including 46 doctors, nurses and other licensed medical professionals, for their alleged participation in Medicare fraud schemes involving approximately $712 million in false billings."[73]

In both years, the illegal schemes were similar to those the feds have been prosecuting for decades: billing for services that weren't needed or provided, paying kickbacks to patients and recruiters, and so on. The bad guys didn't change all that much either. They were HHAs, mental health services agencies, psychotherapists, physical and occupational therapists, DME suppliers, and pharmacists. As Marilyn May, a lawyer who defends clients accused of defrauding the government, observed:

> While the recent nationwide Medicare takedown with charges against 243 people throughout the country garnered lots of headlines—which is, of course, part of the government's enforcement strategy—a closer look at the types of alleged health care fraud cases packaged together under one umbrella shows mostly the same types of garden-variety health care fraud cases that the government has been prosecuting for years. These types of alleged schemes are not new.

She added that these "are the simplest health care fraud cases to prove" and that "[t]he government's simultaneous announcement of charges against large numbers of individual defendants for alleged criminal Medicare fraud is nothing new."[74]

Simply stated, the endless stream of arrests and convictions is a sign of failure, not of success. Criminals keep using the same types of schemes to steal money from taxpayers year after year. As May wrote, "the more things change, the more they stay the same."[75] Only ignorant members of the general public are fooled into thinking that the government has a handle on fraud. In reality, it's caught up in an eternal game of Whac-a-Mole.

As if to punctuate the point, in mid-July of 2017—just after this chapter was revised for what we thought would be the last time—a new nationwide fraud sweep was announced in which 412 people, including 115 doctors, nurses, and other practitioners, were arrested and accused of taking the government for $1.3 billion.[76] This wasn't a takedown of an enormous criminal gang whose elimination would make a sizable dent in the fraud problem. It was the culmination of investigations into hundreds of separate frauds, most of which were small. One involved the operator of a drug treatment center in Florida who offered addicts gift cards, plane tickets, and other goodies—including drugs—to get their insurance numbers. Another was carried out by a cardiologist in New York who had a kickback arrangement with a medical diagnostic company. A third involved a father-and-son pair of psychologists in Texas, who supposedly billed $300,000 in illegal charges over a period of four years. Other suspects were accused of doling out opioids, billing for drugs that were never purchased, or selling prescriptions for cash. These are the same sorts of cons that have bedeviled the health care system for years.

The real point of the announcement is discouraging, but simple. We are losing a never-ending game of Whac-a-Mole to thousands upon thousands of fraudsters, who are collectively robbing taxpayers blind. When Attorney General Jeff Sessions said that the 2017 sweep "again highlights the enormity of the fraud challenge we face," he was repeating an observation that has been made many times before and that is certain to be made again. As long as the federal and state governments keep doling out hundreds of billions of dollars to health care providers, the moles will always win.

## CHAPTER 13: BAD BUSINESS

### Pass the Ketchup, Please

There are seven deadly sins, and Las Vegas exists to provide one convenient location to sample all of them. The Heart Attack Grill is the place for gluttony.[1] Its voluptuous "nurses" serve food that will kill you if eaten too often. There's the 10,000 calorie Quadruple Bypass Burger, a banquet built with 4 half-pound beef patties, 20 strips of bacon, and 8 slices of American cheese. Pair one with an order of Flatliner Fries (fried in lard) and a Chocolate Butterfat Shake, and you've got Vegas's version of a Happy Meal.

Too much happiness can be lethal. Some of the Heart Attack Grill's most loyal customers learned this the hard way. While being interviewed on a business-oriented news program, "Dr." John Basso, the owner, held up a plastic bag that contained the ashes of a recently deceased patron who was also a spokesman for the Heart Attack Grill. Basso challenged other restaurants to be as candid about the dangers of their menu items as he is about his.

The Heart Attack Grill's business model is unusual. Normally, killing customers—or even harming them—is a bad idea. But health care providers that harm patients can make more money by doing so. They get paid once for delivering services that injure patients and a second time for treating the injuries they inflict. This may explain why health care providers harm patients so often.

How often? The matter is subject to disagreement, but, as *Scientific American* reported, "every time researchers estimate how often a medical mistake contributes to a hospital patient's death, the numbers come out worse."[2] A decade ago, the Institute of Medicine made front-page news when it conservatively estimated that medical errors killed 44,000 to 98,000 hospitalized patients each year.[3] Just four years later, Health-Grades, a private organization that rates health care providers, doubled the count, putting the annual death toll at 195,000.[4] Then, in 2013, the *Journal of Patient Safety* published a meta-analysis of prior studies that said "preventable harm to patients" causes more than 400,000 premature deaths per year.[5] (A 2016 study by researchers at Johns Hopkins University School of Medicine broke the upward spiral of estimates by putting the tally of error-related deaths at 250,000.)[6] If we accept the highest estimate, medical errors are the third-leading cause of death in the United States. Only heart disease and cancer kill more often.[7] Even if we use the lowest estimate, medical errors are still the eighth-leading cause of death in the United States, just behind diabetes and just ahead of suicide.

Fortunately, most injured patients survive. Of course, that means that the total number of injuries substantially exceeds the number of fatalities; "serious harm [is] 10- to 20-fold more common than lethal harm."[8] More than 6 million patients may be injured each year.[9]

In 2011, *Health Affairs* published a series of articles that collectively paint a portrait of medical injuries and their associated costs. One group of researchers found that adverse events occurred in a shocking 33.2 percent of hospital admissions, ten times as often as previously thought.[10] Another study estimated that medical errors generated over $17 billion in direct medical costs in 2008 alone.[11] A third study (based on the amounts people would pay to avoid risks to their health) found that medical errors entail annual social costs ranging from $393 billion to $958 billion.[12]

It has been clear for decades that medical injuries result in increased health care utilization. In 2007, an article published in the *Journal of the American Medical Association* estimated that quality problems in outpatient care and medical errors *alone* necessitated "116 million extra physician visits, 77 million extra prescriptions, 17 million emergency department visits, 8 million hospitalizations, [and] 3 million long-term admissions," in addition to almost 200,000 deaths.[13] How much larger would those figures be if we included hospitalized patients?

## HOSPITALS ARE BUSINESSES RUN POORLY

Is it possible that these figures are as high as they are because errors generate revenue and profits for health care providers? Apart from an occasional monster, health care providers don't deliberately harm patients in order to make more money. They claim to take adequate precautions and remind us that bad things happen to their patients because their patients are sick. This is the Reverse Lake Wobegon Effect in action. For decades, it was the conventional wisdom regarding hospital-acquired infections (HAIs), which, according to a 2007 estimate by the Centers for Disease Control, afflicted 2 million patients a year, killed nearly 100,000, and cost over $25 billion to treat.[14] Hospitals claimed they could do little to reduce these numbers because sick patients with weakened immune systems were easy prey for opportunistic bacteria.

The Quality and Safety Research Group at Johns Hopkins Hospital, led by Dr. Peter Pronovost, put the lie to this claim by proving that hospitals can protect patients from HAIs easily and cheaply. His team focused on infections suffered by patients with a central line who are treated in an intensive care unit (ICU). A central line (also called a central venous catheter) is used to give fluids and medication to critically ill patients in an ICU. It is typically inserted in the neck. As we discussed in the Introduction, an infection of the central line, called a CLABSI, for "central line–associated blood stream infection," is often lethal. As Dr. Pronovost and his team observed, "Each year in the United States, central venous catheters may cause an estimated 80,000 catheter-related bloodstream infections and . . . up to 28,000 deaths among patients in [ICUs]."[15]

CLABSIs are almost entirely preventable, and the cost of preventing them is low. When inserting central lines, physicians and hospital staffers need only follow a simple, five-item checklist. They must:

1. Wash their hands with soap;
2. Clean the patient's skin with chlorhexidine antiseptic;
3. Put sterile drapes over the patient's body;

4.  Wear a sterile hat, mask, gloves, and gown while inserting the catheter; and

5.  Apply a sterile dressing after the central line is inserted.[16]

They also have to avoid putting central lines in the groin and remove them at the earliest opportunity. That's it. No special knowledge, expensive drugs, or fancy technology is required. As Dr. Atul Gawande, the health services researcher and author of a book on the benefits of using checklists in health care remarked, "These steps are no-brainers; they have been known and taught for years."[17]

And these steps work not just at fancy academic medical centers, but everywhere. Pronovost's group tested their checklist at 103 ICUs in community hospitals in Michigan. Before the trial, their average CLABSI rate was 7.7 infections per 1,000 catheter-days. After 18 months using the checklist, the average was down to 1.4 infections per 1,000 catheter-days. That's a decline of 82 percent. The median infection rate was 0, meaning that at least half the ICUs reported no CLABSIs at all.[18]

Gawande described the Michigan experiment this way: "The results were stunning. . . . Over 18 months, the program saved more than 1,500 lives and nearly $200 million."[19] The improvement was so dramatic that Michigan's "average I.C.U. outperformed ninety per cent of I.C.U.s nationwide."[20]

The obvious question—obvious to us, at any rate—is: why weren't Michigan hospitals protecting intensive care patients from CLABSIs before Pronovost showed up? Why weren't hospitals everywhere doing so? When inserting central-line catheters, health care workers nationwide weren't taking precautions that were known to work. Worse still, some hospitals had adopted checklists, but their personnel often failed to comply. In interviews conducted by the American Association of Critical Care Nurses, two nurses told of their experiences with physicians who refused to follow established protocols.

Inserting central line at bedside in ICU. Used checklist but surgeon refused maximal sterile barrier and in fact, ridiculed me and hospital staff for instituting (this precaution) when there is no "proof" it works.

Hospital does not allow RN to stop procedure so it was inserted without maximal sterile barrier. . . .

A cardiovascular surgeon was putting in an arterial line at the bedside. We have a checklist that must be completed for line placement that includes full barrier, washing hands, etc. The M.D. refused the sterile gown, mask, hat, and drape, and used only sterile gloves. The nurse offered the full barrier again telling him that all lines were put in with full barrier in our unit. He continued with the procedure. The bedside nurse did not feel empowered to stop the procedure. She later took the problem to the unit manager. No action was taken.[21]

These stories are far from unique. Before the Michigan experiment got underway, Pronovost asked nurses at Johns Hopkins to spend a month observing doctors and to record how often they completed each step when inserting central lines. "In more than a third of patients, [the doctors] skipped at least one."[22]

Nor is the failure to follow known patient-protecting protocols limited to central lines. As Gawande observed, it occurs in many treatments:

A large body of evidence gathered in recent years has revealed a profound failure by health-care professionals to follow basic steps proven to stop infection and other major complications. We now know that hundreds of thousands of Americans suffer serious complications or die as a result.[23]

We know what works, and what works may be simple and inexpensive. But there is a widespread and deadly lack of implementation.

Again, Pronovost's experiment proves the point. Michigan ICUs brought down their CLABSI rates because Pronovost went to great lengths to ensure that hospital personnel always took all five steps. When the Michigan Health and Hospital Association invited him to try out his checklists, he didn't move to implementation directly. Instead, he asked personnel at participating ICUs to gather data on their own infection rates.

They found [that] the infection rates for I.C.U. patients in Michigan hospitals were higher than the national average, and in some hospitals

dramatically so. Sinai-Grace [Hospital, in inner-city Detroit,] experienced more line infections than seventy-five per cent of American
hospitals. Meanwhile, Blue Cross Blue Shield of Michigan agreed to
give hospitals small bonus payments for participating in Pronovost's
program. A checklist suddenly seemed an easy and logical thing
to try.[24]

Pronovost's efforts to get ICU personnel to buy into his experiment
didn't stop there, either. Participating hospitals had to appoint project
managers, who would roll out the checklists and be point persons for
compliance; they had to empower nurses to stop doctors who missed
steps (which was a radical realignment of authority); and they had to
assign senior executives to visit their ICUs, listen to complaints, and
solve problems.

The last step was truly extraordinary. Senior executives never show
up at the sharp end of hospitals—the areas where patients are treated—
but Pronovost was right to bring them in. Many ICUs had logistical
problems. For example, few had adequate supplies of chlorhexidine soap
or full-body sterile drapes at hand. Administrators could solve these
problems and did so once senior executives were fully engaged. Hospitals convinced a medical supply manufacturer to put all the needed supplies into a single kit. Hospitals in Michigan bought the kits and ensured
they were readily available in the ICU.

Why did the Michigan experiment succeed? Before the experiment
started, CLABSIs occurred far too often because hospitals hadn't
even identified, much less solved, a business problem: how to deliver
high-quality services consistently. They needed to design, implement,
and monitor a process so that it worked correctly over and over and over
again.

We say that this is a *business* problem because every type of business confronts it. If you want to compete with Starbucks, Einstein Bros.
Bagels, or even the local coffee shop down the street, you'll have to
serve thousands of cups of coffee, each of which must be fresh, hot, and
brewed correctly. To do that, you'll need ingredients, coffee recipes,
clean equipment, and trained employees. You'll also need a process that
brings everything together. Your ingredients—coffee, creamers, syrups,

sweeteners, stirrers, disposable cups, and so on—will have to be in the right places when needed. They will also have to be stored in ways that preserve their freshness. Your employees will have to use the right ingredients in the proper proportions, check brewing temperatures and times, throw out old coffee, and keep everything clean and in good working order, while providing service that is fast and friendly. To maintain quality day in and day out, you'll have to monitor everything, hire "secret shoppers" to sample the wares, assess customers' satisfaction, discipline or fire workers who fail to follow directions, and so forth.

A person who runs any type of business will quickly discover that it's *hard* to deliver high-quality goods, services, and experiences to large numbers of customers consistently over long periods of time. Consistency doesn't happen by accident; it requires planning, implementation, and monitoring. It also requires feedback and learning. Few things work right the first time. Every mistake provides an opportunity to improve, so mistakes have to be identified and studied. Processes may have to be revised or redesigned many times before "getting it right" becomes automatic.

Many health care providers have problems with logistics. When Pronovost started his work at Johns Hopkins, one of the country's great medical centers, doctors took all of the steps on the checklist only 38 percent of the time. Hopkins' CLABSI rate was a shocking 19 per 1,000 catheter-days—"one of the worst records in the country."[25] Compliance was low partly because doctors had to "go to eight different places to get all the items needed . . . caps were stored in one place, masks in another, gowns in yet another. To make things even worse, many items were altogether missing."[26] Johns Hopkins was exposing patients to deadly risks because the hospital with some of the best doctors in the world was bad at business.

At least Johns Hopkins knew what its CLABSI rate was. Many providers have no idea how well they are doing relative to others. They think they're above average—until an external review shows that they're not. For example, the staff at the Saint Raphael Hospital in New Haven, Connecticut, thought they were doing a good job of preventing HAIs. The hospital's ICU had a checklist protocol in place and an infection preventionist on its staff. Then the state of Connecticut began to require hospitals to report infections and released its findings. Turned out, Saint Raphael's ICU had one of the worst HAI rates in the state. "[W]hen we started comparing to our colleagues, to our neighbors," said Diane Dumigan, the infection preventionist, "we realized we were the outliers. It was an 'aha' moment."[27]

For-profit businesses don't like this sort of "aha" moment. The department head who finds out that *Consumer Reports* just ranked his company's products a standard deviation below the competition knows it's going to be a bad day. Indeed, by the end of the day, more than one person at the company may be out of a job. That's why successful businesses monitor error rates, benchmark themselves against their competitors, and take other steps to ensure quality.

Because hospitals rarely take these steps, outcome quality can vary enormously from one to another. "In the first comprehensive study comparing how well individual hospitals treated a variety of medical conditions, researchers found that patients at the worst American hospitals were three times more likely to die and 13 times more likely to have medical complications than if they visited one of the best hospitals."[28] The findings should put to rest forever the belief that all providers are above average, or even that all are roughly the same. Paraphrasing Dr. Barry Rosenberg, one of the study's coauthors, a *New York Times* reporter observed that, "if someone has a heart attack, the closest hospital could have a death rate of 16 percent, compared with one a little farther away, where the rate was 4 percent."[29]

Rosenberg's study didn't connect individual hospitals to their results, and it seems likely that few hospitals know where they stand.[30] Why? For most health care entities, unlike most non–health care entities, they simply can't make money by measuring or improving quality.[31] A coffee shop owner knows that quality is a key to success. Happy customers will buy lots of coffee and tell their friends about the great place they found. Unhappy customers will take their business elsewhere and publish negative comments on Yelp. In the health care sector, the connection between quality and revenue or profit is far weaker. Sometimes, there is no link because no one knows whether particular providers are good or bad. Sometimes, the connection is upside-down, meaning that providers' revenues and profits are higher if they do a rotten job.

Regulators don't monitor quality either. Although facilities that receive federal funding are subject to government oversight, "the law allows hospitals, ambulatory surgery centers, home health agencies and hospices to pay private, national accrediting organizations for such oversight instead." These private accreditors "often [miss] serious deficiencies found soon after [their reviews] by state inspectors," who examine a sample of hospitals and other facilities each year. They also keep their findings secret. When CMS floated a proposal to require accreditors to release reports about errors and other quality problems at specific facilities, hospitals and accreditors vehemently objected, arguing that disclosure would "adversely affect the collaborative efforts of accrediting bodies and healthcare organizations to improve patient safety and engage in continuous quality improvement."[32] As is always the case with such arguments, they offered no evidence supporting this claim—and the available evidence indicates the opposite.[33]

But CMS found the argument to be persuasive, and it abandoned the proposal. The head of the Leapfrog group, which advocates for quality and transparency in health care, criticized CMS's decision to back down:

> This is disgraceful, unfair to patients as well as employers and other purchasers of health care. . . . The public deserves full transparency on how the health care industry performs. Instead, transparency has been sacrificed to accommodate special interests that lobby to avoid disclosing embarrassing information about health care quality.[34]

Does anyone doubt that the outcome would be different if health care providers were treated like ordinary businesses?

## HOW PAYERS MADE HURTING PEOPLE A GOOD BUSINESS PLAN

Don't believe us that providers often fare better financially when they treat patients poorly? Consider CLABSIs again. In 2013, Pronovost published a study of billings for infected and uninfected patients in matched physical condition, all of whom spent time in the ICU at Queen's Medical

Center in Honolulu, Hawaii.[35] For patients with private insurance who contracted CLABSIs, the charges averaged $495,000. The bills for uninfected patients were only one-fifth as large: $100,000. Infected patients generated much larger profit margins too: $55,000 per patient for those with CLABSIs versus $6,500 per patient for the uninfected.

This staggeringly large profit differential meant that Queen's Medical Center had "no incentive to invest in prevention."[36] Indeed, if Queen's Medical Center had taken steps to prevent CLABSIs, it would have lost money. Stated differently, hospitals have a "perverse incentive to have more line infections," because the system pays more for patients with CLABSIs than for those who remain uninfected.[37]

This problem—that providers cannot make money by measuring or improving quality—is not limited to central lines and CLABSIs. Gawande's research group at the Harvard School of Public Health recently published a study of the billing records for over 34,000 hospital inpatients, each of whom had one of nine common surgical procedures in 2010. More than 1,800 patients, 5.3 percent, experienced at least one potentially preventable complication, such as an infection at the surgery site or a pulmonary embolism. The patients with surgical complications generated $8,084 more in profit on average after the hospitals' variable costs were netted out. Privately insured patients with complications were especially profitable, generating an average of $39,017 more in profit.[38] Another study of a Michigan hospital found that every 1 percent decline in surgical complications cost the hospital $1.2 million.[39] Finally, a 2016 study found that patients who had major surgery at low-quality hospitals cost Medicare thousands more than those treated at top-ranked hospitals because they required more postoperative care and were more likely to be readmitted.[40]

Perverse incentives like these permeate the health care sector. In one study, four programs designed to improve quality of care (by managing high-cost pharmaceuticals, improving diabetes management, reducing smoking, and providing workplace wellness programs) all ended up costing providers money.[41] As three economically minded commentators observed in the *New England Journal of Medicine*, "It's hard to create a favorable [return on investment] for reducing volume in a system dominated by fee-for-service payments for delivering care."[42] Our politically controlled payment system pushes providers to increase volume and punishes them for reducing volume, even when the services they eliminate are low quality or harmful. Even the most conscientious provider is unlikely to pursue money-losing quality improvements with enthusiasm.

Perverse incentives may also explain why it took the staff at Miami's Jackson Memorial Hospital (JMH) almost *20 years* to gain control over an epidemic of HAIs caused by *Acinetobacter baumannii*.[43] These infections are incredibly dangerous. *A. baumannii* is antibiotic resistant. Patients who contract it have an "all-cause" mortality rate of roughly 40 percent.[44]

JMH's staff finally reduced its HAI rate by changing the hospital's culture, not by applying sophisticated medical knowledge. Weekly emails to the hospital's C-Suite, including maps that "showed not only how the infection was spreading but who was spreading it," finally got the administration to take action.[45] Once supported from above, nurses got serious about protecting patients. They spoke up when they saw people doing things that were "dangerous for infection control, such as failing to wash their hands or not cleaning the patient rooms properly." They became "much pickier about their rooms being cleaned," and demanded re-cleanings when rooms "[weren't] up to snuff." They maintained "zero tolerance" for doctors who violated infection-control practices and reminded physicians to take off their lab coats and wash their hands before examining patients. Infection rates plummeted.[46]

When a report of the results of JMH's anti-infection efforts was submitted for publication, one reviewer observed that the article was "more management than science and entail[ed] organizational culture change."[47] Exactly. Many of the most important problems of the health care sector are business problems, not medical problems. They persist because our politically controlled, third-party payer system has taken away any "business case" for improving quality. That's probably why JMH's C-Suite took as long as it did to address the epidemic of HAIs that was stalking its ICU. It's great that infections were finally brought under control, but it shouldn't have taken two decades to build a medical culture that protected patients from an avoidable peril.

Why do these perverse incentives exist? The problem is *not* that doctors, physicians' assistants, nurses, or other medical personnel intentionally and deliberately injure their patients. The dedication of health care professionals, who often work under difficult and unpleasant conditions, is awe inspiring. The problem is that health care providers operate in environments that do not subject them to financial pressures to improve and often pressure them not to improve. Fee-for-service payment arrangements—the kind of payment arrangements that government encourages and that lobbyists for health care providers defend—reward providers for quantity not quality, including services that are unnecessary, ineffective, or even harmful.[48] Unsurprisingly, quality is often mediocre or worse. Inconsistent quality is not a medical problem. It is a business problem, and it requires business solutions. But, if investing in quality leads to lower revenue and profits, few will measure quality or improve it. Absent a business case for quality, quality won't be measured and faulty delivery systems will remain unchanged. When it comes to delivery systems, health care is like any other business. Providers respond to incentives, and they need better incentives to improve.

Many health care professionals and medical ethicists will find these assertions jarring, if not reprehensible. They draw a sharp distinction between health care providers and businesses of other types, and they believe that people trained in medicine should have the final say over how health care businesses function. Doctors, nurses, and other medical professionals should not have laypersons interfering with their judgments or telling them how to work.

This view has two problems. First, it has been an epic failure. Patients are routinely hurt because quality problems go unaddressed. Medical professionals have been in charge of service delivery for a century, yet the evidence of high rates of preventable injuries and deaths is overwhelming. Second, this view fails to recognize the limits of medical training. Medical professionals study biology, chemistry, physiology, and pathology. They also have extensive clinical training. These experiences give them a leg up when it comes to diagnosing illnesses, selecting treatments, and performing procedures. But they receive little or no training in quality improvement. Ask a newly minted doctor what "Six Sigma" means and you'll probably get a blank stare. You'll get the same response if you ask about W. Edwards Deming, Joseph M. Juran, or James Reason, the lions of the quality improvement movement. Medical schools do not teach students how to reduce error rates by designing reliable delivery systems.

To the contrary, medical schools are famous for breeding attitudes that are antithetical to quality improvement. Instead of treating medical errors as opportunities to discover and address defects in delivery systems, medical schools teach doctors to criticize themselves and the people around them for being imperfect. Instead of learning how to draw on other providers' knowledge, doctors often intimidate nurses and other assistants, causing valuable information to be ignored. The culture of medicine is famously punitive. It is also contemptuous of outsiders who lack medical degrees.[49]

The results are plain to see. Medical errors and preventable adverse outcomes are everywhere, as are unrealized opportunities for quality improvement. As one quality improvement researcher put it, in health care, "the low-hanging fruit isn't just low-hanging fruit; the fruit is lying on the ground, and we have to be careful not to trip over it."[50]

## Anesthesia Docs Got It Right

The history of anesthesia safety demonstrates the value of bringing in outsiders to improve quality. "In the 1970's and 1980's . . . 1 in 6,000 administrations of anesthesia resulted in death; and serious brain injuries were even more frequent." Then, over about a decade, the mortality rate dropped "to one in 200,000 administrations"—a 97 percent reduction.[51] Why? Because the leaders of the American Society of Anesthesiologists "set out to systematically identify and address the root causes of mistakes."[52] One of their most consequential decisions was to invite Jeffrey B. Cooper to study their errors and identify equipment-related causes.[53] Cooper wasn't a doctor. He was an engineer trained in critical incident analysis, and he had given a talk entitled "The Anesthesia Machine: An Accident Waiting to Happen" in 1974. By making anesthesia safer, Cooper helped protect millions of patients from harm. Even though he wasn't a doctor, he showed anesthesiologists how to consistently deliver high quality and safe care.

## You Can't Improve without Our Permission

One would hope that regulators, particularly those at the U.S. Department of Health and Human Services (HHS), would welcome efforts to make health care safer. But not always. Federal regulators at HHS's Office for Human Research Protection (OHRP) shut down Pronovost's Michigan experiment in 2007 because they believed that the use of checklists qualified as human subjects research and that the experiment had been carried out without review by an institutional review board (IRB). The IRB would have required the informed consent of the patients and the hospital personnel involved.[54] OHRP's action delayed similar experiments at ICUs in New Jersey and Rhode Island that were in the early stages of implementation.

Of course, hospitals could have continued to use their existing, defective procedures without obtaining IRB approval. That wouldn't have been human subjects research or, indeed, research of any kind. It would, however, have infected thousands of patients every year and killed many of them. Hospitals could also have implemented checklists on their own, and that would have been fine too. Again, that wouldn't have been research. But when hospitals, wanting to do better but not knowing how, brought in an academic consultant to systematically measure their error rates and show them how to do better, that was somehow dangerous human experimentation requiring bureaucratic review and informed consent.

Gawande, who condemned the OHRP's action, noted the likely consequences of OHRP's approach:

> If the government's ruling were applied more widely, whole swaths of critical work to ensure safe and effective care would either halt or shrink: efforts by the Centers for Disease Control and Prevention to examine responses to outbreaks of infectious disease; the military's program to track the care of wounded soldiers; the Five Million Lives campaign, by the nonprofit Institute for Health Care Improvement, to reduce avoidable complications in 3,700 hospitals nationwide.[55]

Of course, research scientists should treat human subjects properly when evaluating the effectiveness of treatments and procedures. But efforts to get providers to take known patient-protecting steps simply don't require the type of oversight IRBs provide. Fortunately, after being pressured by patient safety advocates, OHRP reversed course.

Patients desperately need there to be better incentives for providers to improve health care delivery. Gawande observes:

> there are hundreds, perhaps thousands, of things doctors do that are at least as dangerous and prone to human failure as putting central lines into I.C.U. patients. It's true of cardiac care, stroke treatment, H.I.V. treatment, and surgery of all kinds. It's also true of diagnosis, whether one is trying to identify cancer or infection or a heart attack. All have steps that are worth putting on a checklist and testing in routine care. The question—still unanswered—is whether medical culture will embrace the opportunity.[56]

We'd bet on "probably not." When ICUs in Michigan cut CLABSI rates to near zero, hospitals lost hundreds of millions of dollars in revenues. Unless we improve providers' incentives, so they can actually make money by improving quality, we expect errors and other quality problems will keep harming and killing patients.

That's the prediction of Drs. Gawande and Pronovost too. Despite the remarkable results the Michigan experiment produced, despite the successes other experiments with checklists in hospitals have achieved, and despite the common use of checklists in other industries, the health care sector has yet to deploy them in a systematic way, let alone require their use the way the airlines do. In a 2007 interview, Gawande asked Pronovost how long it will take for doctors and nurses to use checklists routinely. Pronovost's reply: "At the current rate, it will never happen."[57]

## WHEN BUSINESS LEADS, CULTURE WILL FOLLOW

In the end, though, we think that Gawande misdiagnoses the problem by blaming the culture of medicine. "If someone found a new drug that could wipe out infections with anything remotely like the effectiveness of Pronovost's lists," he wrote,

> there would be television ads with Robert Jarvik extolling its virtues, detail men offering free lunches to get doctors to make it part of their practice, government programs to research it, and competitors jumping in to make a newer, better version. That's what happened when manufacturers marketed central-line catheters coated with silver or other antimicrobials; they cost a third more, and reduced infections only slightly—and hospitals have spent tens of millions of dollars on them.

But hospitals wouldn't use checklists, he said, because "the prospect pushes against the traditional culture of medicine, with its central belief that in situations of high risk and complexity what you want is a kind of expert audacity. . . . Checklists and standard operating procedures feel like exactly the opposite, and that's what rankles many people."[58]

Of course there'd be rapid adoption of an infection-killing drug. Hospitals would buy it for $100 and charge patients $1,000. We bet that silver-coated catheters were a bonanza too. Whatever hospitals paid for them, they almost certainly billed insurers considerably more. That's why hospitals were in no hurry to use checklists in 2007. Error reduction reduced their revenues. If government allowed error reduction to be profitable, checklists would be in use everywhere.

Hospitals made it a priority to take the recommended infection-preventing steps when, in 2008, the federal government and private payers stopped paying them more for treating patients who suffered HAIs and other preventable events and errors.[59] The question is why, for so many decades, American hospitals allowed high HAI rates to persist while claiming there was nothing they could do about them. At least "Dr." Basso is honest about the perils of eating at the Heart Attack Grill.

# CHAPTER 14: AN OFFER YOU CAN'T REFUSE

## You Wouldn't Want Us to Hurt Anybody, Would You?

In *The Godfather*, Michael Corleone tells his fiancée the story of how his father, Vito Corleone, made bandleader Les Halley "an offer he couldn't refuse." Either Halley would release singer Johnny Fontaine, Vito Corleone's godson, from his contract or Luca Brasi, Corleone's hitman, would put a bullet in Halley's brain. Not surprisingly, Halley caved.[1]

Metaphorically speaking, lobbyists for health care providers regularly make similar offers when dealing with public officials. Consider how they handled electronic health records (EHRs), which advocates believe can improve medical treatments and reduce spending. When CMS urged providers to adopt EHRs, the industry said it would do so when the feds paid it to. Translated into Corleone-speak, the answer was: "Make it worth our while and we'll adopt EHRs. Otherwise, we'll stick with paper records, which will injure and kill thousands of patients and waste billions of taxpayers' dollars. You decide which one you want us to do."

The threat worked. In 2009, Congress passed the Health Information Technology for Economic and Clinical Health (HITECH) Act, which made billions of dollars in federal subsidies available to pay providers that adopted EHRs. As of late 2015, the United States had shelled

out over $31 billion in bonus payments—more than twice the amount
that EHRs are expected to save over the 10-year budgetary window.[2]


## WE DID BETTER! AT LEAST, YOU CAN'T PROVE WE DIDN'T!

Did the $31 billion buy anything of value? Astonishingly, the answer
isn't clear. In mid-2015, the *Journal of the American Medical Informatics
Association* published a study of "the physician EHR diffusion curve"—
the rate at which doctors deployed the new technology. The authors
found no statistically significant effect of the HITECH Act subsidies on
EHR adoptions. More doctors were using EHRs at the end of the period studied than at the beginning, but the authors failed to find that the
HITECH Act subsidies sped up the implementation rate. In their words,
their "analyses suggest that the external stimulus on physicians . . . had
ambiguous effects on the overall adoption rates. Somewhat like the 'cash
for clunkers' subsidies in the automobile industry, the HITECH subsidies may have only contributed to inevitable adoptions."[3] If this study is
correct, after providers threatened the feds, they got an extra $31 billion
to do what they were going to do anyway.

   This problem is not unique to the HITECH Act. When the government doles out quality improvement grants, it's often hard to know
whether providers improve, much less whether they improve faster than
they would have on their own. For example, the Affordable Care Act
(ACA) earmarked $1 billion for quality improvements. As the dollars
were being spent on various projects, industry cheerleaders bragged that
tens of thousands of health care–induced injuries and deaths had been
avoided, saving almost $12 billion. Once again, it would be nice to know
why providers had to be paid extra to avoid harming and killing patients.
But an even worse problem is that the claims of dramatic improvement were unverifiable, as patient safety advocates quickly pointed out.
Dr. Pronovost observed that the hospitals that received federal dollars
to implement pilot projects used quality measures that were "of low
validity, with data varying among sites and limited quality control."[4]
The projects also lacked control groups, making it impossible to tell how
patients would have fared without the expensive programs.[5]

Why didn't the bureaucrats who handed out the money standardize the collection of data? Dr. Pronovost didn't speculate, but an obvious possibility is that they didn't want good data. If the $1 billion was never intended to help patients but was instead a bribe to buy hospitals' support for the ACA, then good data would only have embarrassed everyone by showing that the funded experiments were duds. Positive yet unreliable data enabled everyone to claim victory and celebrate.

## YOU WANT EVEN MORE THAN $3 TRILLION?

The idea that the public should pay extra for health care improvements is deeply ingrained. In *Crossing The Quality Chasm*, a landmark publication by the Institute of Medicine that was supposed to set out a path for quality improvement, the first suggestion was that Congress kick-start the effort by plunking $1 billion into a Health Care Quality Innovation Fund.[6] Why $1 billion rather than, say $1 million? Because health care policy wonks are accustomed to big budgets. For a measly $1 million grant, they won't even do lunch.

An outsider might reasonably think that paying even $1 million more for quality improvement is stupid. Americans already spend more than $3 trillion a year on health care. That's far more than any other developed nation, whether measured in the aggregate or per person. Are we really supposed to believe that's only enough money to buy mediocrity? Isn't it more than enough to cover the cost of EHRs and other quality-enhancing technologies?

The idea that we should pay extra for quality improvement seems especially galling when one remembers that we don't pay non-health care businesses extra to make their goods and services better. Imagine Starbucks telling its customers, "Give us $5 now and we'll come up with a better cup of coffee later." Other businesses fund improvements with their own money or with money they get from investors, who expect to get it back and then some.

Consider consumer electronics. In 1999, the average price of a 20-inch flat screen TV was $1,200. In 2011, the same TV cost only $84, 7 percent of the price tag 13 years earlier, without even accounting for inflation. Picture quality was much better too.[7] Why the huge improvements? Because *manufacturers* spent billions of dollars on flat panel and manufacturing technology. Early on, the machines that printed flat panel circuits could only handle sheets of glass that were 18-inch squares. Today, they can work with sheets the size of garage doors. Ramping up wasn't cheap. Flat panel fabrication plants built in the mid-2000s cost $1.5 billion to $2 billion apiece.[8]

No one paid flat panel manufacturers extra to bear this expense. They used their own money to sponsor research and development and to underwrite capital improvements. Why? Because they faced stiff competition. The manufacturers knew they'd lose customers if they fell behind the curve. They also sought to gain market share by creating a technological edge. Manufacturers upgraded their technology because they wanted to prosper. No payments from the Treasury were necessary.

Competition does motivate health care providers to implement some improvements. Every hospital wants the latest high-tech tool for performing cardiac procedures, firing protons at prostate tumors, and delivering other profitable services. Fear of losing customers may have something to do with this. But notice that these are quality improvements that involve providers doing more and billing more. Providers rarely implement quality improvements that involve them delivering more while charging *less*. Our politically controlled, third-party payer system punishes them for doing that, even though doing so would make consumers much better off.

The American Hospital Association contends that hospitals must be paid directly to adopt quality-improving technologies because they differ from other businesses:

> Implementing new technology is costly to hospitals while the benefits—both financial and non-financial—accrue somewhat to hospitals but primarily to payers and patients. Contrast this to other industries where most technology directly improves productivity, generates savings and thus builds profitability for the entity that invested in the new technology.[9]

Hogwash. In competitive markets, *every* business that innovates in ways that increase workers' productivity, reduce costs, or make their products better shares the gains with consumers. Consumers benefit by paying lower prices or by enjoying products more. Competitive markets are uniformly tough on sellers, all of whom feel constant pressure to offer customers more for their money. When it comes to making consumers better off by operating more efficiently, hospitals are neither unique nor even especially interesting. We should recognize the American Hospital Association's statement for what it is: an explicit admission by a hired lobbyist that the lack of market discipline has left its member-hospitals uninterested in improving quality of care.

The real reason that health care providers can force the government to pay them to improve is that poor performance usually costs them little or nothing. Mediocrity may kill businesses of other types, but it seems to have little or no impact on health care providers. As David Goldhill observed in *Catastrophic Care*, "the reason hospitals kill so many patients is that they can—killing patients doesn't mean they have less loyal customers or that their profits decline."[10] Hospitals with high infection rates keep on treating patients and making money. Cardiac surgeons prosper even when their patients die at above-average rates. General practitioners who misdiagnose illnesses or overprescribe antibiotics do fine financially. Health care providers can pick and choose which improvements they will make because they face little competitive pressure to improve.

When it comes to other businesses, competition is brutal. Remember Oldsmobile? In the 1980s, the flagging brand adopted the slogan "Not your father's Oldsmobile." The ad campaign backfired, and General Motors shuttered the brand. And you're not buying Renaults, Yugos, Plymouths, Geos, Opels, Suzukis, Isuzus, Daewoos, or Daihatsus either. Competition drove all these brands out of the U.S. market. Chrysler and General Motors are still in business, but both nearly bought the farm during the financial crisis and were only saved by politicians who forced taxpayers to bail them out.

The auto sector is hardly unique. Everywhere one looks, competition dooms companies that underperform. Remember Kodak? Once upon a time, its yellow film boxes were ubiquitous. Paul Simon wrote a chart-topping song about the joys of Kodachrome. But, as digital cameras became cheaper, demand for film, paper, and other Kodak products fell so drastically that the company failed. Its former rival, Polaroid, also tanked. What about airlines? Pan Am and TWA are dead and gone, along with Eastern Airlines and many others. Other famous companies that are dead and buried include Montgomery Ward, Tower Records, Circuit City, Woolworth, and Borders Books.

The turnover rate in the health care sector, by contrast, is low. As Professor David Dranove, of the Kellogg School of Management at Northwestern University, observed:

> Entry is the engine that drives economic progress. Entrants bring new technologies to manufacturing and new service models to sales. Threatened by entry, incumbents strive to innovate and improve customer service. . . . [I]n a typical manufacturing industry, fully one third of established firms are replaced by entrants within five years. . . . Turnover in the service sector is likely even higher.
>
> If entry is the engine that drives change, the health care sector is out of gas. Turnover in the health care sector is slow to nonexistent. Ask yourself, who are the biggest health insurers today? In nearly all states, the answer is the Blues. Who were the biggest health insurers 50 years ago? The Blues. Now name the biggest hospital in your home town and then look up historical data to find the biggest hospital in your town in 1960. Odds are good it is the same hospital.[11]

Other researchers agree. The authors of a 2008 *Health Affairs* article observed:

> Most innovation-intensive industries . . . regularly undergo major changes, including wholesale cycling of industry leadership. But the U.S. health sector has been strikingly ossified, with the same industry leaders (academic hospitals and university medical centers) that led a generation or more ago continuing to hold leadership status today. Disruptive innovation is fueled by entrants, yet the U.S. health care market has managed to either exclude or cripple realistic challenges posed by newcomers with innovative organizational forms.[12]

Health care providers can safely underperform because new entrants find it hard to challenge them.

## BARRIERS TO COMPETITION

Why can't new entrants compete? There are many reasons. Start with innovators who might compete on the basis of price. Retail outlets like Costco, WalMart, and Amazon thrive because buyers want to save money. But patients whose medical bills are largely or entirely covered by private insurance, Medicare, or Medicaid don't care about prices. They are responsible only for copays and deductibles, so that's where their financial interest ends. Because their out-of-pocket expense is fixed, they have no reason to prefer low-cost providers. They may even prefer high-cost providers whose services come with more creature comforts. It's no skin off their backs because their insurers cover the charges.

Insulating patients from the cost of care also reduces the pressure on providers to improve quality. After David Goldhill's father died unnecessarily from a hospital-acquired infection, he wrote:

> Imagine my father's hospital had to present the bill for his "care" not to a government bureaucracy, but to my grieving mother. Do you really believe that the hospital—forced to face the victim of its poor-quality service, forced to collect the bill from the real customer—wouldn't have figured out how to make its doctors wash their hands?[13]

Third-party payment insulates inefficient, high-cost, established health care providers from low-cost competition.

Price-cutting innovators must also overcome patients' tendency to equate low cost with low quality. The phrase "you get what you pay for" is not always true. Better quality goods and services often cost more. But in the health care sector, the connection between price and quality is far weaker. Indeed, it can be inverted, with better providers charging less than inferior ones.

Patients don't know this, so they use price as a signal of quality. In 2012, *Health Affairs* published a study of more than 1,000 employed adults who were given information about health care costs. A substantial minority of the participants "shied away from low-cost providers. . . . Even consumers who pay a larger share of their health care costs themselves were likely to equate high cost with high quality."[14]

Patients' wariness of cheap providers makes it hard for innovators to compete on price.

Now consider innovators who might compete on the basis of quality. Patients should care about quality because their health is on the line. Unfortunately, many quality differences are hard for patients to assess. Consider hospital-acquired infections (HAIs), discussed in Chapter 13. Many patients don't know about HAIs. Even fewer know how their hospital stacks up against other hospitals. And no one knows how to balance the risk of contracting an HAI against any of the other relevant attributes (i.e., quality of the surgeon and nurses, service quality, distance from one's home, and so on). Most patients just go where their doctors send them.[15]

Unfortunately, high-quality innovators can't rely on doctors to point patients in their direction either. First, doctors have no financial incentive to prefer new entrants. Because the law prohibits payments for referrals, new entrants find it extremely difficult to disrupt existing referral arrangements, even when they offer better service at a lower price. Unless high-quality innovators can offer more and better in-kind benefits to referral sources, their ability to attract patients will be limited.

Second, like patients, doctors themselves often have difficulty identifying the best providers. They base their referrals on reputations, friendships, and past experiences. Unfortunately, all of these measures correlate poorly with quality. Even when high-quality innovators spend the money needed to show physicians that they have built a "better mousetrap," referral sources are free to ignore the information.

Consider where doctors send patients who need coronary artery bypass graft (CABG—pronounced "cabbage") surgery. Since the early 1990s, New York and Pennsylvania have issued report cards on surgeons who perform these operations.[16] The report cards reflect the surgeons' risk-adjusted mortality rates—that is, the rates at which their CABG patients die after adjusting for the patients' pre-surgery physical condition. Risk adjustment means that surgeons whose patients are unusually old or unusually sick are not penalized relative to those whose patients are younger or healthier. Send two identical CABG patients to cardiac surgeons with different mortality rates, and the patient who goes to the surgeon with the higher mortality rate will be more likely to die.

The report cards provide a great deal of information about the performance of cardiac surgeons. They are also easy for physicians to access. The states send them to cardiologists in hope of influencing their referral decisions. But doctors rarely use them. Surveys conducted in the mid-1990s found that cardiologists in both New York and Pennsylvania ignored the report cards when referring patients for CABG procedures. A study published in 2004 also found no change in referral patterns.[17] The authors speculated that referring cardiologists remained loyal to particular cardiac surgeons because they had "incentives to direct their patients to specific hospitals" or because of "collegial relationships that are hard to break."[18]

The failure of CABG report cards to influence referral practices was again documented in 2006, when *Health Affairs* published a study finding that New York's annual ratings had no impact on hospitals' or surgeons' shares of the market, even though they were good predictors of expected outcomes for patients.[19] Finally, in 2013, a team of prominent public health researchers surveyed New York cardiologists again. Over half of the doctors considered the report card data "not important or minimally important." Three-quarters said the report cards had little or no effect on their referral decisions. "Seventy-one percent . . . did not discuss the report cards with a single patient."[20]

Maybe physicians don't pay attention to this kind of information for ordinary patients, but they must behave differently when treating VIPs, right? Guess again. When former president Bill Clinton needed heart surgery in 2004, his doctor sent to him a hospital with a proven record of mortality *twice* that of other hospitals in New York.[21] Perhaps this information was fully disclosed to President Clinton, and he made an informed decision to receive care at a facility where his predicted likelihood of dying was twice what it would have been elsewhere, but it seems more likely that the subject never came up.

CABG report cards are not alone in having little impact on referrals. Similar report cards have been prepared by multiple public and private entities, including CMS, the Agency for Health Care Research and Quality, the Joint Commission, the National Committee for Quality Assurance, the American Heart Association, the American College of Cardiology, the Society for Thoracic Surgeons, the American College of Surgeons, *Consumer Reports*, the Leapfrog Group, and *U.S. News and World Report*. There is little evidence that any of these rankings influence referrals. If new entrants can't rely on superior quality to change doctors' behavior and generate a flow of patients, they aren't going to enter the market in the first place.

INSURANCE PAYMENTS REFLECT MARKET POWER, NOT QUALITY

We have already explained that prices don't correlate with quality in the health care sector. Payments by insurers don't correlate with quality either. The Rhode Island Health Insurance Commissioner hired Xerox to study that issue, using data from inpatient and outpatient visits to general hospitals in Rhode Island during 2010. Prior studies had found that payments varied widely and that insurers paid large, prestigious hospitals more, regardless of quality. The new study found that payment levels varied substantially among hospitals and that, "If there is a correlation between quality and payment, it is neither strong nor obvious."[22]

Similar results were observed in Massachusetts, where studies by both the Massachusetts attorney general and the Massachusetts Division of Health Care Finance and Policy found huge price and payment variation for health care services.[23] The Massachusetts Health Policy Commission concluded, "Higher prices are not generally associated with measures of higher quality of care or hospital costs."[24]

The news that quality has little or no impact on payments won't surprise industry insiders. The Massachusetts Health Policy Commission noted that "quality measures do not factor heavily in price negotiations" between insurers and health care providers.[25] Instead, leverage is the key. A study published in *Health Affairs* in 2014 reported that

> High-price hospitals . . . tend to be larger; be major teaching hospitals; belong to systems with large market shares; and provide specialized services, such as heart transplants and Level I trauma care. High-price hospitals also receive significant revenues from nonpatient sources, such as state Medicaid disproportionate-share hospital funds, and they enjoy healthy total financial margins. Quality indicators for high-price hospitals [a]re mixed: [they fared] much better than low-price

hospitals . . . in U.S. News & World Report rankings, which are largely based on reputation, *while generally scoring worse on objective measures of quality, such as postsurgical mortality rates.* Thus, insurers may face resistance if they attempt to steer patients away from high-price hospitals because these facilities have good reputations and offer specialized services that may be unique in their markets.[26] (emphasis added)

Big, prestigious hospitals and practice groups can threaten to take their patients and go elsewhere, so insurers treat them well. Smaller hospitals and practices have less bargaining power, so they get short-changed, even when their services are better and less expensive. For these reasons, it is not surprising that the Massachusetts Health Policy Commission concluded that "much of the variation in inpatient hospital prices is likely unwarranted and reflects the leverage of certain providers to negotiate higher prices with commercial insurers."[27] Third-party payment keeps consumers ignorant, and hospitals are using the loyalty of ignorant and cost-insensitive consumers to rob everyone blind.

According to a published report, a 2016 study of New York hospitals also found that hospitals associated with systems that have large market shares "tend to be higher-priced as a result of the[ir] power . . . in contract negotiations."[28] Some hospitals were 2.7 times more expensive than others in the same region. And although hospitals often contend that they need higher payments from private insurers to offset underpayments by Medicare and Medicaid, the study disproved that claim. Hospitals that extracted larger payments from private insurers treated *fewer* patients covered by these government programs. Finally, "hospitals with higher prices did not necessarily have higher quality," and lower-priced hospitals were often no worse.[29]

Maybe the problem is unique to the Northeast, and the rest of the country is more sensible? Nope. Consider North Carolina, a state with great university hospitals attached to Duke and the University of North Carolina. These institutions can extract top dollar from insurers by threatening to leave their networks unless paid to stay.[30] But North Carolina also has many smaller hospitals located in rural areas. Those hospitals can't steer big patient populations toward or away from insurers. Lacking leverage, they get bargain-basement rates. When "[a]sked why some hospitals [in North Carolina] charge so much, Gerard Anderson, director of the Johns

Hopkins Center for Hospital Finance and Management, said, 'Because
they can. It's not any more sophisticated than that.'"[31]

The same goes for physician practice groups. Those with strong reputations and lots of patients receive larger payments than others. Because
leverage and payments are connected so strongly, hospitals are consoli-
dating and buying physicians' practice groups. Maggie Mahar, a financial writer and health care policy analyst, commented on these trends.

> Across the nation, hospitals have been consolidating, and when they do,
> they flex their market muscles. Few insurers are big enough to stand up
> to them. . . . Large specialty practices with a presence in the community
> enjoy market leverage [too]. And when physicians are employed by
> hospitals . . . those institutions use their market heft to lift doctors' fees
> by as much 30 or 40 percent. The "bounce" can be even greater. . . .
> "Blue Shield of California said that after one group of physicians based
> in Burlingame, Calif., came under the umbrella of the powerful Sutter
> Healthsystem in 2010, its rates for services increased about 140%. The
> insurer said it saw a jump of approximately 95% after a Santa Monica,
> Calif., group became part of the UCLA Health System in January 2011."[32]

We discussed some of the reasons why a hospital's acquisition of a physician's practice can result in increased payments in Chapter 9. But the larger
point regarding market entry is simple. The health care sector is a rough-
and-tumble world where bargaining power matters and the strong players
control large patient flows. This makes the sector hard for new entrants to
break into. Upstarts with small numbers of patients are paid less than existing health care providers even when their services are of higher quality.

In sum, established health care providers have little to fear from new
entrants because innovators have difficulty competing with them on quality or price. For the same reason, established providers can comfortably
deliver care that is mediocre or worse and can take a pass on technologies
that would help patients by improving quality or reducing cost. No matter
what they do, patients will keep coming and payers will keep paying. It's a
very cozy arrangement, for everyone but the taxpayers and injured patients.

That's why providers keep making offers that legislators, insurers,
and patients can't refuse. They don't even need Luca Brasi to enforce the
threat. Don Corleone would be proud.

# PART 2. MISTREATMENT: WHY OBAMACARE FAILED AND WHAT WILL SUCCEED

In Part 1, we identified the problems that Obamacare should have tried to fix. The list was long: Open-ended reimbursement for patented pharmaceuticals, regardless of price. Excessive use of medical treatments. Providers' conflicts of interest. The routine delivery of ineffective and unproven treatments. Games that providers play to maximize their revenues. Charges that bear no relation to costs. Surprise bills and other out-of-network rip-offs. Widespread quality problems tied to dysfunctional business models. Political corruption. And an ocean of fraud.

Part 2 explains why Obamacare failed to fix these problems and describes what we should do instead. Although Obamacare's proponents claimed to have drawn upon every good idea that experts had to reduce health care spending, the program didn't try to address any of the problems described in Part 1. It imposed no limits on drug prices, on the use of unproven medical treatments, or on surprise medical bills. It did almost nothing about fraud. In fact, Obamacare really did just one thing: it expanded access to politically controlled third-party payment arrangements—private insurance and Medicaid—and made them more comprehensive. It should have been obvious to everyone that these changes, which brought millions of new people and billions of new dollars into the system, would cause spending to rise. If the object was to bend the cost curve downward, Obamacare was designed to fail.

From a fiscal perspective, the coverage-expanding component of Obamacare was rotten to the core. As Chapter 15 explains, the health care cost crisis is driven by third-party payment and always has been. Here's how it works, in seven easy steps:

1. Health insurance and public programs like Medicare and Medicaid stimulate demand for more and more expensive health care.
2. Increased demand for more and more expensive health care drives up prices.
3. Rising prices inspire fear in consumers, who worry that they won't be able to afford health care when they need it.
4. Fearful consumers demand more health insurance, insurance that covers more things, and more lavish public programs.
5. Tax preferences for employment-based health insurance add fuel to the fire, by encouraging people to buy more insurance and more comprehensive insurance than they otherwise would.
6. More and more comprehensive health insurance and more lavish public programs stimulate demand for more and more expensive health care.
7. Return to Step 2.

This vicious cycle continued until the first decade of the 21st century, when private health care coverage became so expensive that millions of people could no longer afford it. Then the Great Recession hit, cost millions of people their jobs and their insurance, and demand was depressed even further. For a while, it seemed that health care spending would moderate on its own.

Obamacare got the vicious cycle going again. By requiring people to carry comprehensive insurance coverage, subsidizing premiums, and expanding Medicaid enormously, it reignited the fire. That's why, if the program remains intact and is funded as it was in the past, national health expenditures are projected to grow by 5.6 percent per year over the next decade and to consume 20 percent of the GDP by 2025.[1]

Whether Obamacare will remain in place and be funded is, of course, what everyone wants to know. As we noted in the Introduction, Republicans control both houses of Congress and the White House, have attacked Obamacare repeatedly, and have repealed the penalties on those who don't purchase insurance. Even Democrats, who want to preserve Obamacare, acknowledge that the program has significant flaws that need to be fixed.

The question is, then, squarely raised: What should come after Obamacare? Chapter 16 considers the leading proposals offered by both the left and the right and finds them wanting. The list includes more tax preferences for more people and single payer/"Medicare for All." None of these reforms would do anything to fix the problems we identified in Part 1. To the contrary, all are likely to make some of them worse. If and when Americans get serious about controlling health care costs, they will eliminate tax preferences that drive up aggregate demand by making medical services seem cheap. They will also stop hoping that the government will fix problems instead of creating them.

Chapter 17 identifies reforms with real potential to make American health care cheaper and better. We begin with reforms that consumers can implement on their own. As more and more people purchase policies with high deductibles or are priced out of the insurance market entirely, millions of consumers will have to buy health care directly. Many of these people will go looking for deals. They will turn to retail health care outlets that are convenient, effective, and affordable. As demand increases, retailers will be happy to expand. Initially, they will displace old-style providers as fully as the law allows. Then, they will exert pressure on legislators to loosen the constraints. They will win political battles here and there, and as they do, the case for protecting incumbent providers from competition will crumble and collapse.

Norms will change too. As consumers grow accustomed to buying health care directly, they will increasingly wonder why they ever frequented old-style providers or used insurance to pay them. When it feels natural to go to Walmart or Costco for health checkups, blood tests, eye exams, inoculations, and other medical procedures, the game will be over. Eventually, we predict, the retail health care sector will integrate vertically, and companies like CVS Health and Costco will start running hospitals, nursing homes, and assisted living facilities. Then price, quality, and access to medical services of all types will vastly improve.

Chapter 18 explains that, in the meantime, consumers can save money by breaking local cartels. The hospital near you won't offer a competitive price for the surgery you want because the people who run it think they have a lock on your business. You can show them that they're wrong by having your procedure performed at a world-class hospital or surgery center in India, Mexico, Singapore, South Korea, or Europe. By doing so, you'll cut the price in half and enjoy a nice vacation, even after accounting for the cost of airfare. If you don't want to go abroad, you can also get a good deal by traveling domestically. Just call up the Surgery Center of Oklahoma and they will quote you a package price for a joint replacement that will save you thousands. Or give WeightLossAgents.com a buzz and they will give you a bargain price for gastric sleeve surgery in Miami.

And here's the really good news. You may not have to travel at all. Just tell the folks at your local hospital that you need to save money and have decided to have your surgery elsewhere. They may suddenly see a need to compete and drop their price.

What about pharmaceuticals? We need to provide incentives for drug companies to innovate and develop new treatments. But we don't have to pay them whatever they ask. That's an invitation to get taken. We need a new deal for pharmaceuticals, and fortunately there is one. Chapter 19 explains how prizes can generate innovations without the marketing exclusivity and high prices that come with patents. Chapter 19 also shows how we should address the problem of price spikes for generic drugs.

What about fraud and abuse? All human systems depend on minimum standards of integrity and fair dealing—and must also detect and punish those that misbehave. For too long, we have allowed criminals and con artists to loot the health care system. As Chapter 20 explains, we need to raise the costs of bad behavior by making greater use of whistleblowers. We must also enlist consumers in the battle against fraud, by switching to first-party payment in most contexts and by routing dollars through consumers when costs are borne by insurers or taxpayers.

Of course, there will always be a role for health insurance. As we discuss in Chapter 21, we expect almost everyone will want coverage against catastrophes. Policies that cover only catastrophes are much cheaper than the soup-to-nuts policies that Obamacare forced everyone to buy. More people will be able to buy such insurance, especially after widespread direct purchasing of routine medical treatments exerts strong pressure on providers to charge less.

That said, it is inevitable that some people will be too poor to buy what they need. If we want to help the poor, the first thing we should do is shift to direct purchasing arrangements that have significant power to make health care cheaper. As Chapter 22 explains, lower prices help poor people the most because they are the most price-sensitive consumers. We should also encourage poor people to save what they can and supplement their ability to buy what they need by giving them cash or restricted vouchers. Finally, we should maintain a thin safety net for people who fall through the cracks, but we should require everyone, including the very poorest, to pay for some of the benefits they receive. People tend to undervalue and overuse things that are free.

# CHAPTER 15: HEALTH CARE IS EXPENSIVE BECAUSE IT'S INSURED

## THIRD-PARTY PAYERS DON'T CARE ABOUT YOU

Third-party payers dominate health care. Like Medicare and Medicaid, some of these payers are public, while others—including insurers like UnitedHealth Group, Anthem, Aetna, Humana, Cigna, and the many Blue Cross/Blue Shield companies—are private. Public payers are political operations, so they naturally care about political things, like maximizing their budgets and keeping members of Congress happy. Private payers are like other businesses. They want to maximize their profits. These are not criticisms. Government agencies are supposed to care about politics, and businesses are supposed to care about their finances.

But there is a deeper point. Helping patients and consumers isn't the top priority for third-party payers of either type. This goal matters to them only when, by pursuing it, they can get what they really want: money, bigger budgets, reelection, or something else they care about. Unfortunately, helping patients and consumers only occasionally makes payers better off. Payers rarely care about the well-being of patients or consumers.

To see why, start with Point #1: *Payers want health care to be expensive.* The reason is simple. If medical services were cheap, we wouldn't need Medicare, Medicaid, or private insurers to bear the cost for us. In 2016, the median family with two adults and two children spent almost $17,000 on housing and about $8,300 on transportation, without any help from insurance companies.[1] If medical services predictably cost only a similar amount each year, people could pay for them directly too. This would make consumers and patients happy, but third-party payers would be sad. The need to route more than $1 trillion through the Medicare and Medicaid programs would vanish. The need for private insurers would diminish too.

We can't expect Medicare, Medicaid, or private carriers to put themselves out of business. Rick Scott, the governor of Florida and the former CEO of a scandal-plagued health care company, hit the nail on the head when he asked, "How many businesses do you know that want to cut their revenue in half?"[2] None. "That's why the health care system won't change the health care system," Governor Scott rightly concluded.[3]

If you've grasped Point #1, you should find it easy to understand Point #2: *The more expensive health care becomes, the happier payers are.* The more medical services cost, the more people will want the protection from risk that Medicare, Medicaid, and private insurers provide. Suppose that all of the services a person might reasonably expect to need in an emergency—everything from transportation by ambulance through postsurgery rehabilitation—could be had for $1,500. Spending money on health care is never fun, but many people could afford to bear the risk of having to spend $1,500 themselves. Many people with insurance have deductibles larger than that, and a deductible is just a provision for direct payment.[4] But if an emergency were likely to generate costs in the $15,000 range—ten times as much—insurance would be much more attractive. Many people would think it indispensable. And pretty much everyone would reach that conclusion if the expected cost of emergency medical care was $150,000, an amount that only the super rich could afford to pay out of pocket. The more health care costs, the more consumers will want the protection from risk that third-party payers offer.

Expensive health care also directly benefits the politicians, political appointees, and career bureaucrats who are in charge of Medicare and Medicaid, including the members of Congress who trade influence for political contributions and other support. They want the budgets for these programs to be as large as possible. Bigger budgets mean greater power and more goodies to dole out. Insurance executives also prefer larger companies to smaller ones. These business titans care mainly about their compensation, and the size of executives' pay packages correlates strongly with the size of the companies that employ them.[5]

Because expensive health care makes third-party payers' services essential, their business model depends on fear. They need patients and consumers to be terrified that health care expenses will ruin them. Consequently, they won't work to change the system in ways that would put consumers at ease.

## A Vicious Cycle

Until the second half of the 20th century, doctors and hospitals opposed the government's efforts to stick its nose into their business. Although few people alive today know the history, organized medicine bitterly opposed the creation of Medicare. Dr. Donovan Ward, the head of the American Medical Association (AMA), declared that "a deterioration in the quality of care is inescapable." Similarly, the president of the Association of American Physicians and Surgeons stated that it would be "complicity in evil" for doctors to participate in Medicare.[6] The AMA even hired Ronald Reagan to read a speech on the threat that socialized medicine posed to the American way of life and sent copies of the recording to every doctor's office in the United States.[7]

Today, doctors are Medicare and Medicaid's biggest fans. Opposition morphed into support when they realized that, with the government footing the bills, they could raise their rates—which they immediately did. As Harvard economist Martin Feldstein observed way back in 1970, "after [the] introduction of Medicare and Medicaid, physicians' fees rose at 6.8 per cent per year in 1967 and 1968 in comparison to a 3.2 per cent annual rise in the [consumer price index]."[8] Government programs put money in doctors' pockets, so organized medicine did a 180-degree turn.

Physicians should have guessed that government-run third-party payment arrangements would make them rich. From 1945 to 1965, the fraction of the U.S. population with some form of health care coverage more than tripled, rising from 22.6 percent to 72.5 percent.[9] Doctors benefited enormously. Their charges rose at 1.7 times the rate of inflation. As Professor Feldstein dryly observed, "There appears to be a tendency [on the part of physicians] to increase prices when patients' ability to pay improves through higher income or more complete insurance coverage."[10]

The effect of insurance on hospitals' charges was even more pronounced. Again, Feldstein did the pioneering research. He opened *The Rising Cost of Hospital Care* by observing that "A day of hospital care in 1970 cost . . . five times as much as in 1950"—a staggering increase, especially because "the general price level of consumer goods and services [rose] less than 60%" over the same period. From 1966 to 1970, the last five years Feldstein studied, hospital prices rose annually by almost 15 percent. Why? The main driver was the growing availability and generosity of public and private insurance.[11]

Over the two decades Feldstein studied, the fraction of hospital care paid for by some form of insurance rose markedly. In 1950, the split between insurance and patient responsibility was roughly 50–50. If a hospital day cost $600, the insurer paid $300 and the patient paid $300. By 1968, insurers were picking up 84 percent of the cost.[12] This meant that, at $600 per day, the insurer paid $504 and the patient only $96.

The shift of financial responsibility to insurers was so dramatic that patients actually paid less even as hospitals raised their rates. Suppose that, from 1950 to 1968, the cost of a hospital day trebled, from $600 to $1,800. In 1950, the patient's share would have been $300. In 1968, it would have been only $288. As wages rose and people became wealthier, hospital care seemed like a better bargain than ever, because more and more of its cost was being borne by insurers.

The portion of hospital spending borne by public and private third-party payers kept increasing throughout the 20th century, and total health care spending rose right along with it. In recent research, Amy Finkelstein, a professor of economics at the Massachusetts Institute of Technology, estimated that the spread of insurance was responsible for about half of the six-fold increase in real health care spending per capita that occurred from 1950 to 1990.[13] In other words, insurance caused health care spending to triple. From 1965 to 1970 alone, Medicare drove up real outlays on hospital services by 37 percent. Similar increases were found across all age groups. When insurance inflates demand, prices rise across the board and everyone suffers.

## THE EVIL GENIUS OF INSURANCE: MAKE HEALTH CARE CHEAP AT THE POINT OF SALE

It's easy to see why insurance stimulates demand. At the point of sale, people don't spend their own money. This makes medical services seem cheap or even free, so people naturally want more of them. And, just as naturally, they care very little about the total cost of the services they use.

The average price of a total knee replacement is about $31,000.[14] That's about what you'd pay for a new Audi Q3, a small luxury cross-over SUV. But the average patient who undergoes a knee replacement pays less than 10 percent of the total, say, $3,000. The rest is covered by insurance. If the same arrangement existed in the auto market—call it "new car insurance"—you could buy a $31,000 Audi Q3 for $3,000. So you'd happily take one—or maybe several—even if you would never pay $31,000 out-of-pocket for this particular car.

Insurance generates demand for medical treatments in the same way. You pay a monthly premium over which you have little control, often because the dollars are withheld from your salary. And, once that money is spent on insurance, it isn't coming back, whether or not you actually use any health care. However, you do get to decide whether to have knee replacement surgery or not. The evil genius of health insurance is that, at the point of delivery, it encourages patients to overconsume by making medical services seem cheap. Financially, your knee replacement surgery is the equivalent of a $3,000 Audi Q3. Even if you would never spend $31,000 of your own money on a knee replacement, as long as you value the benefits of the procedure more than $3,000—which is far less than its actual cost—you will willingly go under the knife. And the price stays high because few consumers shop for bargains or refuse knee surgery because of the price.

What's true for you is also true for the millions of other people who carry insurance. You get to buy an Audi Q3 for $3,000 and so do they. Over time, the country will be flooded with new Audis and all of these new Audi owners will impoverish each other. Premiums will have to rise, because the money to pay for all the new Audis has to come from somewhere. Finally, as insurance-driven demand for Audis increases, Audi will increase its prices and aggregate spending will go through the roof.

The problem just described exemplifies what social scientists call a "prisoners' dilemma." Millions of people do something—here, buy insurance that heavily subsidizes medical services at the point of sale— that they think will make each of them better off. But collectively they wind up worse off than they would have been if they had each paid for their own health care. Without insurance, the only people who would have had knee surgery would have been those willing to pay $31,000 for it, just as in real life, the only people who buy Audi Q3s are those willing to part with the same amount of cash. Demand would have been much lower, and prices would have been too.

### STUDIES OF INSURANCE-INDUCED DEMAND

Insurance without a significant point-of-service copayment will inflate the demand for medical services. The total cost of a doctor's office visit might be $200, but an insured person who parts with only the $30 copay won't care. He or she will visit the doctor whenever it's worth spending $30 to do so, even if the value doesn't approach $200.

Doctors understand this, as a recent dispute from Down Under makes clear. Hoping to rein in spiraling costs, a commission appointed by the Australian government raised the possibility of imposing a $6 copay for visits to doctors' offices. Six dollars doesn't sound like much, but it was a large increase from the prior copay—$0. Retirees would have been exempt from the charge, and families would have had to pay it only after seeing a doctor 12 times a year. Despite the trivial size of the copay and the exemptions, the Australian Medical Association condemned the proposal. Why? Because any charge, even a small one, would cause people to see their doctors less often.[15]

In the language of economics, the Australian Medical Association recognized that demand for medical services is elastic. Demand falls when prices rise, and it rises when prices fall. If a patient's cost at the point of service went from $0 to $6, some patients who would gladly consume free medical services would stay home. They would regard their health concerns as being too minor to spend $6 on. Their doctors would then lose the much larger payments for these patients' office visits that the government provides. Although the Australian Medical Association framed the issue around denial of necessary medical treatment, it was really just trying to preserve the flow of money to its members.

Not all medical services are like office visits, though. Consider joint replacement surgery, which we discussed above. The pain, loss of time, and required postoperative physical therapy should discourage anyone from having a knee replaced on a whim. Can the decision to have surgery really be analyzed in the same terms as the decision to buy a car? And what about medical procedures that aren't discretionary, such as emergency surgery for a gunshot wound? Isn't demand sometimes fixed, instead of price dependent?

Absolutely. There are thousands of medical procedures, and the elasticity of demand surely varies across them. But discretionary calls occur often, so there is enough elasticity for insurance to increase health care consumption and spending substantially.

Clever studies have examined the impact of insurance on health care consumption.[16] Several papers focus on Oregon's decision to expand Medicaid in 2008. Oregon allowed anyone who met the eligibility criteria to apply, but it received far more applications than it could accept. So it randomly chose a subset of applicants to receive Medicaid coverage. This created a natural experiment, that is, an especially good opportunity to study the impact of insurance on health care utilization. Because the applicants who received Medicaid (the "winners") were chosen at random from the same pool as those who did not (the "losers"), any differences in health care utilization between these two groups could be chalked up to insurance.

The first article from the Oregon experiment in the medical literature appeared in the *New England Journal of Medicine* in 2013.[17] The researchers determined that "Medicaid coverage increased annual medical spending . . . by $1,172" per household. In other words, the winners used about 35 percent more medical services than the losers. Having Medicaid coverage made only a modest difference in the winners' health, however, although it did reduce financial strain.

A follow-up article examined emergency room usage. Remember the sales pitch for Obamacare? It was supposed to save money because insured people and people covered by Medicaid would see cheaper primary care physicians instead of getting basic medical care at more expensive emergency rooms. That's not what happened in Oregon. The winners used emergency rooms 40 percent *more* often than the losers did. The increase was for "a broad range of types of visits, conditions, and subgroups, including increases in visits for conditions that may be most readily treatable in primary care settings."[18] When people are insured, they use *all* types of medical services more often. A subsequent article on the Oregon experiment reevaluated the earlier findings using an additional year of data. The results were the same. "Newly insured people will most likely use more health care across settings—including the [emergency room] and the hospital."[19]

Another clever study focused on senior citizens and evaluated the impact of qualifying for Medicare on health care utilization.[20] It compared people ages 62–64 to people who were 65. Because the two groups were so close in age, the health status of their members was similar. One might have expected the slightly older group to use a bit more medical care per person, but not much. In fact, hospitalizations, visits to doctors' offices, and the use of prescription meds all spiked at age 65. Why? Because that's when people become eligible for Medicare. The older people used lots of Medicare-financed health care that the people in the 62-to-64-year-old bracket, many of whom lacked insurance, wouldn't (or couldn't) pay for themselves. It is hard to come up with better evidence that the demand for medical treatments is, in fact, quite elastic.

In sum, third-party payment and the cost of health care feed on each other. Back in the 1940s, far fewer people were insured. Consequently, most health care was paid for out of pocket. This kept health care affordable. Then employer-sponsored health care became common, which stimulated demand and caused spending to rise. In the mid-1960s, Medicare and Medicaid extended coverage to tens of millions of additional people, and demand for health care went through the roof. Because supply was limited and third-party payers were footing the bills, prices rose accordingly. This stimulated the demand for insurance even more, triggering greater consumption of medical services, higher prices, and—again—increased demand for insurance.

Feldstein, the Harvard economist, described the cycle more than 40 years ago:

> The price and type of health services that are available to any individual reflect the extent of health insurance among other members of the community. . . . [P]hysicians raise their fees (and may improve their services) when insurance becomes more extensive. Nonprofit hospitals also respond to the growth of insurance by increasing the sophistication and price of their product. . . . Thus, even the un-insured individual will find that his expenditure on health services is affected by the insurance of others. Moreover, the higher price of physician and hospital services encourages more extensive use of insurance. For the community as a whole, therefore, the spread of insurance causes higher prices and more sophisticated services which in turn cause a further increase in insurance. *People spend more on health because they are insured and buy more insurance because of the high cost of health care.*[21] (emphasis added)

As we explained above, the vicious cycle works through fear, and also by making medical services free, or nearly so, at the point of delivery. Remember the $3,000 Audis? The more we route payments through third-party payers, the less we bear the real cost of services at the point of delivery and the more we consume.

The connection between third-party payment and health care spending will be obvious to anyone who bothers to look. In Figure 15-1, the line shows the ratio between the amounts that consumers paid directly for health care and the amounts that were spent by Medicare, Medicaid, and private insurers (left-side axis). The line starts out at about

**Figure 15–1.** The Less We Rely on Ourselves, the More We Spend: Relationship between Direct Financial Responsibility for Medical Expenditures and Per Capita Health Spending

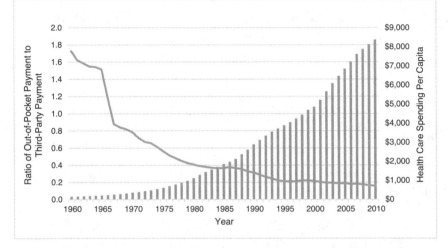

Source: Centers for Medicare and Medicaid Services, "National Health Expenditures by Type of Service and Source of Funds: Calendar Years 1960 to 2015," available at https://www.cms.gov/Research-Statistics-Data-and-Systems/Statistics-Trends-and-Reports/NationalHealthExpendData/NationalHealthAccountsHistorical.html.

1.80, meaning that in 1960 consumers paid $1.80 out of pocket for every dollar spent on medical services by a third-party payer. Then it declines steadily, so that, by 2010, for every dollar a payer shelled out, a consumer spent less than 20 cents. The decline in direct, personal financial responsibility was especially pronounced in the mid-1960s, when Medicare and Medicaid were introduced. The vertical bars show annual health care spending per capita (right-side axis). It rises from a few hundred dollars in 1960 to over $8,000 per person in 2010. As direct payment falls, per capita spending rises. The more heavily we rely on third-party payers, the more we spend.

OBAMA VS. STEIN

Herbert Stein, another prominent economist, is credited with coining Stein's Law: "If something cannot go on forever, it will stop." The vicious cycle described by Feldstein is no exception. Its eventual end is assured. As insurance-induced demand makes medical services more expensive, the price of insurance has to rise. As coverage costs more, employers will be more reluctant to offer it as a benefit and people will be less eager to buy it on their own. Over time, rising prices for health care will slow, stop, and perhaps even reverse the spread of insurance. As the pool of insured consumers starts to shrink, demand for medical services will weaken and the flow of money into the health care sector will grow less quickly than before.

The tipping point that signaled the end of the cycle appears to have been reached at the start of this century. That's when private coverage took a nosedive. From 2000 to 2010, the number of people with private insurance fell from 205.5 million to 196 million.[22] Because the U.S. population grew steadily over that period, the number (and share) of the uninsured increased dramatically. In 2000, about 13 percent of Americans lacked insurance coverage. In 2010, about 16 percent did.[23] In raw numbers, by the end of the decade, 50 million people were uninsured.[24]

The result is shown in Figure 15-2.[25] From 2002 to 2011, the annual rate of increase in health care spending steadily declined. In 2002, Americans spent almost 10 percent more on medical services than they did in 2001. From 2009 to 2012, the year-over-year increase was less than 4 percent.

The declining generosity of employer-provided coverage contributed to this trend. Workers who managed to hold onto their health care coverage in the 2000s found that the terms of coverage were less generous. Especially during the financial crisis, when businesses of all sorts struggled to make ends meet, insured workers found that they were picking up more and more of the costs of medical services through copays, deductibles, and annual payment limits. According to one estimate, "rising out-of-pocket payments . . . account[ed] for approximately 20 percent of the observed slowdown" in the growth of health care spending.[26] In combination, the increase in the share of health care spending that had to be paid for out of pocket and the Great Recession made consumers more cautious about throwing additional money at health care providers.

**Figure 15-2.** Yearly Increase in Total National Health Expenditures (1990–2015)

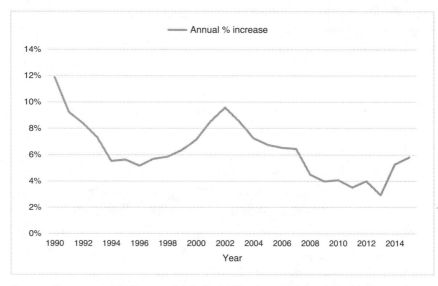

Source: Centers for Medicare and Medicaid Services, "National Health Expenditures by Type of Service and Source of Funds: Calendar Years 1960 to 2015," available at https://www.cms.gov/Research-Statistics-Data-and-Systems/Statistics-Trends-and-Reports/NationalHealthExpendData/NationalHealthAccountsHistorical.html.

From the perspective of the American health care system, which takes for granted that the flow of money will constantly increase, declining growth rates were intolerable. From the perspective of academic health policy experts, the decline in the number of insured was a calamity too. The experts equate insurance with access to medical services, and they equate medical services with good health. That is why both the industry and the academics are big fans of Obamacare, which sought to require all 50 million uninsured Americans to obtain coverage or participate in Medicaid. Forcing 50 million Americans to use third-party payment arrangements would have helped restore the vicious cycle, at least for a while. Once covered, the newly insured would demand even more health care, causing the growth in health care spending to resume its rapid rise and driving more dollars to health care providers.

Seen in this light, Obamacare was a ticket to more years of sizable spending increases. That's why "drugmakers, insurers and hospitals . . . helped bankroll the law. . . . Big business . . . agree[d] to various taxes, fees and reimbursement cuts, and it expects to see a return on investment as newly insured people use its products and services."[27] Health care providers needed new customers. They got millions of them by supporting Obamacare. The insurance mandate, which required people to carry insurance or pay a fine, was the key to keeping the party going. Yogi Berra once quipped, "If people don't want to come out to the ball park, nobody's gonna stop 'em." Obamacare showed that the government *could* stop people from staying home and force them to go to the game.

And, once everyone got there, they were given health insurance with all the bells and whistles. As of 2014, health insurance plans had to take everyone, including people known to have health problems that require expensive treatments. They also had to provide unlimited benefits. An individual who needed $5 million a year in health care would get it. After all, it was somebody else's money—and it could be used to buy almost anything imaginable. Obamacare required insurers to cover ambulatory services, emergency services, hospital care, maternity and newborn care, mental health and substance abuse counseling, prescription drugs, rehabilitative services and devices, laboratory services, preventive and wellness services, chronic disease management, and pediatric services. And the list could always be broadened to accommodate any important constituency, as it was when women and providers complained about the omission of routine mammograms. Obamacare was a smorgasbord, and the menu would predictably become richer and more varied over time as Congress pandered to special interests.

Obamacare also used generous subsidies to help keep the cycle going. The subsidies came in two forms. Premium tax credits for people with incomes up to $97,000 for a family of four ensured that monthly insurance premiums would not exceed specified levels, ranging from 2 percent to 9.5 percent of income. Cost-sharing reduction subsidies lowered insured patients' out-of-pocket costs attributable to deductibles, coinsurance, and copayments for covered services.

Signs quickly emerged that Obamacare was also subject to Stein's Law. As waves of people bought insurance and millions more enrolled in Medicaid, premiums started to rise and government spending increased substantially.[28] The Obamacare exchanges attracted a population whose members were unusually sick. Many of them had previously been enrolled in states' high-risk pools. Some had been denied coverage because of pre-existing conditions. As costs rose, insurers had to raise prices for everyone. This encouraged healthy people to drop their policies. And as they opted out, the pool of premium-payers shrank, became sicker on average, and led insurers to raise prices again. Regardless of who won the 2016 presidential race, the cycle would continue until Obamacare failed or Congress bailed everyone out by massively increasing the Obamacare subsidies.

Medicaid's budget also ballooned. Writing in early 2016, Brian Blase, a researcher at George Mason University, observed, "No major area of federal spending has increased more dramatically since President Barack Obama took office than Medicaid."[29] From 2008 to 2015, total spending on Medicaid grew by 43 percent, or $168.2 billion. The growth had several drivers, including the Great Recession, which put millions of people into poverty, Obamacare's Medicaid expansion, and the fact that new enrollees in Medicaid tended to use medical services in larger amounts. These increases would have been even larger had all 50 states expanded Medicaid, as Obamacare originally intended. Obamacare's Medicaid expansion was primed to create fiscal havoc no matter who won the 2016 election.

### INSURANCE MAKES MEDICINES MORE EXPENSIVE

Shortly after taking office, President Trump declared war on the pharma sector. Drug companies were "getting away with murder," he said, and he threatened to allow Medicare to reduce drug costs by negotiating lower prices.[30] Several pharma execs responded by promising to limit annual price hikes to 10 percent.

To the average American, whose wages have been stagnant for years, a promise to raise prices by "only" 10 percent must have sounded like a pledge to continue gouging. Why 10 percent instead of the rate of inflation, which was much lower? Why raise prices at all instead of cutting them? Most drugs on the market today were invented years ago. Apple can't charge more for old iPhones. Ford can't charge more for trucks built in prior model years. Why should pharma companies be able to charge more for last year's drugs?

Some pharma execs disregarded the 10 percent pledge. Jeffrey Aronin, the CEO of Marathon Pharmaceuticals we met all the way back in Chapter 1, announced that his company would charge $89,000 a year for deflazacort, a treatment for muscular dystrophy that had long been available in other countries and that cost about $1,000. Marathon had gained a monopoly on U.S. sales of deflazacort by obtaining U.S. Food and Drug Administration approval for the medication under the Orphan Drug Act, and Aronin was bent on exploiting it.

When accused of price gouging, Aronin used a well-worn gambit to deflect criticism. He said that most of the money to pay for the drug wouldn't come from patients—it would come from insurance companies. Aronin knew that most Americans hate insurance companies and wouldn't care if drug makers ripped them off. They feel for patients, though, so it was important to emphasize that patients' costs would remain the same.

Aronin was just trying to get the press off his back. But his comment brings an important issue to the surface. When a loss occurs, insurance *is* supposed to enable people to obtain certain goods and services that are too costly for them to afford. For example, few homeowners have enough money to rebuild a house that burns down. That is why most homeowners can and do protect themselves against the risk of fire by buying homeowners' insurance. Health insurance has the same effect when people fall ill. It pays for expensive drugs that people might otherwise be unable to purchase. This is known as the liquidity benefit of insurance.

But insurance *is not* supposed to make the goods and services that policyholders require cost more, or to be the rationale for opportunistic price increases. The fact that an insurer rather than a homeowner is paying to rebuild a house should not affect the price of nails, wood, roofing shingles, or labor. Nor should the price of medications reflect the identity of the buyer. A drug that ordinarily sells for $1,000 shouldn't fetch the absurd price of $89,000 just because a patient's insurer, rather than the patient, is footing the bill. Price increases attributable to the identity of the buyer are part of the moral hazard effect of insurance.

There is a widely held impression that drug manufacturers do charge more for their products when insurers are on the hook. As three prominent professors at Northwestern University's Kellogg School of Management observed, "it is difficult to imagine that Gilead would charge anywhere near $84,000 for Sovaldi," the breakthrough drug for hepatitis C, "were it not covered by insurance." If that is right, they continued, "the existence of insurance for this product has clear implications for access and pricing."[31]

The Kellogg researchers tested a model that, they hoped, would help them learn whether "the unprecedented high prices of new prescription drugs depended on the liquidity benefits of insurance," whether consumers would be better off if these drugs were not insured, and whether insurance enabled pharma companies to charge more than new drugs were worth. Their data consisted of prices for oncology drugs before and after the creation of Medicare Part D—the prescription drug benefit—in 2003.

Their results reveal a sizable influence of insurance on drug prices. Among their many findings were "two reactions to the passage of Medicare Part D. First, the manufacturers of oral chemotherapy products increased their prices. Second, these manufacturers were now able to command prices that exceeded many estimates of the value that they create." In short, "the passage of Part D is associated with a large increase in the average launch price of oncology products," an increase that could not be justified on the basis of the tendency of these drugs to extend patients' lives.[32]

One possible implication is that the prices insurers pay for drugs could exceed the value of those drugs to the patients who receive them. Of course, the prospect of charging high prices to insured patients may have motivated Gilead to develop Sovaldi too. We discuss the need for incentives to innovate in Chapter 19.

In theory, pharmacy benefit managers (PBMs), companies like ExpressScripts and ProCare RX that serve as intermediaries between drug makers, insurers, and pharmacies, could bargain prices down to competitive levels by offering manufacturers access to lots of customers. In fact, PBMs can and do exert downward pressure on prices. But there are also concerns that PBMs may gain by keeping drug list prices high (raising consumers' copays),[33] and by providing insurance coverage for prescriptions that would be cheaper were they purchased for cash. There are also allegations that PBMs are using "gag clauses" in their contracts with pharmacies to hide these facts from consumers.[34]

The real question is why we need PBMs at all. Patients who buy over-the-counter drugs pay low prices, and they do not deal with PBMs. In the retail sector, competition does all the work, for free. PBMs exist only because, by using insurance to pay for drugs instead of buying them directly, we have created a market niche for them.

Clearly, insurance is a gamechanger. It enables patients to acquire new drugs that they could not afford on their own and leads drug makers to strategize to maximize the dollars they collect from insurers. These opportunistic pricing strategies make insurance more expensive—possibly too expensive for many people to afford—and may even enable drug manufacturers to capture more value than they create. It also creates a need for PBMs to serve as middlemen—and no one likes middlemen.

The title of this chapter asserts that health care is expensive *because* it's insured. That's generally true, but not always. Some medical treatments would be expensive regardless. Everyone already knows that. What few people understand is that causation runs from insurance to cost too. Insurance makes health care more expensive than it would be if people paid for it themselves. Americans would purchase fewer medical treatments and would pay much less for them, if not for the existence and government encouragement of excessive insurance.

# CHAPTER 16: BLIND ALLEYS AND LOST CAUSES

## OBAMACARE IS DEAD—LONG LIVE OBAMACARE-LITE

When the 2016 election gave the GOP control of all three branches of government, it seemed a foregone conclusion that Obamacare would be repealed. The House of Representatives had previously voted to abolish all or parts of the law multiple times, and repeal was a central plank in Donald Trump's presidential campaign. Trump even floated the idea of convening a special session of Congress on his inauguration day to eradicate his predecessor's signature domestic accomplishment.

It now seems that Obamacare will remain in place longer than the Republicans led everyone to believe. Although the House passed the American Health Care Act (AHCA) on the second try, the Senate, which is more closely divided, has so far shown itself to be incapable of passing even a minor overhaul of the law apart from the repeal of the individual mandate in 2017. This surprising turn of events has many causes, two of which seem especially potent.

The first is opposition among voters, who like certain benefits of Obamacare (if they don't have to pay for them, that is), especially the provisions that guarantee coverage for people with pre-existing conditions, lower insurance premiums for the near-elderly, and make coverage available for children on their parents' policies until the age of 26. People concerned about the loss of these benefits converted town hall meetings with their

Republican representatives into shouting matches that ranged from angry to almost violent. Patient advocacy groups, including the American Association of Retired Persons, the American Heart Association, the March of Dimes, the Cystic Fibrosis Foundation, the National Multiple Sclerosis Society, and a host of others also heaped scorn on the AHCA, claiming that it would throw the poor, the near-elderly, and the sick to the wolves for no better reason than to reduce the tax burden on the rich.

The second major cause is the opposition of the medical establishment, which has hundreds of billions of dollars in revenues at stake and is using all of its political muscle to protect the flow of cash. Every trade association whose members benefit financially from Obamacare opposed the AHCA, including the American Medical Association, the American Hospital Association, the American Academy of Pediatrics, the Federation of American Hospitals, the American College of Cardiology, the American Academy of Family Physicians, and the American Nurses Association, to name but a few. They opposed the bills that were placed on the Senate's agenda too.[1]

Opposition from entrenched interests is hard for politicians to overcome. It may be the most important reason that Obamacare did not attempt to tackle any of the problems we identified in Part 1. A serious effort to rationalize the payment system would threaten health care providers, pharma companies, and the rest of the medical establishment with the loss of hundreds of billions of dollars in revenues a year. Given that one-third of all medical spending is wasted, the stakes for providers could conceivably be $1 trillion. A threat of that magnitude would unleash a maelstrom that few politicians have the courage to confront. Realistically, one cannot expect Republicans or Democrats to take the steps that are needed to make American health care better and cheaper.

That would be true even if American voters were open minded. They are not. Millions are palpably fearful that they will have to pay far more for insurance or will lose their coverage entirely if Obamacare is repealed. The GOP's members in Congress should have expected this and attempted to put voters at ease. Instead of rushing to abolish Obamacare, they should have developed a plan for protecting vulnerable individuals and embarked on a year-long effort to educate the public. Obamacare wasn't built in a day, and the GOP should not have tried to build its replacement that quickly either. But it threw caution and common sense to the wind. The House raced to enact the AHCA in the shortest possible time and attached no importance to educating the public or learning from it. Many Republican representatives were so reluctant to discuss health care policy with their constituents that they refused to attend public gatherings arranged for the purpose. The Senate rushed the process too, at times moving so quickly that even its members did not know what proposals would be put before them.

Good ideas were casualties of the process. The chief problem with Obamacare was that it was more of the same. It mostly just increased the role of third-party payment in the health care system by expanding Medicaid and making it easier (as well as compulsory) for people to obtain private insurance in the individual market. To combat the pathologies of the health care system, the AHCA needed to be very different. It wasn't. Instead, it was "Obamacare-lite." Being hell-bent on scoring a legislative victory as quickly as possible, the GOP cobbled together a bill that would pass—and the bill that emerged preserved many of Obamacare's core features. Whether the AHCA would make American health care better and cheaper didn't matter nearly as much to House Republicans, so thorough-going reform of the payment system wasn't even attempted.

The AHCA would have kept several key provisions of Obamacare. It would have preserved the provisions allowing adults to keep children on their parents' policies until the age of 26. It would have preserved the provisions that forbid carriers from denying coverage to persons with pre-existing conditions and from charging sick people more. It would have preserved provisions requiring consumers to purchase coverage with unlimited annual and lifetime benefits.

The AHCA would also have tinkered with but not abandoned other Obamacare provisions. It would have converted Obamacare's income-based subsidies to smaller age-based subsidies. It would also have retained Obamacare's community rating of premiums by age while increasing the maximum ratio between the charges for the oldest and youngest enrollees from 3:1 to 5:1.

The AHCA and Obamacare differ in four major ways. First, the AHCA would have frozen and slowly wound back the Medicaid expansion. Starting in 2020, it would have limited funding for the program to a per capita amount times the size of the covered population (rather than having the federal government match whatever the state spends). Second, it would have eliminated Obamacare's individual mandate (which penalizes individuals who don't purchase a minimum level of coverage) and employer mandate (which requires businesses with a certain number of full-time workers to offer coverage as a benefit or pay a tax). Third, it would have allowed insurers to offer less comprehensive coverage packages in states that obtain waivers, rather than requiring them to sell policies that provide the minimum package of benefits that the federal government deems essential. Fourth, it would have raised the annual contribution limits for tax-exempt health savings accounts (HSAs) from $3,400 to $6,550 for individuals and from $6,750 to $13,100 for families. These changes were designed to keep the Obamacare insurance program going while enabling Republicans to say they repealed it.

These are not pathbreaking changes. Anyone who scours the AHCA in hope of finding a big idea with significant potential to pressure health care providers to offer better services at less cost will be disappointed. But only in a small, libertarian corner of the health care policy world was the AHCA criticized for being too much like Obamacare. In the mainstream, it was harshly condemned for cutting Medicaid and for changing the individual mandate and Obamacare's subsidies in ways that would cause millions of Americans to drop their insurance. When the Congressional Budget Office predicted that 28 percent of the nonelderly population would be uninsured by 2026—roughly the same percentage as before Obamacare—centrist economists and policy analysts were mortified.[2]

Because our goal is to make American health care better and cheaper, we have little sympathy for the mainstream critique. It strikes us as a bad idea to give 325 million Americans the means with which to buy all the mediocre, unnecessary, harmful, and overpriced medical treatments they want, while also funneling hundreds of billions of dollars to providers and criminals who commit frauds.

Even so, we too think that the House's version of the AHCA is deficient. Like Obamacare, the bill leaves the payment system mostly intact. It preserves the incentives and tax advantages that distort consumers' spending habits by making medical services and insurance seem cheap relative to goods and services of other kinds. It changes Medicare not at all, and it reforms Medicaid in a way that is bound to disserve the poor. Once states start receiving fixed payments per Medicaid beneficiary, their incentive will be to maximize the number of beneficiaries while minimizing the services that each beneficiary receives.[3] It would be far better to give the money to poor people directly and let them decide how to spend it.

We are also dismayed that the Republicans flubbed the opportunity to change the national conversation about health care by educating the public. Having grown up with Medicare, Medicaid, private insurance, the U.S. Veterans Health Administration (VHA), and other existing arrangements, millions of Americans hold two related beliefs. One is that medical services are too complicated and too expensive for consumers to buy directly. The other is that the more we rely on third-party payment arrangements, the better. Both beliefs are wrong, and the occasion of repealing Obamacare was the GOP's opportunity to explain why. Simply stated, providers perform better and charge less when consumers buy medical treatments directly, and health care can and should be sold in competitive markets. The GOP should have carried this message to voters and left Obamacare in place while explaining it. The message would have played well too. According to a survey taken by the Kaiser Family Foundation in late 2016, the public's top health care–related priorities were "lowering the amount individuals pay for health care [and] lowering the cost of prescription drugs."[4] Fully 67 percent of the respondents said that making health care cheaper should be a top priority for the next administration. Repealing Obamacare ranked much farther down on the list.

Unfortunately, the GOP spent no time educating voters. It rushed to repeal Obamacare without even formulating a program that would work better, let alone taking the time to explain why. That strategy left unchallenged the conventional beliefs that insurer- and governmental-control of health care purchasing are necessary and desirable. The GOP thus ceded the terms of the public conversation to mainstream thinkers, who took full advantage and pummeled the party severely.

## Don't Tempt Me

Suppose you wanted to lose a few pounds. Which would you do: Go through your pantry and toss out the junk food and snacks, or go to the grocery and buy more? We hope you'd know better than to surround yourself with temptations.

When it comes to medical care, overconsumption is an enormous problem. In Chapter 6, we showed that pretty much everything the health care sector has to offer is overused. But, instead of doing what you'd do if you were on a diet, the government keeps tempting people to use more. It offers special inducements to buy health care by exempting the dollars that are used from taxation. This makes medical treatments seem cheap in comparison to other things, like cars, housing, energy, and transportation, so people spend more of their wealth on health care than they would if all types of purchases were taxed equally.

The tax breaks the federal government offers for medical consumption are huge. In 2015, all tax preferences related to health care collectively cost the federal government about $360 billion in revenues that would otherwise have been collected through income and Social Security taxes.[5] The exemptions relating to dollars spent on health insurance account for the bulk of this amount, making them the largest targeted preferences in the federal tax code.

People age 65 and older receive a large tax break too, because the federal government doesn't tax Medicare benefits as income. Although many seniors think they paid for Medicare in full, Medicare actually doles out far more in benefits than the average senior kicked in during his or her working years. A typical one-earner couple can expect to receive Medicare benefits worth $427,000 after paying in only $70,000. A two-earner couple fares slightly worse. They get $427,000 in benefits at the price of $102,000 in Medicare taxes. But that's still a bonus of $325,000.[6]

Medicare Part B, which covers doctors' services, is an excellent value for seniors too. Congress initially set the premiums to cover 50 percent of the program's expected cost. But Congress effectively reduced that share, so Part B premiums now cover only 25 percent of spending on physician services. The balance—75 percent of Part B spending—is an untaxed gift to the program's beneficiaries, paid for out of general tax revenues.

If Medicare were an ordinary investment, these outsized returns would be taxed at the beneficiaries' marginal rates. But they aren't, so health care consumption gets yet another tax preference. The "total tax benefit to Medicare beneficiaries [was] $67 billion in 2013" and has grown by billions of dollars since.[7]

Everywhere one looks, the tax system encourages health care spending. Why? Two reasons. One is the belief that health care is special and that dollars spent on it should be privileged in a way that dollars spent on goods and services of other types are not. This belief is unwarranted. *Health* may be special, but money used to purchase insurance and medical treatments is not. Americans preserve and improve their health and their children's health by spending money on food, water, shelter, clothing, electricity, education, sanitation, gym memberships, and many other things. For most of us most of the time, these other expenditures affect our health far more than dollars spent on insurance or health care.

Investments in public health also often impact our health more than medical treatments. Many of the increases in life expectancy and quality that Americans have enjoyed over the years are due to investments in sanitation, personal hygiene, anti-smoking campaigns, housing, policing, and regulations like mandatory seat belt laws—things not ordinarily thought of as health care.

Markets deserve an extraordinary amount of the credit for improvements in Americans' health too. By offering employment opportunities that raise people out of poverty and by delivering pure foods and other high-quality items at affordable prices, markets have contributed greatly to Americans' well-being.

In short, health may be special, but medical treatments and insurance are not. Expenditures on them should be taxed like everything else.

The second reason for the preferential treatment of expenditures on health care insurance is that elected officials use the tax system to buy support. Politicians who want votes and contributions from homeowners, realtors, builders, and bankers can get both by letting people use tax-free dollars to pay the interest on home mortgages. Likewise, those who want support from health care businesses, senior citizens, and workers can gain by throwing tax breaks at them.

Of course, tax breaks cannot reduce the aggregate tax burden. The money that the government spends has to come from somewhere. Tax breaks just move the burden around. And by doing that, they also distort purchasing decisions by making medical services seem cheap.

Consider the exemptions from the federal income tax that apply to dollars that are withheld from workers' wages and put into HSAs or that are combined with employers' contributions and used to pay workers' insurance premiums. Although they seem to make health care cheaper, they really just encourage spending. When a worker funds an HSA or buys insurance through her employer, she saves the amount that she would have paid in taxes on the earnings involved. This makes medical services cheaper for her, so she puts more money in the HSA or buys more comprehensive insurance coverage than she otherwise would. (Our progressive tax system compounds the problem, by making the subsidy worth more to people who make more, but leave that problem aside.) But the Treasury loses the same amount the worker saves. To cover the same amount of government spending, the tax burden on other workers has to go up. And those workers return the favor when they use their pre-tax earnings to fund their HSAs or to pay their insurance premiums. Then the first worker's taxes rise, and she bears part of their costs. The shell game of tax preferences moves money around, but it doesn't save any money.

To the contrary, tax preferences actually increase medical spending because health care prices rise in response to the increase in demand they induce. This is why the real winners in this rigged game are the providers and insurers who take workers' money. Start with insurance. Because wages used to pay premiums are tax favored, more workers buy coverage than otherwise would and the coverage they buy is more comprehensive. Everyone also wants insurance to pay for more and more things so that the value of their tax preference will increase. This is a clear win for insurers, who can charge more when demand and use increase.

Health care providers gain too. Tax exemptions encourage workers to purchase more insurance, and better-insured workers use more and more expensive medical treatments. The aggregate effect of tax exemptions on medical spending is enormous, as economists Martin Feldstein and Bernard Friedman figured out decades ago: "because the growth of insurance has been the primary cause of the exceptional rise in health care prices, it can with justice be said that the tax [preference] has been responsible for much of the health care crisis of the past decade."[8] The problem has since been compounded by the rise of health reimbursement arrangements, flexible spending accounts, and HSAs. When politicians try to make health care less expensive, they instead make it more expensive.

To summarize, tax preferences exert a powerful upward pressure on prices and spending. We could save hundreds of billions of dollars just by treating insurance and health care like ordinary purchases. We should eliminate all tax preferences for health care.

The AHCA doesn't do that. Instead, it retains all existing tax exemptions, creates tax credits that are available only to people who buy insurance, and raises the ceiling on contributions to tax-exempt HSAs. The latter, at least, is a mixed blessing rather than an unalloyed negative. Because consumers decide how dollars put into HSAs are spent, HSAs encourage direct purchasing. They also create incentives for consumers to be more prudent about medical consumption. They provide a tax preference for money that consumers save, rather than only for money they spend. The fact that the tax benefits of HSAs increase after people reach age 65 (at which point the penalty for nonmedical withdrawals disappears) and that HSA funds are inheritable provide further incentives for HSA holders to be prudent consumers. At the same time, however, the tax advantage attached to HSAs does motivate overconsumption by making medical goods and services seem relatively cheap. This leads people to buy health care instead of other things they would value more, such as housing, energy, education, or transportation. The best that can be said about HSAs is that they make a horrible tax policy less horrible.

When it comes to health care, Americans need to go on a diet. By preserving existing tax advantages and adding new ones, the AHCA encourages us to binge.

## UNIVERSAL COVERAGE

Michael Cannon, the insightful libertarian health care policy analyst, who also happens to be our editor for this book, harshly criticized the GOP for backing the AHCA. He argued that the bill would not stabilize insurance markets but would cause voters to hold Republicans accountable when they collapsed. He feared that passage of the AHCA would produce "the sort of wave election Democrats experienced in 2008, when they captured not just the House and the presidency, but a filibuster-proof, 60-vote supermajority in the Senate." If that happens again, Cannon predicts, the Democrats will roll out "a single-payer system," which is what they've really wanted all along.[9]

Although a wave election seems unlikely—the combination of two interminable wars, the Great Recession, and America's first black major-party presidential nominee makes 2008 unique in American history—Cannon is surely right that the Democrats will enact some form of universal coverage, if given the chance. Supporting "Medicare for All," which Sen. Bernie Sanders and other prominent Democrats have endorsed, appears to be becoming a litmus test for Democratic candidates.[10] The idea appeals to Democratic voters. A 2017 poll taken by the Pew Research Center found that "[m]ore than eight-in-ten Democrats and Democratic-leaning independents (85%) say the federal government should be responsible for health care coverage."[11] Medicare is the largest health care program controlled by the federal government. It would be a simple matter to expand it to all Americans by eliminating the existing age requirement. (Funding the enlarged program would be much harder, of course.)

Medicare is an example of a single-payer system, but it is not the only possible approach. Under Medicare, the federal government pays for services, but it does not own the hospitals or medical practices that provide them. The VHA, whose health care program provides comprehensive coverage for eligible veterans, does both, as do the military departments that serve active-duty personnel. Although some commentators have suggested that VHA facilities be converted into a government-run health care delivery system for the poor,[12] the idea that such a system might service the medical needs of the entire population enjoys no political support.

A so-called "public option" is more popular. With this approach, the government provides insurance to anyone who wants to purchase it. Consumers could still purchase insurance from private insurance companies. In effect, the government competes with those companies. In theory, a public option could provide catastrophic or comprehensive coverage, but it would likely tend toward the latter.

Whatever the model, the main argument for universal coverage is that it's cheaper. Its proponents contend that it generates fewer administrative costs than private insurance arrangements and that it maximizes the government's ability to bargain with providers over prices. Senator Sanders' statement endorsing Medicare for All makes both assertions.

> Creating a single, public insurance system will go a long way towards getting health care spending under control. The United States has thousands of different health insurance plans, all of which set different reimbursement rates across different networks for providers and procedures resulting in high administrative costs. . . . Health care providers and patients must navigate this complex and bewildering system wasting precious time and resources.
>
> By moving to an integrated system, the government will finally have the ability to stand up to drug companies and negotiate fair prices for the American people collectively. . . .
>
> Reforming our health care system, simplifying our payment structure and incentivizing new ways to make sure patients are actually getting better health care will generate massive savings.

In addition, Senator Sanders predicts that adopting Medicare for All would "save the American people and businesses over $6 trillion over the next decade."[13]

Many informed people believe some or all of these assertions. Elisabeth Rosenthal, the doctor-turned-*New-York-Times*-reporter who has produced a raft of informative articles on health care, is one of them. In her 2017 book, *An American Sickness*, she repeats the mantra that "Medicare uses 98 percent of its funding for healthcare and only 2 percent for administration."[14] Rosenthal also chides private insurers for being less efficient. Diane Archer, special counsel and co-director of the Health Care for All Project at the Institute for America's Future, made the same points years before. In a 2011 column entitled "Medicare is More Efficient than Private Insurance," she asserted that "administrative costs in Medicare are only about 2 percent of operating expenditures" while the same activities cost private insurers 17 percent of their revenues.[15] The members of the growing army of left-leaning thinkers who support Medicare for All regard the proposition that Medicare is efficient as an established fact.

Unfortunately, what the consensus really shows is that a lot of smart people are thinking about efficiency in a really dumb way. It makes no sense whatsoever to assess Medicare's efficiency by comparing its administrative spending to its total budget.

The most obvious problem with this measure is that it rewards Medicare for squandering taxpayers' dollars. Suppose that Medicare incurred $30 million in administrative costs while paying out $1 billion in claims. Total spending would be $1.03 billion, and the ratio of administrative spending to total program dollars would be roughly 3 percent. Now suppose that, by spending an additional $30 million on audits, Medicare could discover that half of filed claims are fraudulent and pay nothing on them. With that additional money invested in fraud prevention, Medicare's administrative spending would rise to $60 million and its payments on claims would fall to $500 million. The ratio of administrative spending ($60 million) to total program dollars ($560 million) is now 11 percent—almost four times higher than before. Medicare looks *less* efficient even though it saved $470 million ($500 million saved on fraudulent claims minus $30 million spent on claim audits) that would otherwise have been squandered. On the measure that Sanders, Rosenthal, and Archer employ, the less care Medicare takes to prevent fraud and the more money it lavishes on criminals, the more efficient it looks.

On their measure, Medicare would look less efficient even if it saved the $500 million paid out on fraudulent claims *for free*. To see this, just reduce the dollars Medicare pays out from $1 billion to $500 million while leaving its administrative expenditures at $30 million. Now Medicare's administrative cost ratio is about 6 percent ($30 million/$530 million), *twice* what it was when Medicare paid the fraudulent claims in full. A measure that makes Medicare look worse when it saves money for free is absurd.

A correctly designed efficiency index would put dollars paid out on valid claims in the denominator and dollars spent on everything else in the numerator. This would enable one to see how much it costs Medicare to pay out $1 to a bona fide medical provider for a treatment that was appropriately rendered to a patient. When one slots the numbers this way, the picture of Medicare's efficiency that emerges is both more accurate and far bleaker. In our original example, where Medicare spent $30 on administrative claims while doling out $1 billion, half of which was consumed by fraud, the ratio of other spending to dollars paid out on valid claims is 106 percent ($530 million/$500 million). In other words, for every $1 that was appropriately doled out on health care, Medicare spent $1.06 on other things.

On our efficiency measure, investments in money-saving anti-fraud measures have the right effect: they make Medicare look more efficient, not less. If Medicare spent the additional $30 million needed to eliminate fraud, the ratio of other spending to dollars paid out on valid claims would fall from $1.06 per $1 to 12 cents per $1 ($60 million/$500 million = 12 percent). In other words, the cost of paying a dollar of valid benefits would fall by 87 percent [($1.06 − $0.12)/$1.06]. And, if Medicare could somehow save the $500 million in fraud dollars for free, the ratio would be even lower—6 cents per $1 in valid benefits paid out ($30 million/$500 million =6 percent).

It should now be clear that the advocates of Medicare for All are using a nonsense measure to assess Medicare's performance. Fraud, waste, and abuse are enormous problems for the program. They are estimated to consume one-third of its budget, as we discussed in Chapter 7. Considering that loss alone, Medicare spends 50 cents on such overhead for every $1 it pays out on appropriate care. To make matters even worse, fraud, waste, and abuse persist because the U.S. Centers for Medicare and Medicaid Services spends too little money policing the system it oversees. Proponents of Medicare for All treat the paltry amount that Medicare spends on administration as evidence of superior efficiency when it actually reflects the government's staggering profligacy with taxpayers' money.

The measure used by Sanders, Rosenthal, and Archer has another serious defect. It says nothing about Medicare's administrative costs per enrollee. The omission is important because Medicare for All would greatly increase the number of people Medicare oversees. Today, Medicare covers about 56 million seniors.[16] If Medicare for All were enacted, the program would cover all 323 million Americans. That's about a six-fold increase.

On a per-enrollee basis, Medicare's administrative costs exceed those of private insurers. Robert Book, who wrote about this subject in 2009, contends that, in 2005, "Medicare's administrative costs were $509 per primary beneficiary, compared to private-sector administrative cost of

$453 [per enrollee]." Nor was 2005 an unusual year. The imbalance favored private insurers across the 2000–2005 period.[17] Because Medicare's administrative cost per enrollee is higher, expanding the program would not save money.

The appearance of superior efficiency arises because Medicare pays out far more dollars per patient than private insurers do. Its relatively old and infirm beneficiaries tend to receive more expensive treatments than the general (insured) population.[18] According to Book, Medicare spent $11,000 per beneficiary in 2014, more than double the amount, $4,600 per covered person, that private carriers did.[19] The fact that Medicare spends more on treatments per enrollee does not mean that it is more efficient.

Consider an example. Suppose that a third-party payer spends $100 managing claims relating to Patient A, who winds up receiving $1,000 worth of medical treatments. For this patient, the ratio of administrative cost to dollars paid out is 10 percent. Now suppose that the same payer spends the same $100 managing claims for Patient B, whose care costs $10,000. The ratio for this patient is only 1 percent. But the difference does not indicate that the payer handled Patient B more efficiently. It is a simple consequence of the fact that Patient B received more expensive medical treatments.

When one focuses on administrative cost per enrollee, one sees that Medicare's seeming efficiency advantage would disappear if the program were enlarged to cover the entire U.S. population, as advocates of Medicare for All propose. If the program were to expand, hundreds of millions of younger and healthier people would enter it. These people would tend to need treatments that cost less than those used by Medicare's current beneficiaries. The ratio of administrative cost to benefits paid out per enrollee would increase substantially, and Medicare's make-believe efficiency advantage would disappear.

On any sensible measure of efficiency, Medicare scores poorly. Because Medicare for All would spend more per enrollee than private carriers do, Book predicts that adopting it would increase total administrative costs by $12.5 billion a year.[20] If fraud losses were considered, the increase would be tens or hundreds of billions of dollars larger.

Finally, consider Senator Sanders' contention that Medicare for All would enable the government to negotiate fair prices for prescription drugs and other medical treatments. Again, this is a belief that many people share, including the 16 Democratic co-sponsors of Sanders' bill. But it too is laughable. To see this, just ask why Medicare doesn't bargain over prices already. The program spends more than $630 billion a year, so its financial clout with doctors, hospitals, and drug companies is enormous. But, throughout its entire existence, Medicare has been a price-taker. It has never bargained over prices. Congress forbids it.

The reasons for this are simple. First, health care providers exert great influence on Congress, and they don't want Medicare playing hardball with them over money. When Medicare was on the drawing board in the 1960s, the Democrats needed the industry's support. They got it by handing doctors and hospitals the keys to the federal treasury, that is, by agreeing to pay them whatever they billed. If Medicare for All is to become a reality, the Democrats will have to strike a deal with the devil again. The threat of using Medicare's leverage to obtain lower prices for drugs and medical treatments will be the first thing to go.

Second, if Medicare is ever going to negotiate over prices effectively, it must be willing and able to walk away from the bargaining table when a seller's demand is too high. But Medicare cannot say no. The first time it tries, a political firestorm will erupt and cries of "rationing" and "death panels" will fill the air. Remember the attack on the U.S. Preventive Services Task Force that followed its negative assessment of mammograms, and Congress's race to reverse that decision? No sensible Medicare administrator would risk a repeat of that experience by refusing to pay for an effective drug or treatment because of its price. Health care providers will know that, when bargaining with Medicare, they're playing a stare-down game with an opponent who always blinks.

## OTHER INDUSTRIALIZED COUNTRIES DO IT, WHY CAN'T WE?

Medicare for All and other single-payer programs would bring most of the health care sector under the federal government's control. Putting government in charge of another $2 trillion worth of economic activity will seem like a good idea only if one ignores what has happened during the half-century that the government has run Medicare, Medicaid, the VHA, and other programs. History provides no basis for believing that the government will ever improve quality, reduce spending, or get fraud, waste, and abuse under control. Yet Medicare for All's proponents persist in thinking that the government will magically run an enormous single-payer program better than it has ever run any other health care program before, if and when it takes over the entire health care economy.

Senator Sanders is one of these magical thinkers. Despite having seen firsthand how corrupt and inept the federal government is, he supports the creation of a comprehensive Medicare for All program that would "cover the entire continuum of health care, from inpatient to outpatient care; preventive to emergency care; primary care to specialty care, including long-term and palliative care; vision, hearing and oral health care; mental health and substance abuse services; as well as prescription medications, medical equipment, supplies, diagnostics and treatments."[21] His optimism shines through especially clearly when he compares the United States to other countries: "Other industrialized nations are making the morally principled and financially responsible decision to provide universal health care to all of their people—and they do so while saving money by keeping people healthier. Those who say this goal is unachievable are selling the American people short."[22]

It's far from clear that our government can perform these tasks. Relative to governments in other developed countries, the U.S. government appears to be unusually subject to pressure from special interests and uniquely incapable of rationing. It also often behaves as though it is run by idiots. Its saving graces have been that, for most of this country's history, the government has been comparatively small (when measured in terms of the fraction of GDP it takes in through taxes) and relatively protective of property rights.[23] By massively increasing the size of the federal government, single-payer optimists like Senator Sanders would eliminate these advantages.

Nor is it clear that the United States should want to follow other developed nations. From 2003 to 2009, per capita spending on health care, measured in real dollars, rose at an average annual rate of 2.47 percent in the United States. The median rate for all Organisation for Economic Cooperation and Development (OECD) countries was higher: 3.1 percent.

From 2009 through 2013, in the aftermath of the Great Recession, the average annual increases were smaller and nearly identical: 1.5 percent for the United States and 1.24 percent for the OECD.[24] Thus, all developed countries are experiencing rising spending, including those that currently spend much less per capita than the United States. Universal health care does not appear to be a recipe for keeping spending growth low.

Senator Sanders contends that his Medicare-for-All plan would be a bargain. His website puts the cost at "$1.38 trillion per year." It also boasts that his plan would "cost over $6 trillion less than the current health care system over the next ten years."[25] These claims are implausible on their face. They require one to believe that, even though tens of millions of Americans who are currently uninsured or underinsured will be given comprehensive coverage, spending on health care will decline. There is no precedent for this. In the past, whenever the reach of third-party payment arrangements has expanded, spending has risen. The same thing has happened every time Congress has waded into the health care swamp. For example, as Obamacare was phased in from 2013 to 2015, national health expenditures rose from $2.9 trillion to $3.2 trillion. The Medicaid expansion alone added $100 billion in spending per year, and it would have cost far more if all states had opted into the program.[26]

It is true that Obamacare cut Medicare payments to some providers. That was possible only because the program offered health care providers $2 in government subsidies for every $1 in cuts. Even left-leaning pundits like Jonathan Chait[27] and Ezra Klein[28] acknowledged that the Medicare cuts imposed by Obamacare would not have been possible without the more-than-offsetting increase in spending generated by expanding Medicaid and covering the uninsured. Spending an additional $2 to achieve $1 in cuts is not a recipe for cost control.

When thinking about costs, one must also remember that Senator Sanders' soup-to-nuts Medicare for All plan is far more generous than Obamacare was, and even more generous than the universal coverage plans used in other developed countries. As the Health Policy Center at the Urban Institute observed, Sanders' plan promises "comprehensive first-dollar government-financed health insurance for all Americans, with no benefit limits."[29] Obamacare does not come close to that. In fact, "no health care system anywhere in the world provides everyone with unlimited care," as Michael Tanner, the prolific libertarian policy analyst, points out.

> [M]any of the [foreign] systems [that American single-payer advocates] admire are neither single-payer nor free to patients....There are frequently co-payments, deductibles, and other cost-sharing requirements. In fact, in countries such as Australia, Germany, Japan, the Netherlands, and Switzerland, consumers cover a greater portion of health-care spending out-of-pocket than do Americans.[30]

With no deductibles or copays to encourage people to use medical services prudently, consumption and spending would both increase. When the Health Policy Center at the Urban Institute crunched the numbers in 2016, it concluded that, with immediate implementation of Sanders' program, "national health expenditures would increase by a total of $518.9 billion (16.9 percent) in 2017, and by $6.6 trillion (16.6 percent) between 2017 and 2026."[31] Chris Conover, a health policy researcher at Duke University, estimated that Sanders' plan would cost 40–49 percent more than advertised. To raise the revenues needed to fully cover the rise in spending, federal taxes would have had to increase by 71 percent.[32] The impact on the economy would have been terrible—a 12.8 percent reduction in after-tax income for all Americans and a 9.5 percent decline in GDP, according to the Tax Foundation, a nonpartisan group.[33]

Not surprisingly, Senator Sanders rejects these assessments. They err, he contends, by "underestimat[ing] the savings in administration, paperwork, and prescription drug prices" that his plan would generate.[34] It is remarkable that anyone could be so utopian after spending a lifetime in politics. The U.S. government has never reduced spending on health care, but Senator Sanders believes that, if Congress enacted Medicare for All, suddenly—magically—it would.

# CHAPTER 17: THE RETAIL SECTOR WILL SAVE US—IF WE LET IT

## MARCH MADNESS

If health care operated more like retail, lots of things would be different. There would be advertising and periodic sales. Loss leaders would get people in the door. Providers would open early, stay late, and compete for patients by offering services that are cheaper, better, and faster. Parking would be free and convenient. Providers would bundle goods and services to facilitate one-stop shopping. Many of these things are happening already in the part of the health care sector where consumers control the money.

Dr. Doug Stein, a Florida urologist, does vasectomies: 50 a week; 200 a month; 2,500 a year; more than 31,000 in his career.[1] To attract patients from across the state, he advertises on billboards and works out of multiple locations. He also advertises his price—$590. For his trouble, he pulls in about $300,000 a year—not the highest salary for a physician, but far more than most Americans make.

In advertising for patients, Dr. Stein is far from unique. One can find billboards touting vasectomies in many states. Occasionally, advertisements also appear on TV. In an especially creative effort to bring patients into its offices, Virginia Urology (VU) takes advantage of men's love of sports. Want an excuse for sitting on the couch and watching the NCAA March Madness basketball tournament for three days? Get a vasectomy. VU will

give you a note explaining that you need time off from work and a special recovery kit, which includes a free pizza. And your wife won't nag
you either. She'll be thrilled that she no longer needs to worry about
birth control. If VU's tactic sounds silly to you, don't go into advertising. Demand spikes every year when the tournament gets underway.[2] The
campaign is so successful that other doctors are copying it.[3]

Dr. Stein, the Florida urologist, also brings in patients by having sales.
Men who visit his clinics on days when he trains other physicians get $100
off.[4] In Indiana, the Valparaiso Vasectomy Clinic also offers vasectomies at
half off: "Get one side done & the other is FREE," its billboard screams.
Never let it be said that urologists lack a sense of humor.

### Why Don't Hospitals Have Sales?

Still, at least vasectomy clinics have sales. Hospitals never do. They don't
offer half-off specials, even though that might be a good way of attracting
patients who are considering elective procedures. And they don't offer
discounts to patients treated by medical students. This is strange because
everyone knows that experience matters. That's why Dr. Stein charges less
when patients are treated by trainees who haven't performed thousands of
vasectomies. He also recognizes a good business opportunity. Vasectomies
are elective procedures. To patients who want them but can't afford his
standard price, the $100 discount may make the difference between having
the procedure or an unwanted pregnancy.

The idea that hospitals should have sales strikes many people as funny.
Our proposal, offered in 2001, that health care providers should be paid
for curing patients, not for performing procedures, did too.[5] We suggested,
for example, that a surgeon should receive a low fee if a patient died on
the operating table or experienced an avoidable complication, and a higher one if the operation was a complete success. Our academic colleagues
scoffed at the idea. Result-based compensation arrangements were almost
unknown at the time, and the success of medical procedures depended on
so many variables, they told us, that doctors and hospitals could not possibly guarantee their work. Today, "pay-for-performance" arrangements—
known by the acronym P4P—are common. Even Medicare and Medicaid

use them. Ideas for reforming the payment system sometimes gain traction quickly, even if they seem nutty when proposed.

Besides, lots of health care providers attract business by offering discounts on their regular prices. Even hospitals do, when insurers and patients are willing to haggle. Sales and the chargemaster-based approach to pricing that hospitals normally employ are both forms of price discrimination, where sellers tailor their charges in light of purchasers' willingness to pay. The difference is that discounts off chargemaster prices are negotiated in secret while sales, which occur in public, convey more information, facilitate competition, and enable consumers to capture more of the gains from trade.

In the retail health care sector, sales are everywhere. Hospitals' opaque pricing practices seem odd by comparison.

### FLU SHOTS AS LOSS LEADERS

Consider the humble flu shot, which many retailers sell for $30 or less.[6] At Costco, they're only $15, a price that barely exceeds the $9–$10 wholesale cost of the medication. But the wheeling and dealing doesn't end there. Some retailers sell flu shots below cost by offering discounts on other items to customers who get them. At Target, an inoculation comes with a coupon good for 5 percent off a day of shopping. Randalls offers 15 percent off groceries. CVS's shopping discount is 20 percent. In 2016, Walmart dispensed flu shots for free. For many retailers, flu shots are teasers, not profit centers. They're ways of luring customers into stores, where they will see other things they want to buy.

Flu shots are simple procedures, but health care retailers offer specials on bigger-ticket items too. Consider treatments for spider veins and other cosmetic procedures. Varicose Vein Solutions, a Chicago clinic, ran a Groupon deal that cut its regular price for spider vein removal by half. Ariba Medical Spa, located in Freemont, California, offered the same deal. Its website also runs specials on Botox injections, Juvederm (another type of anti-wrinkle injection), and other services.[7] Looking further on Groupon, we found deals for laser skin treatments, Botox injections, LipoLaser, and liposuction. Dentists ran specials too, on procedures like routine exams, cleanings, whitening procedures, veneers, Invisalign tooth straightening treatments, titanium implants, abutments, and crowns.

Hospitals offer hundreds of elective procedures, including vasectomies, vein treatments, liposuctions, vaginal rejuvenations, tummy tucks, arm lifts, breast lifts, surgery for droopy ears and ear restorations following earlobe piercings, removal of skin lesions, and Botox and Restalyn injections. But their cash prices are usually hidden and they never have sales. Isn't that *stranger* than our suggestion that providers should compete on price?

### IN THE RETAIL SECTOR, PRICES DECLINE

You may be thinking that the procedures we've discussed to this point are still too simple. Hospitals are places where doctors perform complex, invasive surgeries that require general anesthesia, heart and breathing monitors, and other fancy equipment. The fact that doctors and dentists who sell relatively simple services in the self-pay sector offer discounts may not say much about the pricing practices that hospitals should apply to more serious operations.

The observation that "a vasectomy is a vasectomy" provides one answer to this challenge. A man who wants a vasectomy can get one cheaply at one of Dr. Stein's clinics or much more expensively at a hospital, where a surgeon with far less experience will perform the procedure. The location shouldn't affect the price much, but it does. A survey of providers in New York City uncovered prices ranging from $300 to $3,500. A Planned Parenthood clinic was the cheapest, while a no-needle, no-scalpel procedure performed at the Weill-Cornell Medical Center was the most expensive.[8]

A second answer is that retail outlets also have sales on complex medical procedures. Consider breast augmentation, an invasive surgery performed under general anesthesia. The Coral Gables Cosmetic Center, located in South Florida, once held a summer sale during which it offered breast augmentation surgery with saline implants performed by board-certified plastic surgeons "for just $2,800." The price included implants, anesthesia, blood work, and operating room costs.[9] In late 2013, Westlake

Plastic Surgery, located in Austin, Texas, announced a winter special. Until January 1, 2014, women wanting to look their best at holiday parties would receive "$1,200 off" breast augmentation surgery performed by Dr. Robert Caridi, a board-certified plastic surgeon with over 25 years of experience.[10] The reduced prices—$4,600 for saline implants and $5,600 for silicone—covered all charges, including his fee and the fee of a board-certified anesthesiologist as well as the use of his operating room.

Many breast augmentation, reconstruction, and reduction surgeries are performed at hospitals. But unlike retail providers, hospitals never have sales. Why is that? In the retail segment of the health care market, patients are price sensitive because they spend their own dollars. Low prices attract customers, so retail providers offer discounts and other incentives that bring patients in. Hospitals, by contrast, gear their pricing strategies toward insured patients, the most lucrative ones for them to treat. Insured patients aren't price sensitive because they bear only a small fraction of the cost of the services they receive: about 3 percent of hospital-related costs, on average. That's why hospitals rarely post their prices or have sales.

The contrast between hospitals and retail providers could hardly be starker. Hospitals' prices are industry secrets that are negotiated with insurers behind closed doors. Retailers' prices are publicly disclosed hard numbers that make it easy for patients to comparison shop. The result? Hospital services cost more and more every year, while the cost of retail services holds steady and sometimes declines.

The now-classic example of declining retail prices is LASIK, an outpatient surgical procedure that ophthalmologists perform to improve patients' vision. LASIK isn't covered by insurance, so patients pay for it directly and price competition is fierce. Google "LASIK" and you'll find lots of advertisements from doctors who offer the service. Many ads include information about prices—the very information hospitals claim to be unable to provide about other surgeries. You can also find LASIK Groupons galore, and there are price-comparison websites that help explain doctors' pricing strategies.[11] If you decide to have LASIK, you'll know the cost up front and you won't have to worry about hidden charges or being gouged.

You'll also save money on LASIK if you buy it today because, from 1996 to 2005, the real price of the service fell by nearly 30 percent.[12]

Competition made LASIK *cheaper*, thereby making it more easily available to millions of Americans who would otherwise have done without it or, at least, put it off until they could afford it. In real dollars, cosmetic surgery became less expensive too. From 1992 to 2013, "the price of consumer goods, as measured by the inflation rate, increased by about 64 percent. . . . Yet, during this same period, the price of cosmetic medicine rose only about 30 percent—less than half of the consumer price increase."[13] At the same time, demand boomed. More than 10 times as many cosmetic procedures are delivered today as were performed two decades ago.[14]

Why did LASIK and cosmetic procedures become more affordable? Consumer demand, first-party payment, and competition. As Devon Herrick, a leading commentator on retail health care, explained:

> Doctors who perform cosmetic services quote package prices, and generally adjust their fees to stay competitive. The industry is constantly developing new products and services that expand the market and compete with older services. As more cash-paying patients demand procedures, doctors rush to provide them. There are few barriers to entry in cosmetic surgery. Any licensed physician can enter the field.[15]

When we pay for health care the same way we pay for other services—by spending our own money instead of an insurer's—good things happen: prices fall and quality improves as providers compete for business.

By comparison, over the same period that LASIK and cosmetic surgery became cheaper, the prices of medical services covered by insurers rose at two to three times the rate of inflation.[16] Can you think of a single hospital-provided service whose price, like LASIK, is 30 percent lower today than it was a decade ago? We can't. Prices rise even for services that use old technologies. Computers are faster and cheaper today than ever before, but the same cannot be said for magnetic resonance imaging (MRI), CT scans, electrocardiograms, or ultrasound tests when performed in hospitals.

Competition has also moderated or driven down prices for in vitro fertilization (IVF), a service that helps women get pregnant but that patients must usually pay for directly. In 2010, Marcie Campbell, a St. Louis resident, could not afford the going rate for IVF in her area, which was about $20,000 plus several thousand more for medications. Then Dr. Elan Simckes opened Fertility Partnerships and started offering an inclusive IVF package for only $7,500. Dr. Simckes' thinking was Economics 101—competition among IVF providers would bring prices down. Unfortunately, there are limits on how effective this strategy can be, at least as long as the American Board of Obstetrics and Gynecology caps the number of new doctors that can be trained in the field each year: "The competition in fertility cannot develop if an organization can limit the number of people providing the service."[17]

Naturally, doctors with established IVF practices in St. Louis "felt threatened by the pricing model" and went ballistic. They shouted loudly that patients shouldn't choose providers on the basis of cost and that IVF services shouldn't be treated like an industry. Taking a jab at retail medicine, one of Dr. Simckes' competitors fumed, "This isn't Walmart. Embryos aren't like toothpaste." But what counts in the IVF world is the frequency with which live births occur after embryos are implanted, and on that metric, Fertility Partnerships outperformed the doctor who was complaining.[18]

Fast forward to 2016. Fertility Partnerships is still doing business in St. Louis, but now it has competition. The Missouri Center for Reproductive Medicine (MCRM) offers its inclusive premium package, IVF Gold, for less than $10,000 and also boasts of providing "medication protocols that yield successful outcomes at a cost as low as $1,000."[19] MCRM also offers discounts to military personnel, first responders, educators, and medical-service employees.

Other discounters are also entering the field, and some of them are bundling services even more attractively. Typically, IVF clinics bill for their services separately from the pharmacies they send their patients to for fertility-enhancing drugs. Pharmacies' charges add $3,000–$6,000 to the final tally. WINFertility, a company that "manages the treatment of thousands of infertility patients annually," makes one-stop shopping possible at an attractive all-inclusive price. It deals directly with drug manufacturers, specialty pharmacies, and qualified fertility specialists on a large scale, then includes drugs in its prices, which, on average, are 36.5 percent lower than prevailing unbundled rates.[20]

Embryos aren't toothpaste. But retailers can figure out how to deliver both toothpaste and successful pregnancies less expensively when given free rein to innovate.

## Hospitals Jack up Prices . . . Because They Can

In 2017, *ProPublica* reported that Children's Hospital Colorado charged $1,877.86 to pierce a 5-year old girl's ears. The surgeon who performed the procedure charged the girl's family another $110 for that service, bringing the total to almost $2,000. (The girl's mother, who brought her in for a minor surgical procedure, assumed the doctor was throwing in the ear piercing for free, since her daughter was already under anesthesia.) To add insult to injury, "the surgeon's piercing of one ear was off-kilter so it had to be redone"—which it was, at a shopping mall, for $30.[21]

*ProPublica*'s story is far from unique. Reports of absurd hospital charges are common. After having a cesarean section, one new mother received a hospital bill that included a $39.95 charge for holding her baby against her chest. The hospital labeled the charge "skin to skin."[22] After being bitten on the foot by a snake while taking out the garbage, Eric Ferguson went to the Lake Norman Regional Medical Center, where he was given anti-venom and monitored. The hospital's list price for the medication was $81,000. The discounted price his insurer negotiated was about $20,000. The retail price of anti-venom online? $750.[23]

In 2013, the *New York Times* compared retail charges for five routine supplies and services with the list prices charged by the California Pacific Medical Center (CPMC).[24] In every instance, the retail price was much lower. A pain pill that retailed for 50 cents fetched $36.78 when sold by CPMC. CPMC charged $137 for a bag of IV fluid that cost $1 and $154 for a neck brace whose retail price was $20.

Other price comparisons made hospitals look bad too. A breast-pump kit that cost $543 at the hospital was available for $25 online. A CT scan of the abdomen sold for $4,495 at the hospital versus $400 at an outpatient facility nearby. The hospital priced a blood count test and a blood electrolyte test at $259.06 and $293.25, respectively. The same tests usually cost less than $10 each at independent labs. The hospital billed a vial of skin glue at $181, a tube of antibiotic cream at $125.84, and a vial of local anesthetic at $79.73. These items cost $15.99, $36.99, and $5, respectively, on the internet. And, lest one forget, hospitals buy medical supplies in bulk at wholesale prices.

Want more comparisons? How about charging $18 for diabetes test strips that are available on Amazon.com for 56 cents apiece in boxes of 50, and $24 for niacin pills that cost only 5 cents each at retail drugstores? That's what the Seton Medical Center in Daly City, California, did. It also charged $77 for a box of sterile gauze pads, the retail price of which was probably a few bucks.[25]

These are not isolated examples. Look online and you'll find countless articles reporting that hospitals charged obscene amounts for goods and services that were available much more cheaply at retail outlets. One appeared under the title "How to Charge $546 for Six Liters of Saltwater."[26] The "saltwater" was normal saline solution that hospitals purchased for 46 cents to $1.07 per liter bag then resold to patients for hundreds of dollars. "Some of the patients' bills . . . include markups of 100 to 200 times the manufacturer's price, not counting separate charges for 'IV administration.' And on other bills, a bundled charge for 'IV therapy' was almost 1,000 times the official cost of the solution." Insurers commonly pay hospitals twice as much for artificial joints as the devices cost.[27]

In 2015, *Health Affairs* published a study entitled "Extreme Markup: The Fifty U.S. Hospitals with the Highest Charge-to-Cost Ratios." Using bills filed by almost 4,500 hospitals, researchers compared hospitals' chargemaster rates to Medicare's allowable cost, which "includes both direct patient cost (for example, emergency department, operating room, and intensive care) and indirect general service cost (for example, administration, laundry, and pharmacy)" for all patients, not just seniors. "On average, U.S. hospital charges were 3.4 times the Medicare-allowable cost." As if that wasn't bad enough, the 50 hospitals with the highest charge-to-allowable-rate ratios "charge[d], on average, 10.1 times their cost. This means that they [we]re charging markups of more than 1,000 percent."[28]

Hospitals offer a variety of rationales for their listed prices. They claim to overcharge some patients in order to cover the cost of charity care for others. They argue that their costs are high because they make ancillary services available and offer round-the-clock care. The truth is less pleasant.

Hospitals impose absurd markups because they *can*, and because by doing so they maximize their revenues and their managers' and employees' salaries. As the authors of the *Health Affairs* article concluded, the main causes of high markups are pricing opacity and hospitals' superior bargaining power. Another factor, discussed in Chapter 8, is that Medicare literally rewards hospitals for increasing their chargemaster prices. The predictable result is that many hospital services are cash cows. As Steven Brill writes, "Outpatient care is wildly profitable" and accounts for about $500 billion a year in overspending.[29]

The executives who run companies that deliver medical treatments in the retail sector are not angels, and those who run hospitals are not devils. All are managing their companies in profit-maximizing ways. Retail-medicine executives would probably charge outrageous prices too if they could. *But they can't, because they have to compete with other retailers for cost-conscious patients.* And that's the point.

## Cheaper Hearing Aids Are on the Way

In the retail sector, ridiculous markups are impossible to maintain. Walgreens can't charge $100 for a few aspirin tablets when CVS sells a bottle of 100 pills for $5. To compete with their many rivals, whose prices are low and easy to find, retail pharmacies have to sell medical goods and services as cheaply as they can. This includes prescription drugs, whose prices once were hidden but are now advertised. There are even online price comparison websites that, when given the name of a drug and a zip code, will show the prices at nearby pharmacies.[30]

We're so confident that competition among retailers can make medical goods and services cheaper, we'll go out on a limb. Over the next 10 years, we predict, hearing aids will become better and more affordable. Why? Retailers have broken the lock audiologists once held on their distribution. Today, digital hearing aids are available at Costco, Sam's Club, and Amazon.com, high-volume sellers known for cutting costs. Smaller, more specialized outlets like Audicus.com offer fancier models that cost up to $649—pricey but still far less than most audiologists charge. As more retailers enter the field, prices will become easier to compare and competition will intensify. Bargain-hungry consumers will look for better deals, but they will be interested in quality too. A hearing aid that works poorly isn't a bargain, even if it's cheap. With pressure on both quality and price, retail offerings are bound to improve.

We'll even make a second prediction: audiologists' charges will also fall, or audiologists will lose business. If they keep their prices high, they won't be able to compete with Costco Hearing Aid Centers, which offer similar services—including product demonstrations, hearing tests, follow-up appointments, cleanings, check-ups, loss and damage coverage (with no deductible), warranties, 10 extra batteries, and a 90-day trial period—at no additional cost. Currently, audiologists' charges for ancillary services like these "account for up to 70 percent of the final price of a hearing aid."[31] In the face of competition from retailers like Costco, we doubt that such steep markups will last. It seems likely that audiologists will have to price their hearings aids and services separately and minimize the cost of both.

We are confident that competition will make hearing aids more affordable because retailers have driven down prices for medical services before. Past being prologue, it is reasonable to expect them to do so again.

There is a complicating factor, however. Some insurance plans cover hearing tests and hearing aids. The more insurers are involved, the longer it will take the retail sector to force prices downward because insured patients care less than others about costs.

## Retail Medicine Is Viral

Retail medicine can spread quickly too. Flu shots again provide an example. "Before the H1N1 pandemic of 2009, almost no pharmacists administered flu vaccines. But [in 2012], pharmacists working for Deerfield, Ill.-based Walgreen Co. administered 5.5 million flu shots among the 9 million vaccines they delivered."[32] CVS did 3.5 million more.[33] Although most people still go to doctors' offices to be treated, "about 20 percent of adults received shots at a retail pharmacy [in 2011], up from 12 percent the previous year, according to the Centers for Disease Control and Prevention."[34]

Many more people receive flu shots at mass inoculations staged by their employers, who'd rather get all their workers treated quickly and cheaply than lose work days to doctors' office visits or illness.

The trend away from traditional providers reflects price and convenience. Retailers have lots of locations, see patients quickly and without appointments, are open year-round, and charge bargain-basement rates. MedStar Health, a retail outlet that operates in Maryland, makes sure that its stores are easy to find by locating them near Starbucks coffee shops.

No wonder retail clinics are gaining ground in a host of areas that were formerly the bread and butter of traditional providers, including

- Vaccinations for pneumonia and shingles;
- Screenings for high cholesterol, lipid levels, blood pressure, pregnancy, and colorectal cancer;
- Assessment, treatment, and management of chronic conditions like asthma, diabetes, and hypertension; and
- Treatment of simple acute conditions such as upper respiratory infections, sinusitis, urinary tract infections, allergic rhinitis, influenza, bronchitis, sore throat, inner ear infections, swimmer's ear, and conjunctivitis.

As clinics become better established, they're offering a broader range of services too. WakeMed Health and Hospitals, which operates in Raleigh, North Carolina, responded to cardiovascular patients' desire for convenience by developing a pilot program for deep vein thrombosis testing.

To see how much ground retail pharmacies cover, how quickly they've spread, and where they're likely to wind up in the future, consider CVS, now arguably the country's biggest health care company.[35] Around the start of the 2010s, CVS operated about 650 MinuteClinics in 25 states and Washington, D.C. It also sold tobacco products, which brought in about $2 billion a year. Then, in 2014 and 2015, the company rebranded itself. It changed its name to CVS Health, removed all tobacco products from its stores, made plans to increase the number of clinics to 1,500 by 2017, established a host of relationships with existing health care provider networks, and bought all of Target's pharmacies and in-store clinics for

$1.9 billion. By 2016, CVS Health had 1,135 clinics up and running in 33 states, and "about 50% of the U.S. population actually live[d] within 10 miles of a Minute Clinic."[36] CVS Health literally bet the company that the retail medical marketplace will expand.

CVS Health is making the future happen too. In 2015, it teamed up with IBM, which can help CVS's clinical personnel improve the diagnosis and treatment of health problems by applying evidence-based decision techniques and using data mining to predict patients' likely medical needs.[37] With IBM and CVS working together, millions of people may one day be able to sit in kiosks and use a computer to quickly assess the accuracy of medical diagnoses, the desirability of recommended prescriptions, and the availability of alternatives. The joint venture may be an especially valuable source of information for patients with chronic diseases like hypertension, heart disease, diabetes, and obesity, four leading causes of death and disability that collectively account for more than 80 percent of health care spending.[38]

Target is using similar data-mining techniques to determine which of its customers are likely to be pregnant. It then sends them coupons and ads for things they are likely to need. Sometimes, Target knows about pregnancies sooner than some people might like.

> About a year after [Target began using the] pregnancy-prediction model, a man walked into a Target outside Minneapolis and demanded to see the manager. He was clutching coupons that had been sent to his daughter, and he was angry, according to an employee who participated in the conversation. "My daughter got this in the mail!" he said. "She's still in high school, and you're sending her coupons for baby clothes and cribs? Are you trying to encourage her to get pregnant?"
>
> The manager didn't have any idea what the man was talking about. He looked at the mailer. Sure enough, it was addressed to the man's daughter and contained advertisements for maternity clothing, nursery furniture and pictures of smiling infants. The manager apologized and then called a few days later to apologize again.
>
> On the phone, though, the father was somewhat abashed. "I had a talk with my daughter," he said. "It turns out there's been some activities in my house I haven't been completely aware of. She's due in August. I owe you an apology."[39]

When it comes to the use of technology to improve the delivery of health services, the future is now.

## The Doctor Shortage May Be Organized Medicine's Undoing

Retail clinics provide lots of medical services on a first-party payer basis. Although they accept insurance, patients pay out of pocket one-third of the time. By contrast, patients who visit primary care physicians spend their own money only 10 percent of the time.[40] One should therefore expect retail clinics to give patients more of what they want—quality care delivered efficiently—and less of what insurers want—expensive care that makes insurers indispensable. Consumers' preference for retail providers will likely intensify in the near future, as a strategy that organized medicine has long used to inflate physicians' incomes finally backfires.

For decades, the medical profession has kept the number of doctors artificially low, by preventing new medical schools from opening and limiting the number of graduates. The Association of American Medical Colleges predicts a shortfall of 12,000 to 31,000 primary care doctors by 2025.[41] Most newly minted physicians receive 50 or more job offers during their residencies. Half receive 100 or more.[42] This induced shortage makes doctors wealthier than they would otherwise be.

But the shortage of physicians also means that patients must often wait to be treated. Even before Obamacare added millions of people to the insurance rolls, delays of two to three weeks were common in many cities.[43] Now, as demand for medical services increases, waits will predictably increase too. This signal of unmet demand substantially strengthens the "business case" for retailers to enter the health care market. With tens of thousands of credentialed pharmacists, physician assistants, and nurse practitioners available to see patients after waits of 15–20 minutes, traditional doctors' offices will be easy pickings.

The rise of retail medicine will also erode the norm of going to doctors' offices and emergency rooms for medical treatments. When getting a flu shot, being treated for a urinary tract infection, or having a diabetes check-up at a retail clinic feels normal, people will wonder why they ever wasted their time in waiting rooms, and physicians will struggle to hold on to patients. Urgent care clinics will do the same to hospital emergency rooms. Why put up with the rigmarole, delays, and hidden costs that hospitals impose when an urgent care clinic can handle a minor emergency just as well and is conveniently located in the nearest shopping center?

Massachusetts, the state whose mandatory insurance program, enacted under Governor Mitt Romney, became the model for Obamacare, provides a taste of what is to come. From 2010 to 2012, the typical wait to see a family physician went from 29 to 45 days. Delays are especially long in Boston, where patients often wait two months to see their family physicians.[44] That's why, in the 2010–2012 period, CVS could profitably open 37 new MinuteClinics in Massachusetts, a state that had only 13 retail clinics *total* in 2009.[45] If the medical cartel had done a halfway decent job providing high-quality care conveniently and affordably, retail medicine would never have gotten off the launching pad.

## RETAIL IS HERE TO STAY

Doctors haven't taken the threat from retailers lying down, of course. They first tried to kill the retail clinic movement in its infancy. When that effort failed, they launched a rear-guard action to limit further encroachments.

Since 2007, the American Medical Association (AMA) and state medical societies have called for governmental investigations of joint ventures between retailers and pharmacy chains and for restrictions on the services that retail clinics can provide.[46] They have tried to capture a portion of the profits that retail clinics generate by supporting regulations that require nonphysician providers to be supervised by physicians.[47] They also protect their turf by pushing "scope of practice" recommendations that, if adopted by state legislatures or regulators, would limit what clinics can do.[48]

Doctors don't want competition from other types of providers, either. "Physicians, whom the nurses call 'organized medicine,' are the main people standing in the way of bills that expand the scope of what nurses are allowed to practice."[49] Fortunately, nurses have won recent battles. Twenty-one states have enacted laws that give them what is known as full practice authority, meaning they can prescribe medications and operate without direct oversight from physicians. But the turf war continues. In mid-2017, the AMA's House of Delegates endorsed a measure requiring the organization to oppose efforts by physician assistants to gain the freedom to practice without having to report to physicians.[50] For years, the AMA has fought legislation that would allow pharmacists to prescribe medications too.[51]

Despite these efforts, doctors haven't been able to prevent retailers from expanding. Their appeals to elected officials have faced several impediments. First, the medical industry is split. Although CVS Health and Walgreens operate most of the existing retail clinics, many hospital chains and physician groups are also involved, including big players like the Mayo Clinic, Aurora Health Care, and Sutter.[52] In Oklahoma, MinuteClinic teamed up with OU Physicians, a group of 560 doctors, some of whom became the clinics' medical directors. Providers with stakes in the success of retail clinics don't want them to fold. Second, the big retailers have enough wealth and lobbyists to counter organized medicine's political campaign.[53] Third, doctors' groups have an obvious financial conflict of interest, which makes it easier to dismiss their complaints. As Dr. Sam Unterricht, the president of the Medical Society of the State of New York, candidly admitted, his organization opposes retail clinics because they pose "a threat to physicians financially."[54] "Retail clinics will cost doctors money" isn't a winning public relations message.

Recognizing this, doctors' lobbies have also employed their traditional gambit of purporting to speak for patients. The medical profession contends that retail clinics endanger patients by using simplistic decision and treatment protocols, disrupting doctor–patient relationships, overprescribing medications, and fragmenting the delivery of health care.[55] These assertions have little or no empirical support.

In fact, when it comes to treating minor illnesses, retail clinics often achieve better quality scores than physicians. A 2007 study published in the *American Journal of Medical Quality* reported that retail clinics adhered to established clinical guidelines for the treatment of sore throats 99 percent of the time, a record few family physicians can match.[56] A 2011 study that appeared in the same journal found that children served at retail clinics received similarly high levels of recommended care.[57] A 2013 study found that patients who visited retail clinics generated lower total treatment costs than similar patients who were treated elsewhere.[58] These findings should not be surprising. Retail clinics are staffed by nurse practitioners, who have been shown in many studies to deliver primary care that "is as good as and sometimes better than care given by physicians" and "patients often express higher satisfaction with care delivered by nurses."[59]

The most detailed study of retail clinics, led by researchers at RAND, was published in the *Annals of Internal Medicine* in 2009. It compared the treatments patients enrolled in a large Minnesota health plan received for three medical conditions—otitis media (ear ache), pharyngitis (sore throat), and urinary tract infection—at retail clinics, physician offices, urgent care centers, and emergency rooms. The evaluation covered three dimensions: cost, performance on 14 quality metrics, and receipt of seven preventive services. The conclusion was clear and unambiguous: "Retail clinics provide less costly treatment than physician offices or urgent care centers . . . with no apparent adverse effect on quality of care or delivery of preventive care." How much less costly? Forty to 80 percent less. The comparison to ERs was especially revealing: "In emergency departments, average prescription costs were higher and aggregate quality scores were significantly lower than in other settings." Retail clinics are far better places than emergency rooms for patients with minor problems.[60]

### If You Can't Beat Them, Join Them

If retail clinics are here to stay—and the studies provide no basis for curtailing them—physicians will have to adapt. To hold on to patients, they will have to reduce wait times and cut costs. Many have already taken steps in both directions by bringing nurse practitioners and physician assistants on board. This is all to the good. Newly minted physicians cost more than $1 million each to produce. People educated that intensively should provide high-value services that require the creative application of medical knowledge. They shouldn't spend precious time on problems that other professionals can treat every bit as effectively at far less cost.

Some physician groups have decided to compete with retailers by becoming more consumer friendly. In 2007, HealthCare Partners Medical Group, California's largest private physician practice with more than 500,000 patients, posted its prices for 58 common procedures online. A chest X-ray ran $61, a physical exam for a middle-aged patient cost $140–$160, and flu vaccinations were $15, plus a $31 administrative fee.

Why the shift from secrecy to disclosure? "The move was motivated in part by the rapid advance of walk-in medical clinics at drugstore chains and discount retailers, such as CVS Caremark Corp. and Wal-Mart Stores Inc., where the prices of blood pressure checks and flu shots are as easy to spot as those for rubbing alcohol and cat food." When asked about the move, Dr. Robert Margolis, the practice group's founder and chief executive, replied sagely, "It feels like the right thing to do." Funny how it didn't feel like the right thing to do until retailers started poaching patients.[61]

In 2009, the Surgery Center of Oklahoma (SCO) did the Health-Care Partners Medical Group one better.[62] It posted all-inclusive charges for 112 common surgeries, refused to accept Medicare or Medicaid, and negotiated payment arrangements with employers that bypassed conventional insurers. Drs. Keith Smith and Steve Lantier, SCO's cofounders, adopted this approach after becoming disillusioned by the traditional hospital business model.

SCO is a for-profit business. It keeps its prices low by being efficient. Wait times for physicians and patients are minimized, increasing the number of procedures that can be performed. The staff is lean too. With few exceptions, every employee at SCO is directly involved in patient care. By comparison, Integris Health, a nominally nonprofit organization that runs the nearby Integris Baptist Medical Center in Oklahoma City, had 18 administrators whose compensation averaged $413,000. "One reason our prices are so low," Dr. Smith remarked, "is that we don't have administrators running around in their four or five thousand dollar suits."[63]

The impact on prices is enormous. Integris charged $33,505 for a complex bilateral sinus procedure, which helps patients with chronic nasal infections. This bill covered only hospitalization; the fees for the surgeon and the anesthesiologist were extra. At SCO, the *all-inclusive* price for the same operation is $5,885. Not surprisingly, Integris's bill was loaded with overcharges, including $360 for a steroid available at wholesale for just 75 cents, and $630 for three doses of a painkiller called fentanyl citrate, which all together cost the hospital about $1.50.[64]

SCO deals mostly in cash. Companies that self-fund their workers' health care benefits pay SCO directly, as do patients. Keeping traditional insurers out of the picture helps reduce costs. The same is true for other providers, many of which are starting to offer discounts for cash. Sometimes the discounts are so big that patients are better off bearing the whole cost themselves, rather than using their insurance. Jo Ann Snyder learned this the hard way. A hospital in Long Beach, California, charged her $6,707 for a CT scan. Her deductible and copay brought her share of the bill to $2,336; her insurer paid the rest. She later learned that the *total* price would have been $1,054 if she had paid for the scan in cash.[65] She thought that her insurer, Blue Shield of California, had negotiated a good price for the service. It hadn't.

Other area hospitals offered even better deals. When Chad Terhune, the *Los Angeles Times* reporter who covered Snyder's story, called around, he discovered that the Los Alamitos Medical Center, which listed the price of an abdominal CT scan at $4,423 on a state-run website, had a negotiated rate with Blue Shield of $2,400 and a cash price of $250. All eight of the hospitals contacted reported similarly large discounts for cash, although Los Alamitos had the lowest price overall.

A hospital in Boulder, Colorado, that wanted $600 for a knee X-ray when a patient used her high-deductible insurance policy, charged only $70 when she paid cash up front.[66] When the patient later needed an MRI, the hospital offered her a choice between paying $1,100 with her insurance or only $600 in cash. Regional Medical Imaging in Flint, Michigan, charges $510 for an MRI of the knee when patients use high-deductible plans but only $265 when they pay cash. The perversity of this practice should be evident. In both cases, the patient may bear the entire cost because even the higher charge may fall wholly within a patient's deductible. But even so, bringing insurance into the picture, even if only to get credit against one's annual deductible, increases the price.

When it comes to insurance making things more expensive, generic drugs offer a clean example. Consider what Dr. David Belk, who blogs at True Cost of Healthcare, wrote about pharmacies' charges for amlodipine:

> I'll always ask a new patient about the cost of their medications. A patient might tell me (for example) "I have high blood pressure," and then hand me a prescription he recently bought of amlodipine (a common medication for high blood pressure). So I'll ask, "How much did you pay for this amlodipine?" "Not much," he'll say. "I have insurance, so it only costs me $10 a month."

It only takes a few phone calls to change his view. I'll often start by calling the pharmacy where he bought the medication (CVS for example) and ask, "If someone buys your club card for a $15 annual fee, how much would three months (90 pills) of amlodipine cost? Answer: $12. Next, I'll call Costco and ask: "How much will a full year's supply (365 pills) of amlodipine cost a person who doesn't use insurance?" Answer: $26.49! For a full year!

So, what's going on? Why do patients get such bad deals when they use their insurance?[67]

Elsewhere, Belk answers his own question:

In the last decade most of the patents for these medications have expired, and so now more than 80% of the medicines that are commonly pre-scribed by doctors are generic and very cheap. Medications that used to cost pharmacies $400 for 100 pills (and then were sold to you for a profit) now cost pharmacies anywhere from $1–$10 per 100 pills. That's right: many medicines got more than 100 times cheaper. What they sell them for, though, is their business.

Most pharmacies realized that it wasn't in their interest to tell anyone that drug prices were dropping. With everyone used to using insurance to buy their medication, the pharmacies could just continue to charge the same copay, and make a substantial profit without receiving any payment from the insurance company. In the meantime, the insurance companies were happy because people still bought prescription drug coverage for these medications, believing that they were saving money when, in fact, they weren't. It cost the insurance company nothing so everyone won (except the customer).

The copays are still based entirely on the insurance plan so the same medicine in the same pharmacy might cost $5, $10 or $25 for a months' supply. To see how much of a windfall this is for retail pharmacies, we need only to look at the finances of the two largest retail pharmacies in the US: CVS and Walgreens. Since 2001 both CVS and Walgreens have tripled their total revenue from retail pharmacy sales and doubled their number of retail pharmacies in the US. They were able to fund this growth mostly from the sale of generic prescription medications sold to customers, almost all of whom used a third-party payer (insurance) to buy their prescriptions.

What's more, people might pay several hundred dollars a year to get prescription drug coverage on their insurance, even though that coverage increases the cost of many medications and cost[s] the insurance company nothing. It's like buying a book of coupons that say "one for the price of two" at your local grocery store. You can see why they didn't want to tell you about it.[68]

Other commentators have also discovered that insurance coverage for generic medicines can be a scam.[69] More evidence that the interests of consumers and insurers are not the same.

### PAY YOUR DOCTOR THE WAY YOU PAY YOUR GYM

At retail clinics, patients may see different medical professionals on different visits. One nurse may treat a patient's sore throat, and a different nurse may be on duty when the patient returns for a follow-up visit. This worries Shannon Brownlee, a leading commentator on health policy, who contends that many patients, especially those who are older or have chronic conditions, need ongoing relationships with physicians. Brownlee predicts that retailers will siphon off the easier and more profitable cases that can be handled quickly, leaving the less profitable patients who require extended consultations to primary care physicians. To protect the fragile finances of these doctors' practices, Brownlee wants "state regulators [to] limit the scope of services retail clinics are permitted to provide." Otherwise, "we will watch health care become a commodity, and an ancient and honored profession [will be] replaced by drugstore chains."[70]

Brownlee's recommendation is the sort of top-down, Rube Goldberg solution that only a mainstream health policy analyst could love. Wanting physicians to spend more time with patients who need longer visits, she would prevent millions of people from using retail health care delivery services that are quick, convenient, and cheap. Needless to say, her proposal fails to create the incentives that might make it work. Rather than spend extra time with needy patients, doctors would maximize their gains by handling lots of easy cases and telling everyone else to take a hike. But, even if the proposal would work, shouldn't more direct options be explored before the government curtails the freedom of millions of consumers?

A direct solution exists too. Patients who would benefit from longer consultations can simply pay for that service. They can buy nurses' or physician assistants' time at retail clinics. They can buy doctors' time too. They can even purchase advice for dealing with chronic illnesses online. Direct purchasing will drive down the cost of advice too, for the same reason that prices for simpler stuff fall: because people are spending their own money. When everyone pays directly, everyone gets what they need and no one is forced to use inferior delivery arrangements.

Consider patients who use concierge doctors. By paying a monthly fee, these patients receive unlimited access to basic medical services, just like members receive unlimited access to their gyms. Typically, the fees vary on the basis of age, which proxies for predicted usage. In 2015, Atlas MD, a concierge practice run by Drs. Doug Nunamaker and Josh Umbehr, charged $10 per month for children up to 19 years old, $50 for people who are 20 to 44, $75 for those who are 45 to 64, and $100 for patients 65 and older.[71] "Everything the doctors can do in their office is included in the fee. They also give a lot of advice by e-mail and on the phone."[72] Atlas MD also helps patients by negotiating deals with outside vendors on services the practice doesn't provide. A cholesterol test costs their patients $3, a tiny fraction of the $90 charge that the lab they deal with bills to insurers. An MRI costs $400 instead of $2,000, again the typical third-party charge.[73]

Concierge practices limit their size to ensure that patients will receive quick access to services and unhurried treatments. Doctors associated with Atlas MD are responsible for no more than 600 patients, far fewer than the 1,000 to 2,000 patients a typical family physician sees. The arrangement works well for older people and those with chronic conditions who want to spend more time with their doctors. Consider the case of Scotti and Lois Fullbright, who moved to Wichita, Kansas, to be near their grandchildren.[74] By paying $75 each per month, they "could see the primary care doctors at Atlas MD as many times as they wanted. Now, they get an appointment within a day, and they have unlimited access to the doctors by phone and e-mail."

Some practitioners who operate on the concierge model even make house calls. Heidi Johnson, a pediatric nurse practitioner, visits sick kids at home. This eliminates the need for patients and their parents to travel, only to spend time waiting in a doctor's lobby with other sick children. Johnson charges $80 per visit and does not take insurance. The cost is comparable to the $77 fee patients' insurers ordinarily pay pediatricians and to the charges patients would incur at an urgent care clinic. If more than one child needs attention, Johnson gives a discount, charging just $50 for the second sick sibling she sees on the same visit. All of the prices are listed on Johnson's website. Johnson limits her practice to 1,500 patients, more than normal for a concierge practice; but, judging from her patients' evaluations, she manages the workload well.[75]

Concierge medicine is picking up steam. According to Tom Blue, chief strategy officer of the American Academy of Private Physicians, there were about 5,500 concierge doctors in the United States by 2013, up from 4,400 the preceding year.[76] That's a one-year annual growth rate of 25 percent. Most concierge doctors charge about $100 a month per patient—more than Atlas MD—and have 300 to 600 patients as members.

Concierge practices generate an obvious complaint: only people who are rich enough to pay the monthly fees can afford them. But many people pay more for insurance than Atlas charges, especially when the calculation includes employers' contributions, which are just deductions from workers' wages. Consumer demand may also encourage the creation of low-cost practice groups for people whose incomes are low. Retailers like Walmart have figured out how to provide lots of goods and services to this segment of the population. They may figure out how to deliver health care too, if given the freedom to do so.

Kathleen Stoll, director of health policy at a consumer advocacy group named Families U.S.A., expresses two related complaints about concierge medicine. She worries, first, that because concierge practices provide a limited range of services, patients who experience serious illnesses requiring expensive tests and procedures will be left on their own. She also has unspecified misgivings about patients paying for health care with their own money. "I'm always cautious when it's a cash basis," she said. "Are you somehow being put at risk? I'd have a list of questions."[77]

The first concern is legitimate. Patients who join concierge practices must make separate plans for catastrophic health care needs. They typically do so by purchasing policies with high deductibles. These plans are much cheaper than traditional plans, but they do cost money. The second concern reflects the corrosive impact that widespread reliance on third-party payers has had on health policy analysts. First-party payment—the way people usually pay for cars, houses, food, computers, telephones, and pretty much everything other than health care—works extremely well for consumers. It puts them in the driver's seat by pressuring sellers to deliver the goods and services consumers want at prices they can afford. Our experience with third-party payment hasn't been nearly as good.

## Let Costco Run the Mayo Clinic

It is hard to argue with a straight face that the health care system is run efficiently. So why shouldn't Costco, a members-only retail empire, be able to operate a soup-to-nuts program covering all of its customers' medical needs, including treatments now delivered in hospitals and doctors' offices as well as the basic services walk-in clinics provide? Costco would employ or contract with doctors, just as it currently employs or contracts with the medical professionals who staff walk-in clinics. Billing for most services would be handled internally on a cash basis, but customers with insurance could send receipts to their carriers for reimbursement. Costco would also handle all other logistics associated with the delivery of care.

Presumably, a Costco-run soup-to-nuts medical operation would draw on everything and anything that works: retail clinics for customers' basic needs, concierge services when the special talents of physicians are required, and surgical treatments based on SCO's fixed-price business model. And, if Costco's health care business had to compete with similar operations run by Sam's Club and CVS Health, competition would pressure all three retailers to do something they're good at—minimize prices by squeezing out inefficiencies while delivering services conveniently in surroundings that customers like. In theory, the retail sector could bring spiraling health care costs under control. The question is: Will we let it?

Although the answer should be yes, recent history indicates that the American Hospital Association and other industry representatives will fight tooth and nail to prevent competition. Twenty years ago, physician-owned specialty hospitals were unheard of. In 2000, they accounted for about 1 percent of Medicare spending.[78] Within a decade, though, specialty hospitals had grown so much that they threatened the profitability of traditional hospitals. How did the old-line industry respond? By convincing Congress to put a provision into Obamacare that prevents new physician-owned hospitals from being built and also keeps existing specialty hospitals from expanding.[79]

The restriction is blatantly anti-patient. In 2012, Medicare designated hospitals to receive bonus payments as a reward for quality achievements. The first hospital on the list was Treasure Valley Hospital in Boise, Idaho—a physician-owned facility. In fact, 9 of the top 10 performing hospitals were physician owned, as were 48 of the top 100.[80] Specialty hospitals make up less than 10 percent of all hospitals in the United States, but they dominated Medicare's quality list.

No one knows what the next great innovation in the delivery of health care will be. It could be retail medicine, urgent care clinics, or a personal health "app" that a handful of entrepreneurs currently have on the drawing board. It could come from Amazon, which is positioning itself to break into the retail pharmacy market and may possibly combine efficient drug delivery with telemedicine.[81] But one thing is certain. Old-line providers will fight any innovation that would make health care better or cheaper at their expense. The past is the best predictor of the future, and they've done this time and again.

We don't let local hardware stores decide where Home Depot and Lowe's can open stores. We don't let local appliance stores control the spread of Sears, Kohls, or Best Buy. We don't let local grocers prevent Whole Foods, Trader Joes, or Walmart from invading their turf. And we should not give health care providers veto power over competitive entry.

The evidence that retailers can manage the delivery of medical treatments well is clear. There is no health care cost crisis in the retail sector and never has been. Retailers sell a vast array of health-related products, including pain relievers, antiseptics, toothpaste, dental floss, cold and heat packs, nicotine gum, pregnancy test kits, and treatments for colds, allergies, burns, warts, fungal infections, swimmer's ear, and a host of other conditions, all of which are competitively priced. If you're seriously devoted to good dental health, you can buy a plaque-destroying Sonicare electric tooth-brush for $50. That's about half what the same item cost 10 years ago.[82] Almost every retail pharmacy has a blood pressure machine that customers can use for free. When we buy health care directly at retail, we're treated very well.

The health care cost crisis is a byproduct of the third-party payment system. Imagine what the food business would look like if most people had "grocery insurance." As former senator Phil Gramm sagely observed in one of the epigraphs that begin this book, if we had a system "where 95 percent of what you put in your grocery basket [was] paid for by grocery insurance, you would eat differently, and so would your dog."[83] Americans will be much better off when we buy health care the same way we buy everything else.

# CHAPTER 18: BARGAINS GALORE IN BANGALORE

## Your Passport Is Your Ticket to Lower Prices

In the United States, prices for health care are astronomical. That's a big reason why many Americans seek medical treatments abroad, where the same services are far cheaper. The precise number of medical tourists is not known, but Patients Beyond Borders puts the number at 1.4 million.[1] AARP's estimate is lower—1 million, with dental work "accounting for about a third of all health-related trips, followed by surgeries such as coronary-bypass and bariatric operations, at 29 percent. About 13 percent of American medical travelers seek cosmetic surgery, and 7 percent get orthopedic procedures such as hip and knee replacements."[2]

The amounts medical tourists save by getting treatments abroad vary depending on the procedure and the destination. Many countries, including Costa Rica, India, Malaysia, Mexico, Thailand, and Turkey, offer Americans the chance to cut their medical bills by half or more. A hysterectomy is likely to cost $32,000 in the United States but can be had for only $4,000 in Thailand. A kidney transplant goes for $150,000 here at home but costs only $25,000 in the Philippines. An American couple can expect to spend about $20,000 for a round of in vitro fertilization here but can get the same service in Israel for only $3,500.[3] The more a medical service costs at home, the more Americans can save by going abroad. For big-ticket items, the savings can be large even after deducting the cost of travel.

Of course, quality and safety matter as well. But that's where many foreign health care providers excel. They offer services that are as good as or better than those Americans can get at home. "[M]any hospitals— particularly the larger institutions in Asia and Southeast Asia—boast lower morbidity rates than in the U.S., particularly when it comes to complex cardiac and orthopedic surgeries, for which success rates higher than 98.5 percent are the norm."[4] These aren't fly-by-night operators. "[S]everal major medical schools in the United States have developed joint initiatives with overseas providers, such as the Harvard Medical School Dubai Center, the Johns Hopkins Singapore International Medical Center, and the Duke-National University of Singapore."[5] Accrediting organizations like the Joint Commission International (JCI) and the International Society for Quality in Health Care set standards for many foreign hospitals too. JCI, a branch of "[t]he oldest and largest standards-setting and accrediting body in health care in the United States," even maintains a website where patients can learn whether foreign providers have earned its seal of approval.[6]

Competition motivates all producers to raise their game and get control of their prices. Remember how Americans once thought that domestic cars were the best? Ford, General Motors, and Chrysler nurtured this myth and made it seem unpatriotic to buy a foreign car. But foreign cars were better values, so buyers flocked to them. And, as experience with foreign cars grew, more and more people saw through Detroit's propaganda and the stigma against buying foreign cars disappeared. Now, imports from around the world are available everywhere, and competition has made all cars better, safer, and cheaper.

The truth about American health care is remarkably similar. Quality is often poor, variable, or unknown. Prices are absurd. Many foreign providers offer services that are better or just as good and that cost much less. Wanting to preserve their local monopolies, domestic providers discourage us from going abroad by stoking our fears. But the truth will emerge eventually. And as Americans learn the truth, we'll find the idea of traveling for health care more appealing, and we'll be more willing to embrace it unless we get better service and lower prices at home.

## First-Rate Cardiac Surgery for the Masses

Coronary artery bypass surgery, also known as CABG (pronounced "cabbage"), is used to treat blocked coronary arteries. It is what people are referring to when they say they had a single, double, triple, or quadruple bypass. CABG surgery is a big deal, and hospitals price it accordingly. The world-famous Cleveland Clinic reportedly charges more than $100,000.[7]

CABG surgery is dramatically cheaper—a mere $1,600—at the Narayana Hrudayalaya (NH) hospital in the Indian city of Bengaluru, formerly known as Bangalore.[8] NH is the brainchild of Dr. Devi Shetty, a heart surgeon turned businessman who wants to make health care more affordable for his countrymen.[9] At $1,600, someone who would otherwise have gone to the Cleveland Clinic for CABG surgery would save enough money by going to NH to pay for a multiyear vacation—even after deducting the cost of travel.

NH's low price may lead you to think that it delivers terrible care. In health care, Americans often use price as a signal for quality—and, when something seems too cheap, we are wary. But, NH's "mortality rates are comparable with or better than those in Britain and the U.S."[10] According to a Harvard Business School case study, NH

> was staffed by approximately 90 cardiac surgeons and cardiologists, many with extensive training and experience in top-class international institutions and several of whom had performed more than 10,000 heart surgeries individually in their careers. . . . With their vast experience, the surgeons at NH were able to achieve international standards in their procedures: NH boasted of a 1.27% mortality rate and 1% infection rate in coronary artery bypass graft (CABG) procedures, comparable with rates of 1.2% and 1%, respectively, in the United States."[11]

The case study was comparing NH's mortality and infection rates to those achieved by the *best* cardiac surgery centers in the United States—but many American hospitals experience far more deaths and complications than NH. "Hospitals in California that perform CABG surgery have an average mortality rate of nearly 3 percent (2.91)."[12] No wonder Srinath Reddy, president of the Geneva-based World Heart Federation, observed that NH is proof positive that "[i]t's possible to deliver very high quality cardiac care at a relatively low cost."[13]

## Size Matters

NH's costs are low and its quality is high partly because of its size. At 1,000 beds, NH "is the largest heart surgery hospital in the world." Every year, its surgeons perform more cardiac procedures than the Cleveland Clinic and the Mayo Clinic combined.[14]

American hospital administrators often claim they have to charge insured patients high prices because they have to cover the cost of the charity care delivered to the poor and the uninsured. But about 40 percent of the surgeries performed at NH are delivered for free or at reduced prices to patients who cannot afford the full rate.[15] That's about 20 times the volume of charity care the average American hospital delivers, and NH still keeps prices far lower than U.S. hospitals. NH, which charges paying customers the lowest prices one can imagine, has never turned away a patient for lack of funds. A 2016 news report actually described NH as "cash-rich" and explained that it and other Indian hospital groups are expanding into Africa, where they expect to undercut private hospitals there too.[16] If we're lucky, these entrepreneurial providers will one day colonize the American health care market.

In keeping with our view that retailers hold the key to reducing health care costs, Shetty calls his strategy the "Walmart-izing" of health care.[17] The high volume of procedures reduces the per-unit cost of surgeries, lab tests, scans, and everything else that is necessary to deliver high-quality health care services.

> While other hospitals may run two blood tests on a machine each day, we run 500 tests a day—so our unit cost for each test is lower. And this works with all our processes. Also, because of our volumes, we are able to negotiate better deals with our suppliers. Instead of buying expensive machines [like other hospitals do], we pay the supplier a monthly rent for parking their machines here—and then we pay them for reagents that we buy to run the machines . . . and they are willing to do this because our demand for the reagents is high enough to make up the profits for them.[18]

NH further increases its size and bargaining power by combining orders with a hospital in Kolkata (formerly known as Calcutta). It also embraces new technologies that cut costs, such as digital scans that require neither film nor developing. Finally, NH runs "comprehensive hospital management software for its operations, which help[s] maintain minimum inventory and allow[s] quicker processing of tests."[19]

NH also minimizes its administrative overhead. No overpaid executives are running around NH. Labor costs overall are a much lower share of operating expenses than in U.S. hospitals. "Compared to hospitals in the West which spend up to 60% of their revenues on staff salaries [including surgeons' fees], the comparable percentage for salaries at NH is only 22%."[20] And NH's doctors receive fixed salaries and put in long hours. At NH, cardiac surgeons are workers, not rock stars.

### CARDIAC SURGEONS IN SHORT SUPPLY? TRAIN YOUR OWN

In America, organized medicine artificially limits the supply of specialists, thereby keeping wages high and driving up prices. In India, Shetty is shattering the cartel. NH runs 19 postgraduate programs, offering diplomas in subjects like cardiac thoracic surgery, cardiology, and medical laboratory technology. These programs produce intermediate-level specialists who are ready to operate on patients in much less time. "'India's current situation for training in cardiac care is equivalent to saying you need a degree in automotive engineering to repair cars,' said Shetty. 'Obviously if that were the case, we would not have any moving vehicles since we don't have that many engineers!'"[21]

Cardiac surgery *is* rocket science, and the doctors who perform it must be well trained. Even so, NH has proven that the time and cost of producing competent cardiac surgeons can be drastically reduced. And it's not finished cutting costs yet. Doctors at NH hope one day to be able to perform heart surgery for a mere $800.[22]

### IF YOU BUILD IT, THEY WILL COME

Since founding NH, Shetty has created a network of 23 hospitals that operate in 14 cities under the name of Narayana Health. He has also created a "health city" in Bengaluru that includes, in addition to NH, a 1,400-bed multi-specialty hospital that handles cases involving neurosurgery, neurology, pediatrics, nephrology, urology, gynecology, and gastroenterology.

The campus also houses world–class centers for cancer treatment and bone marrow transplantation.

By comparison to new hospitals in the United States, Shetty builds his on tiny budgets. He observed, "Near Stanford [University in Palo Alto, California], they are building a 200–300 bed hospital. They are likely to spend over 600 million dollars. . . . Our target is to build and equip a hospital for six million dollars and [to] build it in six months."[23]

Not surprisingly, Bengaluru is now an international destination of choice for people who want outstanding health care at an affordable price. NH has performed tens of thousands of surgeries on patients from 25 foreign countries.[24] Other large health care providers compete with NH for business and lure thousands more to India for care. The Fortis Escorts Heart Institute and Research Centre in New Delhi is one of them. It charges $6,000 for open–heart surgery. Unlike U.S. hospitals, which never have sales, Fortis celebrated "Heart Month" by giving patients 10 percent off its regular prices for angioplasty and CABG.[25] And, like NH, Fortis and other competing hospitals have data systems that permit real–time monitoring of service delivery, including deviations from the expected cost of care and variations in clinical practice. Squeezing out inefficient variations helps ensure that all patients receive high–quality care at low cost. As a result, these inexpensive private hospitals "provide world–class service: doctors with training comparable to that of U.S. physicians (many with medical training in the United States), the latest technology and equipment, and infection and mortality rates that compare to those of U.S. hospitals."[26]

The contrast with American hospitals could hardly be sharper. Here, quality improvement is a nightmare. Many administrators have little idea how well or poorly their hospitals are doing. They don't even collect data. U.S. hospitals also refuse to adopt new technologies that benefit patients unless paid extra for doing so. In India, quality improvement is data driven and routine. The reason? Like other consumer–oriented businesses in the United States and elsewhere, private hospitals in India make money by avoiding mistakes:

> Because Indian hospitals compete on both quality and price, hospital managers have instituted quality assurance and improvement as integral to the business models. In a low-price setting, these hospitals must maintain

high-quality services to minimize adverse events, which generally raise the costs of care. Acceptance of financial risk by hospitals within capitated models for care delivery in India has added another driver for quality and efficiency. This concept was aptly summarized by N. Krishna Reddy of Care Hospital, who stated that in this business model, "we can't afford to have complications."[27]

As this example reflects, in a well-functioning market, hospitals have to compete for business—and they have to eat the costs of errors instead of passing them on to insurers. In that market, quality assurance programs that protect patients from complications and medical errors are quickly and seamlessly adopted, because they are good for the provider's bottom line.

NH and its competitors don't try to serve just the poor of India. To attract foreign patients, private hospitals in India "offer more luxurious services for higher prices. . . . Patients can pay more to enjoy more elegant rooms, but the technologies used for procedures are the same for all patients."[28] To ensure that accommodations are up to snuff and that services are packaged the way visitors want, management teams include staff members trained in the hotel industry. Hospitals in other Asian countries are using the same business model. According to a 2015 report by Deloitte,

> Medical care in countries such as India, Thailand and Singapore can cost as little as 10 percent of the cost of comparable care in the United States. The price is remarkably lower for a variety of services, and often includes airfare and a stay in a resort hotel. Thanks, in part, to these low-cost care alternatives which almost resemble a mini-vacation, interest in medical tourism is strong and positive.[29]

How strong is the interest in medical tourism? The global market generates an estimated $50 billion to $65 billion in revenue and is growing at an estimated annual rate of 20 percent.[30] As noted above, Americans are traveling to obtain many types of treatments, including CABG, cosmetic surgery, dental work, cataract removal, joint replacements, bone marrow transplants, bariatric surgery, fertility treatments, and commercial surrogates.[31] Most Americans head to nearby countries like Canada and Mexico. Hungary, India, Malaysia, Singapore, Thailand, and many Latin American countries are also popular destinations.

## COMPETITION WILL CAUSE QUALITY TO IMPROVE

We have said repeatedly and shown in other chapters that the quality of American health care is often poor. Depending on which estimate one believes, medical errors rank somewhere in the top 10 causes of death in the United States.

When assessing the quality of foreign doctors and hospitals, this fact must be kept in mind. They don't have to be perfect to be as good as domestic providers. This is important because patients can experience dangers when traveling abroad. For example, they may be exposed to illnesses that are not problems in the United States. Patients who travel to India may be at greater risk of contracting hepatitis B, for example, and should perhaps receive inoculations for it as a matter of course.[32]

In addition, Americans who are treated abroad may also require follow-up or corrective medical procedures after returning home. Things can go wrong in foreign hospitals, just as they can at home. It is exceedingly difficult to sue foreign providers for medical malpractice.

These problems must be put in context, however. Suing American health care providers for malpractice is no piece of cake either. Although doctors, tort reform advocates, and many politicians proclaim otherwise, the civil liability system in the United States is stingy. Patients lose the vast majority of malpractice trials—75 to 80 percent, according to many studies. The system also routinely sends patients with meritorious complaints home empty handed. The biggest problem with the American medical malpractice system is that it systematically undercompensates patients, with the most severely injured patients faring the worst.[33]

Insurance subrogation is an enormous and growing problem too. When private insurers, Medicare, or Medicaid pay for American patients' medical bills, the payers are entitled to recoup their costs from the patients' tort recoveries. For example, suppose that a patient is injured during surgery and requires follow-on medical treatments that cost $100,000, all of which are paid for by the patient's health care insurer. Then, the patient sues the hospital and collects $150,000 in compensation. The insurer can recoup the $100,000 it paid out from the $150,000 that the patient received, leaving the patient with little in the way of compensation. This is one reason why Americans who are injured by medical malpractice rarely sue. There is often little or nothing to be gained.

When it comes to quality, there are two additional important things to note. First, medical tourists tend to frequent the best institutions that foreign countries offer. Economist David Reisman explains:

> A top-tier clinic in a Third World country will often have better-quality capital and manpower than a second-tier hospital in the USA or the UK. Medical travellers [sic] typically go to the high-standard hospitals. They are seen by an English-speaking specialist and not a houseman. They benefit from a high ratio of doctors and nurses to beds. They are treated with state-of-the-art equipment by local staff just returned from a refresher course. Outside it may be heat and dust. Inside it may be the best that money can buy.[34]

Because top-tier foreign providers have incentives to treat high-profit travelers well, it is easy to understand why surveys consistently find that most people who travel for care are satisfied with the treatments they receive.

Second, tourism encourages all providers—domestic and foreign—to do better. Throughout the world, malpractice lawsuits are hard to win, so they exert little pressure on providers to improve. The signals sent by market forces must therefore be exceptionally strong. But when patients are caught up in local monopolies, as many Americans are, market-generated signals are weak because the patients lack alternatives to their local providers. Anything that helps them go elsewhere will subject local providers to pressure to do better. The end result of medical tourism may therefore be that American patients will receive treatments at home that are better and cheaper.

The pressure exerted by access to foreign providers will be great because, as mentioned already, the ones used by American medical tourists tend to be first rate. For example, the Apollo hospital chain in India has an almost perfect success rate for cardiac surgeries. Only the best American providers, like the Cleveland Clinic, do as well. Apollo's success rates for kidney transplants and bone marrow transplants compare with the Cleveland Clinic's as well. When it comes to ventilator-associated pneumonias, a side effect of surgery to be avoided, Singaporean hospitals outperform their counterparts in the United States. "The medical tourist having treatment at the top" foreign institutions, Reisman says, "has good reason to expect at least the same chance of full recovery that he would have had at home."[35]

## WHICH COUNTRIES CAN UNDERPRICE THE UNITED STATES? ALL OF THEM

A skeptic might think that other countries can sell medical services more cheaply than American providers because they are poorer. Many things are cheaper in India than they are in the United States. Workers' wages are lower. Land costs less, as do buildings and other inputs. But the sad truth is that prices in the United States are so out of whack that even hospitals in wealthy European countries can undercut us.

Consider the case of Michael Shopenn, who needed a new hip. The average price in the United States rose from $35,000 in 2001 to $65,000 in 2011. In 2007, Shopenn received a quote of nearly $100,000. So, instead, he went to Belgium and had his hip replaced for $13,660, including the cost of round-trip airfare.[36] Had he preferred fine wine and foie gras to chocolate, he might have gotten the same deal in Paris, France, and used a small part of the savings to treat himself to a meal at one of that city's storied restaurants.

Figure 18-1 visualizes some of the data from the Deloitte report we referenced above. It shows that, using 2008 prices, Americans could save money on a wide range of procedures by going abroad, despite incurring the travel costs. Because prices for medical services in the United States' third-party payer system are only going up, gains from traveling will likely increase in the future. As they do, more and more Americans will seek health care abroad and the services provided by health care providers will increasingly be outsourced.

In fact, outsourcing is happening already. Some American hospitals use radiologists located abroad to read X-ray films and scans. The images go out over the internet and are read by "nighthawks," a term that describes "American-trained diagnostic radiologists located in India and Australia who provide immediate diagnostic interpretation of CT images obtained in emergency rooms after hours."[37] PlanetHospital, a medical tourism intermediary that monitors hospital certifications, has offered to set up similar arrangements with Indian physicians reading MRIs for $400 to $500.[38]

**Figure 18-1. Average U.S. Inpatient/Outpatient Prices vs. Average Foreign Prices (2008)**

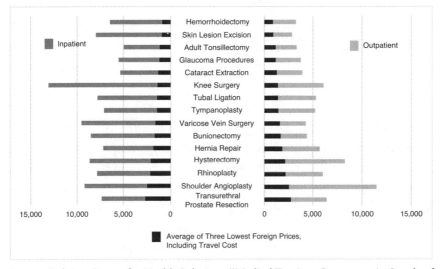

Source: Deloitte Center for Health Solutions, "Medical Tourism: Consumers in Search of Value," 2008.

## GO WEST, OR JUST THREATEN TO

Americans don't have to travel abroad for bargains. They can get them by traveling domestically too. This is so because prices for medical services can vary enormously over fairly short distances. Manhattan is so expensive that health care plans operating there could save money by chartering private jets and sending patients to Buffalo to receive treatment.

To get discounts, patients need only be able to deprive providers of market power by threatening to take their business elsewhere. The benefits of this strategy are not hypothetical. U.S. hospitals attempting to serve the Canadian market have offered large discounts to Canadian patients. Canadians can wait for free health care at home, or they can be treated immediately by paying cash for medical services in the United States. Because Canadians can go wherever they want to receive care, U.S. hospitals have to offer them bargain rates. That's where North American Surgery (NAS) comes in. NAS negotiates discounts with surgery centers, hospitals, and clinics across the United States. A Canadian wanting a hip

replacement who went through NAS would pay $16,000 to $19,000—
more than a hospital in India would charge, but less than half the going
U.S. rate.[39]

Just as Canadians can get good prices by traveling the short distance
to the United States, Americans can obtain discounts by traveling to
neighboring states. A cash-paying U.S. resident who is willing to travel to
another city can "have procedures for up to 75% less than they would pay
if they were treated closer to home."[40] Partly, the discount is for paying
cash, which eliminates the cost of billing an insurer. But it also reflects
hospitals' desire for business that would not otherwise come their way.

Hospitals also offer big discounts to U.S. businesses that are willing
to send their insured employees to other states for care. Consider Carter
Express, a logistic, freight, and transport firm based in Anderson, Indiana.[41]
It saved 23 percent on an employee's surgery for prostate cancer by
participating in BridgeHealth International's domestic medical travel program. BridgeHealth negotiated a lower price with a hospital in Denver and
made the patient's travel arrangements. "Go west, young man" wasn't good
advice just in 1871. In 2018, it can be the ticket to lower-cost health care.

BridgeHealth has a growing number of competitors. One innovative
entrant is MediBid, which enables patients to shop online for lower-priced
medical care, whether local or in another state.[42] According to MediBid's
CEO, out-of-state hip replacements cost $14,450 to $19,000, prices comparable to European rates.

Because most Americans would rather travel domestically than internationally, domestic medical tourism has significant growth potential. The
savings generally run 20 percent to 45 percent of the typical cost of a
procedure, even after travel expenses and intermediaries' fees are paid.[43]

Actual travel isn't even required. Patients can get discounts just by
threatening to go elsewhere. Hannaford Bros., a Northeastern supermarket
chain, learned this when it offered its 27,000 workers the option of getting
hip and knee replacements in Singapore. The company would waive all
deductibles and copayments and cover transportation costs for the patient
and a spouse or significant other.[44] The offer got no takers. No employees
made the trip. But that didn't matter. Simply creating the possibility of
travel was enough. In short order, "several hospitals in Boston [called] to

say they would match the price of the Singapore hospitals."[45] No worker had gone anywhere; merely having access to competitors brought down the price. And the story gets better. While Hannaford was negotiating for lower prices in Boston, a hospital in Maine—Hannaford's home state— also offered to match the Singapore rate.[46]

Many companies are following Hannaford's lead.[47] Walmart, the nation's largest employer, offered insured employees no-cost heart and spine surgeries at leading hospitals across the country, including the Cleveland Clinic, the Mayo Clinic, and Geisinger Medical Center.[48] Employees can go elsewhere, but those who do must be willing to incur significant out-of-pocket costs. Lowe's, the home improvement store, entered into a similar arrangement with the Cleveland Clinic, which agreed to match the price charged by hospitals in India for cardiac surgery.[49]

## SHARE PAINS, GAINS, AND INFORMATION

The strategy of identifying low-cost providers and requiring insureds who use more expensive ones to cover the additional cost is called "reference pricing." A program instituted by CalPERS, the health plan that covers 1.3 million current and former California public employees, showed that reference pricing can reduce costs significantly and in unexpected ways.[50] CalPERS identified 41 hospitals that charged $30,000 or less for joint replacements while meeting objective quality standards. It then told its members that they could obtain surgeries at these hospitals at no cost (other than their usual deductibles) or go to other hospitals and pay any overages themselves. The results were fantastic. Before the program started, the average cost of joint replacements for CalPERS members had risen from $28,636 to $34,742 in just two years. Then, in 2011, it suddenly dropped 26.3 percent, to $25,611. By requiring members to bear the additional charges expensive hospitals imposed, CalPERS did the impossible: it brought prices down. Not only that, hospitals outside CalPERS' chosen 41 dropped their prices by a staggering 34.3 percent. Wanting to attract business, they did the obvious thing: compete on price.

Reference pricing saves money because, in the noncompetitive environment in which health care services are delivered, different providers often charge vastly different amounts for the same services. Prices for minor procedures like vasectomies can vary by hundreds of dollars or even a few thousand within the same geographical area, depending on whether the surgery is performed at a doctor's office, a specialized clinic, or a general-purpose hospital. When it comes to major operations like joint replacements, CABG surgeries, and stent implantations, the differences are even larger.

In theory, patients could put overpriced providers out of business by refusing to use them. In reality, patients who are covered by Medicare, Medicaid, or private insurance don't care all that much about costs, because they aren't responsible for their bills. They're only on the hook for copayments and deductibles. Because the dollars they might save by using inexpensive providers would help only other people, consumers have no real reason to shop.

Reference pricing alters this dynamic. By requiring patients who use overpriced providers to pay extra, it discourages profligacy. It also tells providers who want to hold onto their patients and attract new ones that they will have to compete.

Reference pricing is an incomplete strategy, however, because it is all pain and no gain. It discourages insureds from using providers whose charges exceed the reference price, but it does not reward them for using providers who charge less than the reference price. Even if the reference price seems like a good deal, some doctors or hospitals might be willing to undercut it. It would be to an employer's advantage to learn that these providers exist, but reference pricing arrangements give workers no incentive to find them because workers gain nothing by using them. All of the money saved goes to the employer.

It may help to put the point this way. The reference pricing approach assumes that, below the reference price, employers know more about prices than workers do and can bargain over prices more effectively. Perhaps that's true sometimes or even often. But is it true always? There's no reason to think so. Workers may often learn things that their employers don't know because they meet with providers directly. Employers should therefore treat workers like their eyes and ears and take advantage of the information they gather.

Because workers can deal directly with providers over instances of care, they may have opportunities to bargain for better prices too. Employers could easily take advantage of this possibility by encouraging workers to be good shoppers. They need only give employees a portion of any discounts they obtain on reference prices. For example, if a worker negotiated a deal on a minor operation that reduced the employer's cost by $500, the worker might receive a check for $250. The employer would still be better off, and it would also learn that a provider exists who is willing to deliver a service for less than the reference price.

This isn't just pie in the sky. A company called SmartShopper contracts with employers to provide information and financial incentives to employees, encouraging them to receive care at high-quality facilities that charge less. The *New York Times* reports that SmartShopper gives workers a list of providers in their network and rates them on the basis of quality. It then provides cash incentives to use lower-cost providers: "The incentive size depends on the care being performed and the difference in cost compared with other options. A blood test may garner a $25 reward for a worker picking a lower cost provider. Meanwhile, someone getting bariatric surgery, which can cost upward of $20,000, could get a $500 check."[51]

Sharing the upside with workers will also help foster a virtuous dynamic by enabling an employer to turn its workforce into an army of motivated shoppers. In times when wages are stagnant and the cost of complicated procedures is high, it's easy to imagine workers calling providers in their areas and asking them to beat a reference price. Workers may not even have to make phone calls. Wanting to gain their business, local providers who know that employees share in discounts may advertise their willingness to beat reference prices or publicize their fees. This would reveal information that an employer could use to advantage in the next round of negotiations with the reference provider.

Employers could also help workers shop more effectively by taking two additional steps. First, they could require providers that want to be picked as the reference price benchmark to submit all-inclusive prices, like those posted by the Surgery Center of Oklahoma. Second, they could post the submitted information on websites for use by their workers and others. This would make it easier for employees to ask other providers to price the same bundle, and the information they gather could be posted on the company website as well.

The amazing thing is not that competition works in health care. It reduces prices and improves quality everywhere it is tried. The amazing thing is that the health care sector has stifled competition for decades and, by doing so, has pocketed trillions of dollars while providing shoddy care. This can and should change. By threatening to take their business elsewhere—which may be to providers in other countries, states, or cities—and by acting on incentives to use providers who offer better services for less, American patients can force providers to compete. When they do, health care will quickly become cheaper and better.

# CHAPTER 19: PRIZES, NOT PATENTS

## MONOPOLY: A TERRIBLE WAY TO PRICE DRUGS

Having people pay for most medicines themselves would alleviate many of the abuses that pharma companies commit. The average wholesale price (AWP) scandal discussed in Chapter 3, in which drug companies posted phony list prices that enabled them to take taxpayers to the cleaners, would never have happened. Neither Medicare, nor Medicaid, nor any private carrier would have relied on the phony numbers published in a manual when deciding how much to pay. Prescription drugs would have sold at real retail prices, just like pain relievers, cold remedies, and other nonprescription items. Drug prices would have a natural limit too: consumers' willingness to pay. Manufacturers couldn't charge whatever they want.

A switch from third-party payment to first-party payment would not be a cure-all, though. Pharma companies could still charge monopoly prices for branded drugs under patent because they would still enjoy marketing exclusivity. And even after a drug has gone generic, there are pricing problems that should be dealt with. Any serious plan to control spending on prescription drugs must address both of these problems. We address each in turn.

The first problem requires patent reform, which requires an act of Congress. That makes it exceedingly unlikely to happen. The pharma sector is adept at blocking any proposed legislation that would take money out of its pockets. Consider the fate met by recent efforts to legislate

alternatives to patent monopolies. In 2005, Sen. Bernie Sanders filed the
Medical Innovation Prize Act. It embodied an idea that has been floating
around in academic circles for decades: using prizes to stimulate research
and development of new drugs. The bill went nowhere. The similar bills
that Senator Sanders introduced every two years thereafter also died. And,
when Congress did enact a patent reform law in 2011, it made no provision for prizes. It did not even include a pilot program.

The idea was dead on arrival in Congress because the pharma sector has too much at stake. Citing a white paper produced by the Center
for Economic and Policy Research, the *Huffington Post* reported that
"Americans spent $250 billion on prescription drugs in 2009, but would
have spent just $25 billion had all drugs been sold as generics, meaning
without patent protections."[1] The difference, $225 billion, was the reve-
nue that the elimination of patents would have cost name-brand pharmaceutical companies in just one year. No wonder the U.S. Chamber of
Commerce, the lobby of the corporate sector, also pooh-poohs the idea
of eliminating patent monopolies.[2] It is overwhelmingly likely that existing arrangements will remain in place, in which event "the excess cost of
prescription drugs attributable to patent protection [will] likely . . . exceed
2 percent of GDP before the end of the next decade."[3]

A well-designed prize regime would eliminate the need for drug
monopolies, thereby reducing prescription drug prices to competitive levels.
It would also create incentives for innovation, including incentives to develop
orphan drugs for small populations, and could also be tailored to encourage
drug companies to test the efficacy of old drugs. Finally, if funded openly
by the federal government, a prize regime would place the costs of drug
innovation on-budget, where they would be borne by all taxpayers—rather
than just by the consumers who happen to need drugs (and their insurers).

Because Congress is unlikely to replace patents with prizes, we are reluc-
tant to spend much time discussing how a prize system might be designed.
The matter is a complicated one that would take many pages to address.
A workable prize regime must answer (at least) the following questions:

- Which prizes will be offered?
- How large will they be?

- What criteria must the winner meet?
- How will the existence of a winner be determined?

These are the same questions that the patent system answers, albeit haphazardly and with many unwanted side effects.

To give readers a sense of both the advantages a prize system could offer and the difficulty of designing one, in the discussion below, we use a regime that ties rewards to innovators' documented research costs. A prize system that was actually adopted would have to be more complicated than our example, and there might be a better system that would not tie prizes to costs at all.[4]

## A SIMPLE COST-BASED PRIZE SYSTEM

Before getting into the nuts and bolts, a couple of background points must be made. First, a reward system based on prizes will not work perfectly. Nothing does. A prize system just has to work better than the existing system of patent monopolies, and there are good reasons to think that one would.

Second, a prize system will require public funding and will therefore have to involve Congress. In theory, Congress could wreak as much havoc with a prize system as it has with the patent system. That seems unlikely, however. Under the current system, drug companies' returns on research and development (R&D) come from diverse sources: the budgets for Medicare, Medicaid, the U.S. Department of Veterans Affairs, and other public programs, and from purchases of prescription drugs that are paid for by insurers or consumers. Under a prize system, those returns would all come from one place. Because the process of connecting those returns to innovation would be more transparent, legislators who sought to make the prize formula unduly favorable to the industry would have to expect negative press coverage. The issue of funding any pro-industry increase in prize amounts or other changes would also invite scrutiny.

Finally, a prize system would not do away with patents entirely. Pharmaceutical companies operate internationally, and other countries deal with them in different ways. It may therefore be important for them to obtain patents in the United States so as to be able to register those patents elsewhere or to protect their interests in other ways. Our proposal would let drug manufacturers do that. It would only deny them monopolies on domestic sales of new medications.

Normally, a prize system offers a cash payment for an invention that meets a detailed set of success criteria. The payment can be a lump sum or a variable amount tied to subsequent developments. In the case of a pharmaceutical, the amount paid could be tied to things like the number of units sold at a specified price postdevelopment or the documented increase in life expectancy after several years of use. Details like these would have to be worked out.

A different strategy for incentivizing drug makers would tie the size of the prize to actual, documented R&D costs (including conducting clinical trials) that are incurred. Companies hoping to obtain U.S. Food and Drug Administration (FDA) approval for new drugs would submit confidential periodic filings showing all of the drugs they are studying and the associated R&D costs. When FDA approval for a particular drug was granted, a company would apply for a prize and submit an accompanying final statement of its research costs for the new medication. This final statement would be audited and made available to the public. The company would then receive a check from the U.S. government, the size of which would be a predetermined multiple of the approved research costs.[5] The same approach would govern pharma companies' applications for approval of old drugs and orphan drugs.

This proposal has several important strengths. Transparency is one. Because final cost statements will be audited and available for public inspection, R&D outlays would be on the table for everyone to see. The prize multiplier would also have been set in advance through a public process. Everyone would know why the government cut the check that it did.

The prize regime would also create clear incentives. During the process of setting multipliers, administrators would receive input from a variety of sources, as they do now when regulating public utilities. The expected value of new drugs, the cost of capital, and other considerations that influence the economic rationality of risk taking would all be considered, and the industry would have its say. Once the multipliers were fixed, innovators would know what they stood to gain before investing in R&D. Incentives could also be retuned. If experience showed that certain types of drugs were needed but not being pursued, R&D could be encouraged by making multipliers larger.

Conservatives may object to our proposal on the ground that regulators are unlikely to size prizes correctly. We agree there is a risk of error that, given the well-known phenomenon of industry capture, would likely result in prizes that are too large. But there is a serious public goods problem at the heart of pharmaceutical innovation that must be handled in some way. The problem is that, unless they can gain by developing new products, pharma companies will lack incentives to invest in research. But garnering rewards would be difficult if competitors who bore no R&D costs were free to duplicate new inventions and sell them at lower prices than inventors would be able to charge.

Currently, the patent regime allows inventors to capture profit by using the power of the government to prevent competitors from duplicating their creations and undercutting their prices. (The Unapproved Drugs Initiative and the Orphan Drug Act work the same way. Both stop other manufacturers from continuing to sell.) This is a coercive and messy process. It spawns litigation over the validity of patents and their scope. It encourages the use of strategies like evergreening and pay-for-delay settlements. It encourages consumers to buy cheaper drugs abroad while also requiring the U.S. government to prevent them from doing so by policing imports. It imposes deadweight losses on society and only weakly links inventors' returns to the risks and costs that were incurred. Finally, it enables manufacturers to take advantage of the payment system's inability to impose meaningful limits on the amounts they can charge. A prize system would have none of these shortcomings.

Of course, a prize system would cost taxpayers money, because the dollars needed to fund the prizes would come from them. But, in light of the many problems existing arrangements generate, it seems better to use the tax system to fund prizes than to impose costs as the patent system does. Today, those costs fall on consumers, insured populations, and taxpayers, whose dollars buy drugs at inflated prices for millions of people, support research, and also fund drug-related tax preferences. This scattershot approach has many downsides. It creates problems for people with diseases that require expensive medications. It creates problems for insurers, who must figure out how to deal with these people while pricing insurance in ways that maintain stable risk pools. It creates problems for the public, which shares the cost of developing new drugs only to find itself exploited by drug companies when discoveries pan out. Finally, it creates problems for orphan populations that are too small to motivate drug companies to look for needed treatments. By comparison, taxing people to fund prizes seems simple, straightforward, and fair.

Of course, the big advantage of a prize system would be that, post-invention, prices for drugs would be set competitively. Once the FDA approved a new drug or determined that an untested old drug was effective, all companies would be free to make it. Competition should then force prices downward toward manufacturers' production costs. This is the efficient, pro-consumer price that emerges naturally when markets are competitive.

## How Much Would a Prize System Cost?

The fundamental economic problem in the pharma sector is that it costs an enormous amount to create a safe, effective new drug but only pennies to manufacture the actual pills. (Pharmaceuticals are not unique in this regard; computer software and blockbuster movies from Hollywood share these characteristics.) If drug companies sold pills at their marginal cost, they'd never recoup the billions they spend on R&D. That's not a viable business model, and it would leave patients with a suboptimal level of pharmaceutical innovation.

The existing patent monopoly model enables inventors to recoup their sunk R&D costs by pricing medicines well above the marginal cost of production. As we have seen, this approach has enormous downsides. Of particular interest is that it ties drug companies' returns to their sales, not to the risks and costs they incur. It is the latter attributes that should matter in setting a market price. The combination of R&D costs and success odds define the gambles that pharma companies take when exploring new drugs. When the gambles are good ones, because the expected costs and the odds of succeeding are high, small prizes may provide all the inducement that is needed. By contrast, when the costs are high and the odds are long, the returns on success must be large. Under the existing patent regime, inventors will take these gambles only when they can charge exceedingly high prices or sell large volumes—or, better still, both.

A prize-based approach would provide compensation for sunk R&D costs directly and would remove sales revenues from the picture. An innovator wouldn't necessarily have to sell a drug at all. It would only have to obtain FDA approval.

To create good incentives, the checks cut by the government will have to be large. According to the Pharmaceutical Research and Manufacturers of America (PhRMA), the trade association for the drug industry, its members spent $51.2 billion on R&D in 2014.[6] Because, as other sources report, "95% of the experimental medicines that are studied in humans fail to be both effective and safe," many of the molecules on which that money was spent won't pan out.[7] To enable drug companies to stay in business, a prize regime would have to reward them lavishly when they produce winners. It would have to treat them like trial lawyers who work on contingency and give them bonuses for success.

Exactly how much the government would have to spend cannot be determined with precision. One reason is that PhRMA's numbers may exaggerate the cost of research. As Dr. David Belk has explained, drug companies sometimes treat costs associated with advertising and marketing as R&D.[8] A recent study, which pulled numbers from drug companies' public filings with the U.S. Securities and Exchange Commission, found that, for 10 cancer drugs that were approved by the FDA, the median cost was $648 million and the median revenue was $1.7 billion. The reported median cost was substantially lower than the $2.7 billion that is often said to be the outlay required to bring a new drug to market.[9] An auditing process is needed to ensure the accuracy of the cost figures on which prizes would be based.

The process of estimating the cost of a prize system is also complicated by the existing pharma business model, which causes enormous variation in R&D costs per approved drug. According to Matthew Herper, who writes about medical economics at *Forbes,* some companies spend billions of dollars per new FDA-approved drug while others spend far less.[10] To some degree, this variation reflects the connection between invention and expected sales. If sales were removed from the picture and all compensation for R&D costs came from prizes instead, the pharma sector would reorganize itself. Presumably, companies that perform R&D inefficiently would get out of the business or hire someone else to do it for them.

If the exact cost of a prize system cannot be estimated with precision, we can nonetheless be sure that the government will have to spend billions. But the cost of innovation should still be much lower than it is now. One reason is that existing patent monopolies let pharma companies capture 100 percent of the returns on new drugs even when they bear far less than 100 percent of the R&D–related risk. Taxpayers already bear a large fraction of the cost of drug-related R&D through research grants and other means. But taxpayers currently get little financial return on these outlays because the dollars generated by sales go to drug companies. A prize system would compensate drug companies for only the R&D costs they actually bear. Consumers would keep the rest of the gains.

Another reason is that a prize regime would enable the U.S. government to share the cost of R&D with governments elsewhere. This could be a boon to American consumers. Currently, the United States accounts for over 40 percent of pharma companies' total revenues, even though it contains only 4–5 percent of the world's population.[11] American consumers subsidize drug innovation for the rest of the world, while the rest of the world does little or nothing in return. But, if sales monopolies were eliminated, prices here would fall and subsidization by that means would end. The U.S. government could then reduce the cost of prizes further by negotiating deals with other countries, which could help their own citizens by eliminating their sales monopolies and kick in a few bucks to help with the cost of prizes. Even if those other countries insisted on continuing to free ride, we would still be better off with a prize system than the current approach of combining patents with open-ended reimbursement at whatever price point the drug manufacturer decides to set.

Finally, a prize regime has already been tried in the United States with some success.[12] In 2007, the federal government sought to incentivize drug makers to develop treatments for certain neglected diseases.

It offered a prize in the form of a priority review voucher (PRV) that a successful drug maker could use to shorten the FDA approval time for any drug it had in the pipeline, including one that might be vastly more profitable. Winners could even sell their vouchers to other drug companies that wanted expedited review for their discoveries. United Therapeutics reportedly received $350 million from another drug maker for the PRV it won for developing a cancer treatment for young children.[13] The bounty supplemented other incentives drug makers had to produce the desired medications.

Having touted prizes as substitutes for patents, we emphasize the limits of our approach. We do not recommend, and would not support, a policy of replacing patents with prizes across the board. This is partly because, in most sectors of the economy, prices are subject to a natural ceiling: consumers' willingness to pay. The lack of a similar limit in the health care payment system makes the prospect of adopting a prize regime for new drugs unusually attractive. Competition also appears to be less robust in the pharmaceutical sector than in other areas. As shown in Chapters 1 and 2, drug makers seem to have figured out how to maintain high prices even when branded drugs are close substitutes. Elsewhere, competition by rivals who invent around patents is more likely to minimize the dead-weight losses that patents entail. Finally, we should start small and sort out which of the many competing prize regime designs work best.

### THE MOST EXPENSIVE DRUG IN THE WORLD—FOR NOW

Every time we think we know which drug costs the most, we learn of a new one that costs even more. In 2016, we first learned about Soliris, a treatment for paroxysmal nocturnal hemoglobinuria (PNH) that received FDA approval in 2007. PNH is a rare blood disease that afflicts about 10,000 people in North America and Europe combined. Until Soliris came along, the only treatment for it was a bone marrow transplant, a procedure that wasn't very effective. Soliris doesn't cure PNH but does improve sufferers' quality of life, so doctors prescribe it often.

Soliris is prohibitively expensive. It costs $440,000 a year, and PNH sufferers have to take it their entire lives. One patient, Janet "Bunny" Williams of Albuquerque, New Mexico, has already received more than 200 Soliris infusions at an estimated total cost of more than $13 million.[14]

Why does Soliris cost so much? Partly because it was expensive to develop and partly because manufacturers can charge whatever they want, knowing that insurers and public payers will pay up. Alexion Pharmaceuticals, the company that makes Soliris, reportedly spent nearly $1 billion over 15 years to develop the drug. That's a lot of money, but the returns are far larger. Alexion "reported revenue of $2.6 billion for the drug in 2015 alone." The effect of Soliris sales on Alexion's market capitalization has been astounding. "The company's stock has soared more than 300 percent in the past five years, boasting a faster rate of growth than Apple Inc. over the same period." Alexion's stock price rose 130 percent in 2010 alone.[15]

Whether Alexion bore the amount of risk that it contends is seriously disputed. According to Sachdev Sidhu, a University of Toronto researcher, "the public science is well over 80 or 90 percent of the work. . . . Public resources went into understanding the molecular basis of the disease, public resources went into the technology to make antibodies and finally, Alexion, to their credit, kind of picked up the pieces."[16] Sidhu added that Soliris is cheap to make too. "It probably costs less than 1 percent of the price of the drug to make the drug."[17]

Soliris provides an example of how a cost-based prize system might work. During the 15-year period in which research on Soliris was underway, a condition of eligibility for a prize would have been that Alexion file periodic cost reports with the FDA, along with a final report when FDA approval was sought. The reports would have been audited by an established means. Upon approval being granted, Alexion would have received a prize based on its documented costs and a reward formula that was known in advance. Generic manufacturers would then have been free to make and sell Soliris. Competition would then have driven the price down toward the actual cost of production, and neither members of the orphan population of PNH sufferers nor their insurers would have been gouged. America's taxpayers would have borne the full cost of the R&D, but they had already paid for much of that by supporting university research, and the remaining cost would be spread across all governments that chose to participate in the United States' prize regime. The only losers would have been Alexion's shareholders, who would have received normal stock market returns instead of spectacular ones.

### WHAT ABOUT GENERICS?

A prize system cannot help reduce the prices of generic drugs, which are already off-patent. What can be done to make them less expensive?

Regrettably, the most effective options with which to address generic drug prices require governmental action. For example, many of the problems we identified in Chapter 1 are attributable to insufficient competition in the generic drug market. Substantial price hikes occur and stick because only one company makes a drug or because manufacturers adopt tit-for-tat strategies or play other pricing games. Illegal, anti-competitive conduct may underlie some of these problems. Only aggressive antitrust enforcement can discourage this type of behavior.

The FDA also bears part of the blame. There is a sizable backlog of pending applications from generic drug manufacturers who want to enter the market. Congress should give the FDA the resources it needs to process these applications more quickly. Until that happens, the FDA should reprioritize applications in a manner calculated to bring prices down. Currently, it follows a FIFO (first in, first out) plan. That approach doubtless seems fair to the pharmaceutical companies, but it results in significant consumer harm. A more consumer-friendly approach would move applications for drugs that have experienced significant price spikes to the head of the queue. Approval of new entrants should reduce prices by expanding the number of suppliers. And, once incumbents realize that price hikes will result in new market entry, they may be deterred from jacking up prices in the first instance. In short, the FDA (which after all is the Food and *Drug* Administration) should start paying attention to drug prices—and use that information to inform judgments about the impact of agency action and inaction.[18]

More broadly, it is important to recognize that, because the FDA controls market entry, its actions and decisions can greatly influence the prices at which generic drugs change hands. Policy makers should consider liberalizing access to the U.S. market by relaxing the agency's grip on entry.

Why not let a company that qualifies to sell a generic drug in Canada, England, France, Israel, or some other developed country automatically qualify to sell the same drug in the United States—at least so long as the branded drug has already been approved by the FDA, and the marketing exclusivity provided by the Hatch-Waxman Act has expired? These countries have the expertise needed to protect their citizens from excessive risks and the desire to do so. Instead of requiring companies that meet their standards to waste time and money satisfying the FDA, we could simply waive them in to the U.S. market. The resulting increase in competition would surely benefit consumers.

In the meantime, consumers can expand their choices by engaging in another form of medical tourism: purchasing drugs abroad. They can do this legally by visiting foreign countries and bringing medications back with them. The U.S. Customs Department allows travelers to bring in a 90-day supply of a prescription medication purchased abroad, as long as the traveler has a prescription for the drug and the pharmacy fills the prescription as written. One hitch is that the FDA and the Customs Department don't want travelers to use this option to bring unapproved generic drugs into the country, so these drugs are at risk of being seized. It is not clear how vigorously Customs actually enforces this requirement, particularly against ordinary citizens. Indeed, there may well be a speakeasy norm, where only the loud and obnoxious get their drugs confiscated and everyone else is waved through.

Another option is ordering prescription medications from online pharmacies in other countries, which ship drugs into the United States. Although it is illegal to do so, the practice is flourishing. According to a 2016 report, "[a]s drug prices have spiraled upward, tens of millions of generally law-abiding Americans have committed an illegal act in response: They have bought prescription medicines outside the U.S. and imported them."[19] As WebMD observes:

> Current law says that if Granny decides she can get her heart medications more cheaply in Alberta than in Alabama, she could be busted for either bringing it over the border or having it delivered to her. Does that mean that dear Granny is likely to do a stretch in solitary? Hardly, experts say, because nobody wants to be seen putting the cuffs on elderly

pensioners. Also, they'd have to arrest the governments of the states of Wisconsin, Minnesota, Illinois, Vermont, as well as many city govern- ments and private employers who have turned north for lower-cost prescription drugs.[20]

The list of states that buy drugs for their own purpose in Canada or help others do so is now up to nine, and the cities, counties, and even school districts that do so number in the dozens.[21] Given that they are flouting the law and that millions of Americans are doing so too, the prohibition on buying drugs abroad seems to fall into the same category as the speed limit.

As law professors, we are reluctant to encourage people to break the law. Instead, we repeat the point we made when discussing retail medi- cine. When consumers lead from below, politicians feel pressure to follow. Given the number of people and the number of government entities that are buying drugs abroad, we think it unlikely that Congress will decide to spend the dollars that would be needed to prevent this from continuing. To the contrary, as the number of people who are responsible for their own drug costs continues to grow, foreign purchases will become increas- ingly common and pressure will mount for Congress to call off the dogs. Recent efforts to beef up enforcement, including a crackdown on stores in Florida that help tens of thousands of people purchase Canadian drugs, may push the issue to the front of the policy agenda.[22]

Amarillo Slim was a famous and successful poker player. He is widely credited with the observation, "If you're at a poker table and you don't see a sucker, it's you." The decision to use health insurance to pay whatever price the pharmaceutical manufacturers have decided to ask for makes us all into suckers. Prizes, antitrust enforcement, revisions to the FDA approval process, and self-pay are the best ways we know of to start playing to win.

# CHAPTER 20: PLAYING WHAC-A-MOLE
## TO WIN

•

## A FUTURE GOVERNOR OF FLORIDA?

As we explained in excruciating detail in Part 1, fraud occurs at every conceivable point in the health care supply chain. Drug companies, pharmacies, doctors, nursing homes, hospitals, home health care services, durable medical equipment suppliers, ambulance companies, and patients have all committed health care fraud, as have criminals whose only connection to the system is that they prey upon it. Most of these fraudsters target government-run payment systems, which are easier to rip off than private ones, but private payers must also be on guard. Medicare, Medicaid, and private insurers must all play a neverending game of Whac-a-Mole. The question, which this chapter addresses, is how payers can minimize their losses.

One obvious approach is to identify strategies that work and build on them. The case of Todd S. Farha provides a promising example. Farha, the former CEO of WellCare, defrauded Florida's Medicaid program out of millions of dollars by inflating the amount WellCare spent on mental health services.[1] In 2014, he was sentenced to three years in federal prison. For a Florida fraudster, the punishment was unusually harsh. Compare Farha's fate to that of Rick Scott, who was CEO of Columbia/HCA when it committed one of the largest Medicare frauds in history. While Farha went to prison, Scott went on to become governor of the Sunshine

State.[2] Federal prosecutors had asked that Farha be imprisoned for 20 years. Maybe they feared Florida voters might elect him governor too.[3]

WellCare's scheme worked like this. Under Florida law, companies that provide mental health services to Medicaid patients must spend at least 80 percent of the dollars they receive actually delivering care. They can spend the remaining 20 percent on administrative expenses and other things. If they spend less than 80 percent treating patients, they are legally required to rebate the difference to the state. The object is to discourage providers from shortchanging patients and pocketing the money they save.

WellCare used a simple strategy to circumvent this regulation.[4] It billed for mental health services through its Staywell and HealthEase insurance plans, but it used a subsidiary named Harmony to handle the treatments. To make the books look right, WellCare paid Harmony 85 percent of the billing receipts, thereby seeming to spend more than 80 percent on patient care. In fact, Harmony spent only 60 percent of the dollars it received on treating patients. In other words, WellCare spent only 51 percent (60 percent of 85 percent) of the money it received on patient care and pocketed much of the rest. For example, WellCare documents showed that Florida paid $30 million for mental health services provided in 2005, of which the company spent only half providing care to patients. From 2003 to 2007, WellCare supposedly kept $40 million that it should have refunded.

WellCare's scheme came to light when Sean Hellein, who worked for WellCare as a financial analyst, decided to become a whistleblower. Working with the FBI, he wore a wire and secretly recorded 650 hours of conversations. Some of the statements he recorded were damning. According to a *Bloomberg News* report, Peter Clay, then WellCare's vice president of medical economics, said that providing actual data on payments would "show a 50 percent loss ratio" in all years, the same ratio reported for 2005.[5] A few months after this comment was made, WellCare refunded $1.1 million to the state. It should have repaid at least $11 million more.

All the while, WellCare's profits grew, its stock price surged, and corporate insiders made millions by selling their shares. The company's spectacular success attracted the attention of Carl McDonald, a Wall Street analyst who knew it was too good to be true. In March of 2007, he advised investors that, for WellCare's profit margins to be as large as they were, Florida's Medicaid program had to be overpaying. "It would seem to be only a matter of time before the state figures this out," McDonald wrote.[6] The state never did. Had Sean Hellein not ratted on his employer and donned a wire, WellCare would still be taking Florida for millions.

WellCare's scheme is typical of one classic form of health care fraud. A mainstream provider run by talented people takes a government payer for millions. WellCare wasn't some fly-by-night entity. It was "the largest insurer in Florida's Medicaid program." "The head of Florida Medicaid briefly served on its board and left with $1 million in stock."[7] And Todd Farha wasn't some run-of-the-mill con artist, either. After graduating from the Harvard Business School, he acquired WellCare with the help of George Soros, the billionaire investor, who operated a fund that provided $70 million in seed money.[8]

Sean Hellein held an interesting position.[9] He wrote computer code that identified the most expensive patients on WellCare's Medicare and Medicaid plans. Ideally, insurers use this information to appoint nurses to work with high-cost patients in hope of managing their care more efficiently. Instead, Farha and other WellCare managers tried to force these patients off WellCare's rolls. For example, in 2004, WellCare convinced the parents of 425 premature babies to take their business elsewhere.[10]

Hellein refrained from rocking the boat until 2005, when he learned that WellCare was stealing money from the state. That's when he lawyered up, contacted the FBI, and started wearing a wire in 2006. Despite being understandably nervous, he did his work so well that WellCare's managers rewarded him with $300,000 worth of stock.

The big break came in 2007, when Hellein videotaped a meeting of WellCare's top executives. At the time, Florida's Medicaid officials had demanded an accounting of WellCare's spending on behavioral health services. The managers knew that the company had spent only half the amount reported to the state. So they devised a simple solution: double every charge. "Hellein sat in [a] swivel chair videotaping every speaker. 'You had about 20 people talking about how to defraud the state.'"[11] Afterward, Peter Clay, Hellein's direct report, was upset that the meeting was so large. "You have to be careful," Clay said. "This is fraud."[12]

After the FBI raided WellCare and the company's stock tumbled, Hellein feared that he and his family would be attacked. "A guy who refused to identify himself spent three days sitting in a truck at the end of Hellein's driveway."[13] Others made threatening phone calls or pounded on his front door. So he moved his family to Atlanta and started afresh.

For his troubles, Hellein eventually became wealthy. Under the False Claims Act (FCA), whistleblowers can share up to 30 percent of any monetary settlement that the government negotiates with the wrongdoer. In 2012, WellCare agreed to pay $137.5 million to resolve the civil case, plus $40 million in fines and another $40 million in forfeited fees. Hellein's share was nearly $21 million, which he split with his lawyer.[14] On top of that, WellCare paid another $200 million to settle a shareholder suit.[15] Three WellCare executives (Farha, the chief financial officer, and the former vice president for government affairs) went to jail. Peter "This Is Fraud" Clay, was fined $10,000 and ordered to perform 200 hours of community service.[16]

## WHAT WHISTLEBLOWERS HAVE IN COMMON

In some respects, Sean Hellein was a typical whistleblower. He held a fairly high-level position at the company where the wrongdoing occurred, so he was privy to information that outsiders don't normally possess.

Dinesh Thakur was in a similar situation.[17] Ranbaxy Laboratories, one of the top producers of generic drugs in the world, hired him to be its director and global head of Research Information and Portfolio Management. Upon taking the position, he discovered that Ranbaxy's quality control systems were lacking and that the company was covering up the problem by substituting other manufacturers' drugs for its own in quality tests. After making his concerns known to Ranbaxy's board and getting nowhere, Thakur filed an FCA suit. The U.S. Food and Drug Administration subsequently banned the importation of Ranbaxy drugs and revamped its overseas inspections protocols. In 2013, Ranbaxy paid $500 million to settle with the feds and the states. For his troubles, Thakur was awarded $48.6 million from the federal government's share.[18]

Whistleblowers come in many sizes and shapes, though, and not all are corporate insiders. Richard West was a patient who learned the hard way that his home health care provider, Maxim Health Care, had over-billed Medicaid for assisting him. West, "an intubated, wheelchair-bound veteran [who was] debilitated by muscular dystrophy" was denied Medicaid coverage for additional visits because his yearly allowance had been exhausted. In fact, Maxim had billed Medicaid for 700 hundred hours of services West never received. West filed an FCA suit after complaints lodged with state and federal Medicaid officials and with the U.S. Department of Veterans Affairs produced no results. The resulting investigation uncovered a pattern of billing fraud so vast that Maxim eventually paid $150 million to settle with the federal government and the states. West received $15.4 million, which, like all whistleblowers, he shared with an attorney. However, as if to prove conclusively that no good deed goes unpunished, the state of New Jersey demanded that he repay it for the Medicaid benefits it provided and slapped him with a $900,000 lien.[19]

West was a patient, not a high-level corporate executive, so he was not privy to Maxim's secrets. He didn't know that he was a pawn in Maxim's scheme to defraud Medicaid either. That fact came to his attention only because Maxim got greedy and exhausted his Medicaid allowance too quickly.

Why didn't West know sooner that Maxim was charging for services it never delivered? Because he wasn't Maxim's customer. Maxim sent its bills to Medicaid. The home health care visits were free to West, so, like most patients on Medicaid or Medicare, he had no reason to care about the charges—until he found out that his Medicaid eligibility was exhausted. Then his financial interest suddenly became very real.

That's one thing that most whistleblowers have in common: a strong interest in spotting a fraud. In West's case, the interest derived from his need for additional home visits, which he couldn't afford and for which Medicaid refused to pay. In the case of Sean Hellein, the whistleblower who put the feds onto WellCare, it came from the desire to protect himself from becoming complicit in the company's fraud and possibly going to prison. And, in all cases, the financial interest in revealing fraud is strengthened by the FCA, which entitles whistleblowers to keep a sizable portion of the government's recoveries.

One pharmacy company, Ven-A-Care of the Florida Keys, created a business model based on the inducement provided by the FCA. The owners of Ven-A-Care—Mark Jones, Zachary Bentley, and Luis Cobo—created the company to provide infusion services for AIDS patients but were nearly run out of business after they refused to join forces with National Medical Care Inc. (NMC), a nationwide dialysis company that was heavily engaged in the average wholesale price (AWP) scam.

After licking their wounds, Jones, Bentley, and Cobo decided to learn how NMC was making so much money. They studied drug prices, which they had access to because they were a pharmacy. They hired former FBI agents. They posed as nurses and called NMC dialysis centers to inquire about drug costs. They called Florida's Medicaid office to ask how much it paid for drugs. After building their case, they filed an FCA suit against NMC in 1994. Then, while that case was pending, they broadened their focus and "began looking at how some of the largest pharmaceutical companies were using excessive reimbursements [generated by the AWP scam] as kickbacks to pharmacies and doctors to increase sales."[20] They also looked at the whole range of prescription drugs, not just infusion agents given to patients with HIV. They capped off their investigation by filing FCA suits against dozens of pharma companies.

Jones, Cobo, and Bentley got their first big break in 2000, when NMC paid $486 million to settle the civil case and to resolve criminal charges, to which NMC pled guilty, that also resulted from it.[21] Their cut was $45 million.[22] The payment put them back on their feet and convinced them to make FCA litigation their full-time business. Then settlements with Big Pharma companies began to roll in—at least 24 of them, eventually. Baxter paid $14 million. Bayer paid $38.2 million. Bristol-Myers Squibb plunked down a whopping $515 million. Altogether, these settlements generated about $3 billion, of which Ven-A-Care's slice was a cool $597.6 million.[23] Plainly, it can be more profitable to be a professional FCA plaintiff than a professional pharmacist.

### THE BEAUTY OF PRIVATE ENTERPRISE

The size of Ven-A-Care's reward and the fees earned by other whistle-blowers have generated lots of complaints. Most come from the corporate sector. It hates FCA suits, which forced corporate wrongdoers to fork over $42 billion from 1987 to 2013. That's why the U.S. Chamber of Commerce lobbies constantly for changes that would gut the FCA.[24] No sensible person would give any credence to its complaints. The best sign that the FCA is working well is that businesses in fraud-ridden industries want it to go away.

Corporate America hates whistleblowers for the same reason it dislikes tort plaintiffs: it doesn't control them or the courts. Like tort litigation, *qui tam* litigation—the Latin name given to cases filed by whistleblowers under the FCA—is a species of private law enforcement. Instead of government officials holding wrongdoers accountable through the federal and state regulatory apparatuses, citizens represented by private, contingent-fee attorneys do the job via the courts. And unlike regulators, who are routinely captured and bribed by the industries they're supposed to police, the citizens, lawyers, and judges who figure in FCA lawsuits aren't so easily corrupted. The citizens want justice and financial settlements. Their lawyers want to help their clients recover, because that's how they get paid. And the federal judges who preside over *qui tam* cases tend to be honest. They live and work in a culture that encourages them to base decisions on evidence and law. No wonder corporate wrongdoers want FCA lawsuits to disappear.

The evidence that private lawsuits deter fraud and punish fraudsters more effectively than government regulation is everywhere. The biggest FCA recoveries routinely result from whistleblower suits. For example, in 2013, Johnson & Johnson (J&J) paid $2.2 billion to resolve a variety of drug-marketing allegations. The whistleblowers, who shared $168 million, were all former J&J employees.[25] A whistleblower also turned in Dr. Farid Fata, the monster who lied to patients about the results of their cancer screenings so he could make money by pumping them full of expensive drugs. Fata was thought to have "prescribed over 9,000 unnecessary injections and infusions to at least 553 patients over a six-year span."[26] Despite the length and breadth of his misconduct, neither the Michigan Bureau of Health Professions (MBHP) nor federal fraud watchdogs identified him as a malefactor. To the contrary, the MBHP gave him a clean bill of health even after a nurse who worked for him reported him as a dangerous physician. Fata would have continued to harm patients indefinitely had not Dr. Soe Maunglay, who figured out what he was up to, and George Karadsheh, the practice manager of Michigan Hematology Oncology, reached out to the FBI.

Private actions greatly outnumber FCA cases initiated by the U.S. Department of Justice (DOJ) too. During the 2010–2015 period, whistle-blowers filed 3,963 FCA actions; the DOJ filed 711. That's a ratio of almost 6 to 1. Recoveries make the DOJ look somewhat better. Over the period, private *qui tam* suits grossed $17.5 billion while the DOJ lawsuits brought in $6.7 billion. The numbers are closer, but the ratio is still 2.6 to 1 in whistleblowers' favor. These are the numbers for all *qui tam* suits alleging that someone defrauded the federal government. When one narrows the focus to health care fraud, the superiority of private litigation is even clearer. Again looking at 2010–2015, private whistleblowers brought 2,613 suits versus 189 DOJ-filed complaints (almost 14 to 1) and $13.6 billion in *qui tam*–initiated recoveries versus $1.6 billion in DOJ cases (8.7 to 1).[27]

Why do whistleblowers uncover so many more frauds than the government? One reason is that there are more of them. Every person who works in an organization where a fraud on the public might be committed is a potential informant. Private enforcers therefore outnumber public monitors by at least 100,000 to 1. Another reason is better access to information. No one wants to be prosecuted for fraud, so the people who commit it naturally try to hide it from the government. They can do that easily, but they have a much harder time deceiving corporate insiders. A third reason is that private citizens have better incentives. They care about winning, not about the political agendas that may color discretionary calls at the DOJ, and they can make money on cases that may be too small to attract the DOJ's interest. Private enforcement is more successful than public enforcement because whistleblowers are more motivated, have more eyes and ears, and are more likely to know what's going on.

The complaints of businesses whose goods and services are paid for with public funds seem even less persuasive when one considers that the DOJ reviews all privately filed FCA complaints and exercises considerable control of all FCA litigation. Under the statute, the DOJ can intervene in *qui tam* actions and take them over. It does this about 25 percent of the time, and when it does, the odds of securing a monetary recovery are about 90 percent.[28] By contrast, when the government decides to stay out, dollars are recovered only 10 percent of the time. The DOJ's decision to decline to participate in a *qui tam* action is practically the kiss of death.

## WHY NOT MAKE THEM RICH?

Not all complaints about whistleblowers come from corporate types who dislike the possibility of having spies in their midst. Michael Loucks, a former acting U.S. attorney in Boston, thinks whistleblowers are over-paid. Instead of giving them a percentage of the dollars they recover, he would limit awards to $2 million per case. "The purpose of the [FCA] is to incentivize people to blow the whistle, not to make whistleblowers rich," he says.[29] Because whistleblowers work on contingency—they and their lawyers only get paid when the government recovers money—Loucks' recommendation is fundamentally the same as the recommendation to cap lawyers' contingency fees.

There is, however, an important difference between the two types of payment. Although both are contingent on results obtained, lawyers' fees are set in markets while whistleblowers' fees are fixed by statute. The best the government can do is approximate the fee that is needed to give potential whistleblowers a strong incentive to sue under the FCA. It is hard to know whether the government has set the fee too high, as Loucks contends, or too low, as might also be the case.

A start at resolving this matter can be made by looking at the facts. From 2010 to 2015, whistleblowers in cases involving health care fraud were paid $2.1 billion out of the $13.6 billion that was recovered in the lawsuits they commenced. That's an average fee of 15.6 percent, which the whistle-blowers shared with the lawyers who filed their cases. Typically, the split is 60:40, meaning that the whistleblowers retained about $1.27 billion and their lawyers got the rest. In turn, that $1.27 billion was paid out in 2,613 cases, yielding an average net payment of just over $485,000 per successful, whistleblower-initiated health care fraud case. Because FCA cases often involve multiple whistleblowers, the average take-home per person was even less.

Obviously, there's a great deal of variation around the average payment. Were that not so, the guys who created Ven-A-Care would still be running a pharmacy. But the amounts that whistleblowers typically take home are not that great, especially given that many of them take actions that endanger their careers.

Critics might say, "The average payment is fine. I just want to cap fees so people like the Ven-A-Care guys don't make out like bandits." But what's wrong with making them rich? Before Ven-A-Care's actions put a stop to it, the AWP scam was costing taxpayers billions of dollars a year.[30] At that rate, taxpayers recouped the whistleblowers' fee in just a few months. Doesn't Ven-A-Care show that the FCA's incentive arrangement served taxpayers well?

The market for legal services also provides strong evidence that fee caps are a bad idea. Sophisticated business clients rarely use them when hiring lawyers to handle commercial lawsuits on contingency. Instead, they pay percentages of their entire recoveries, without limit. They also pay more than 15 percent, the average in FCA cases. For example, when NTP Inc. sued Research In Motion Ltd., the company that manufactures the Blackberry, for patent infringement, it promised its law firm, Wiley Rein & Fielding (WRF), a one-third contingent fee. When the case settled for $612.5 million, WRF took home more than $200 million. The fee arrangement used in this case is representative of the market, even though the recovery is unusually large.[31]

One could argue with some force that FCA fees should be lower than those that prevail in the market for legal services because, in the largest cases, the DOJ typically takes over the litigation. That is true, but it does not warrant a change. FCA fees are already lower than private market arrangements by about 50 percent. Besides, why tamper with a good thing? Not only does the FCA deter frauds, the government pays out less than 16 cents on every dollar it brings in. That's an excellent cost-to-return ratio. Given that tens or even hundreds of billions dollars are being lost to fraud every year, shouldn't whistleblower fees be higher than they are?

The FCA is one of the few effective mechanisms for policing fraud in government programs. Given the enormous amount of fraud that still occurs, Congress should strengthen the FCA. Capping whistleblowers' fees would do the opposite by weakening the incentive to turn state's evidence. Why take a gamble on winning $1.2 million, the portion of the $2 million award proposed by Loucks that a whistleblower would keep after paying an attorney, when one can live a peaceful life and possibly even make more money by keeping one's mouth shut? Remember Sean Hellein? He received a $300,000 stock bonus from WellCare while the fraud was ongoing. Working with the FBI was also a nightmare for him and his family. His wife thought he was crazy for rocking the boat. Had the execs at WellCare known that FCA awards were limited to $1.2 million, they might have bought his silence, and that of every other employee involved in the fraud, by spreading the wealth more evenly. Whistleblowers' rewards must be proportional to the fraud. Otherwise, the architects of the largest fraud schemes could always buy the silence of colleagues who are potential whistleblowers.

## FREE THE SCOUNDRELS

Health care fraud is so common and costs the Treasury so much money that all options with any potential to rein it in should be considered. One such possibility would be to grant whistleblowers who were personally involved in frauds immunity from prosecution. The people who know the most about frauds are the folks who commit them. The flow of information to the government would greatly increase if the perpetrators were to step forward. The knowledge that the first person to rat out his or her friends would be immune from prosecution would discourage people from working with others to commit frauds. Every additional conspirator would be another person who, at some point, might think it advisable to turn everyone in. The destabilizing effect would be especially great in corporate America, where the prospect of doing jail time is the only real deterrent.

Giving immunity to scoundrels who turn state's evidence would be a change from existing practice, but not as marked a change as one might think. Lawyers who represent whistleblowers report, "In the vast majority of cases, government prosecutors do not focus on the conduct of the whistleblower. Rather, their investigative efforts are directed toward the planners and architects of the fraud against the government, and particularly on those who benefitted financially."[32] In plain English, immunity grants to small-fry fraudsters who turn state's evidence are already common. It is mainly when the person blowing the whistle was "an architect of the fraud" that prosecutors "almost certainly will not grant immunity."[33] It seems obvious that this limitation discourages high-level participants from reporting. It must also encourage fraud in the first place by reducing the likelihood that high-level conspirators will turn their co-conspirators in.

Insofar as architects are concerned, the deterrent to reporting is even more severe than just described. Under the FCA, when a person who helped plan or initiate a fraud becomes a whistleblower, a federal judge has discretion to reduce "the share of the proceeds of the action which the person otherwise would have received." In other words, instead of the customary 15 percent, a culpable whistleblower's share of the FCA recovery could be much smaller. And, if the whistleblower is convicted of a crime, he or she cannot share in the FCA recovery at all.[34]

It is easy to see why these provisions exist. The desire for justice runs deep in honest people, and it clearly would be unjust if the persons who orchestrate frauds could enrich themselves by turning themselves in. The law doesn't let murderers become their victims' heirs, so it's easy to see why it doesn't let high-level conspirators profit from their misdeeds either.

We know that justice is important. Collectively, we've spent almost six decades teaching law students that justice under law is one of the pillars of civil society. But it is also important to deter criminal behavior, and injustice must sometimes be tolerated to eliminate an even greater injustice. Health care fraud is flourishing. All existing policing mechanisms have failed, including the most potent, the FCA.

The time has come to think outside the box. If we always do what we've always done, we'll always get the results we've always gotten. We should consider letting high-level conspirators off the hook when they rat on their friends. The possibility of giving them ordinary relator shares should also be on the table. Although we describe this approach as "thinking outside the box," it would actually return the statute to the vision of the principal sponsor of the 1863 bill that became the FCA. Sen. Jacob Howard (R–MI) described the bill as relying on "the old-fashioned idea of holding out a temptation, and 'setting a rogue to catch a rogue' which is the safest and most expeditious way I have ever discovered of bringing rogues to justice."[35] If we want to catch more rogues, we should be more open to rewarding the rogues who are willing to turn them in. Otherwise, our efforts at fraud control will amount to "déjà vu all over again."

## MILLIONS OF MALLETS

When it comes to fraud, the health care system is hardly unique. All public programs are rife with fraud. That's why the FCA exists. President Abraham Lincoln called for its enactment during the Civil War because fraudsters were plundering the Union Army's resources. Little has changed since then except the magnitude of the losses. If fraudsters steal more from the health care system than from the Defense Department or the Social Security Administration, it is partly because more dollars pass through it.

The health care sector loses about $1 trillion a year to fraud, waste, and abuse. The government has no hope of winning this game of Whac-a-Mole. It hardly even tries, partly because many of the biggest moles are mainstream health care providers that don't want their actions or their bills carefully scrutinized.

But it is important to see that this game occurs only in the part of the health care sector where third-party payers predominate. There are no comparable stories of fraud, game playing, or predation in the retail sector, where people buy things directly. Nor do any comparable statistics exist regarding dollars lost to fraud, waste, and abuse. No one contends that fraud accounts for 10–20 percent of retail medical spending. Nor does anyone argue that one-third of all dollars spent at retail medical outlets are wasted. There surely are some abuses in the retail sector—no human system is wholly immune—but there's nothing like the corruption that pervades the third-party payer sector.

It's easy to see why. In the retail sector, people spend their own money. Consequently, they have no interest in allowing themselves to be ripped off by avaricious providers or con artists. Nor can anyone gain by ripping off third-party payers. Retail outlets sell lots of durable medical equipment, including wheelchairs of every imaginable description. But there's little or no wheelchair fraud because retailers can't make money by giving away wheelchairs for free. There aren't many overpriced wheelchairs either because shoppers can spend their money wherever they want. High-priced sellers have to offer better quality or more bells and whistles to convince buyers to part with extra cash.

When people spend their own money, they won't pay for services that weren't delivered either. Most consumers are careful when their own dollars are on the line. It's only when someone else is paying the freight that consumers toss their medical bills in the trash without reviewing them. Dollar-conscious consumers won't waste $1,000 on an unnecessary ambulance ride to a dialysis clinic when a taxi costs only $25.

There's also less fraud in the retail sector because consumers have their guards up. A provider who wants a patient to part with money must convince a skeptical purchaser that a service will be beneficial, and the provider also has to deliver. Every consumer is armed with a mallet too. A scammer might rob a few people—but, as the number of rip-offs mounts, so do the number of police reports. Eventually the cops close in. When millions of people have mallets and the inclination to use them, Whac-a-Mole isn't much fun for the moles.

Although switching from third-party payment to first-party payment would quickly end most abuses, progress could be made even without ending Medicare, Medicaid, and other government programs. We need only take advantage of the instinct people have to be careful with their own money. Instead of paying providers for delivering services to patients, government could give money to patients and let them buy what they need. If Medicare and Medicaid gave beneficiaries flat amounts per month or per year, recipients could use the dollars to purchase most medical goods and services at retail. They could also buy coverage for catastrophic health care needs from private insurers. And they would be cost and fraud conscious in both instances.

The prospect of giving money to beneficiaries raises many interesting issues. Won't beneficiaries squander the money on all sorts of things, then show up at emergency rooms, which will have to treat them for free? Aren't they too dumb to buy medical services without help from third-party payers? Won't they fall prey to unscrupulous relatives and con artists, who will part them from their cash? We discuss these questions and many others elsewhere in the book. Here, we'll continue to focus on fraud, waste, and abuse.

If dollars were doled out to beneficiaries instead of being paid to providers, the effect on many criminals would be dramatic. Start with the bandits who submit truckloads of phony bills to Medicare and Medicaid. They'd be out of business immediately. "Pay and chase" would also perish. Other forms of waste and abuse would plummet, as price- and quality-conscious consumers demanded more for their money and questioned inflated charges. Intelligent shopping wouldn't happen immediately, but the incentives for price and quality to become more transparent and for patient-assisting services to develop would all be in place. These behaviors and tools would emerge and mutually reinforce each other, replacing a vicious cycle with a virtuous one that protects consumers.

Criminals would still try to get money from CMS by falsely claiming to be eligible for Medicare, Medicaid, or other federal health care programs. Remember the Russian diplomats from Chapter 12 who got Medicaid to pay for maternity services and postnatal care? There will always be criminals like them. In addition, if the government offers larger cash subsidies to people with low incomes or costly illnesses, as it should, some fraud will occur as people claim to be poorer or sicker than they actually are in order to get more money. The government believes that this already happens to some extent when Medicare adjusts the amounts it pays to insurance companies based on how sick their enrollees are.[36] Wanting to deter it, the DOJ joined a whistleblower suit against a giant insurer that had allegedly "improperly generated and reported skewed data artificially inflating beneficiaries' risk scores, avoided negative payment adjustments, and retained payments to which it was not entitled" in the amount of "at least over a billion dollars."[37]

Yet fraud would be much easier to police in a system where the government gave beneficiaries money. First, the variety of frauds would be greatly reduced. It is easier to police one relatively simple payment to each of Medicare's 55 million enrollees than to police 1 billion claims, each of which could be false or misleading in countless ways. Second, individual beneficiaries could not possibly engage in the massive fraud schemes Medicare currently enables, and professional fraudsters would have far more difficulty collecting the information they need to mount such schemes. Finally, once most Medicare and Medicaid bureaucrats are freed from the impossible task of policing millions of health care providers and scrutinizing billions of bills, there would be more manpower available to focus on the frauds that remain. CMS could also police all of these forms of fraud without incurring the wrath of legitimate providers, who have a huge stake in CMS's easy payment rules.

Catastrophic health insurance would also draw fraudsters, just as private insurance programs do already.[38] But, when private carriers fall victim to frauds, their owners—not taxpayers—suffer. Consider an example. In 2015, Aetna filed a racketeering complaint in which it accused Houston's North Cypress Medical Center of paying kickbacks to referring physicians and of overbilling Aetna to the tune of $120 million. North Cypress returned the favor by claiming that Aetna earned "a good portion of its roughly $500 billion in net revenues" by cheating out-of-network providers.[39] A court will figure out the truth, but regardless of who is right, taxpayers won't have one red cent at stake. A policy of giving money to beneficiaries instead of paying providers would privatize the problem of fraud.

The private sector also has stronger incentives to police fraud than the government does. Ever have to enter your zip code at a gas pump? Ever have to memorize the three-digit code on the back of your credit card? Ever had a credit card purchase stopped in its tracks? Ever received a text message or an email asking you to call in about a suspicious transaction? Ever had an old credit card canceled and a new one issued automatically because the account may have been compromised? Then you know that financial institutions use the latest techniques and approaches to combat fraud. It makes sense to turn fraud control over to the people who actually care about the problem and are best situated to do something about it.

# CHAPTER 21: CATASTROPHIC COVERAGE IS GOOD COVERAGE

## A PRIMER ON HEALTH CARE INSURANCE

Solving the health care cost crisis requires relying less on insurance and paying for more medical treatments ourselves. Because the fear of being uninsured drives many people crazy, we hasten to add that we're not urging people to drop their insurance. Nor do we favor governmental policies that would take insurance away from people who currently have it or that would prevent people who want it from buying it. What we want are policies that would encourage people to use insurance to handle the problems that insurance is well suited for. Right now, health insurance mostly covers the wrong things. It also pays too much (and does so in almost the worst way imaginable) for most of what it covers.

A few seconds of theory show that "health insurance" in modern America isn't really insurance at all. Consider a simplified model of how insurance works in the rest of the economy. In this model, "risks"—that is, the likelihood that losses will occur—come in only two types: low and high. Low risks are unlikely events like having your house struck by lightning. High risks are probable events like needing to buy gas after driving hundreds of miles. The costs that must be borne when risks turn into realities come in only two varieties too: low and high. Low cost is what you spend when you refill your gas tank. High cost is paying to rebuild your house after lightning sets it on fire.

**Table 21-1. Risk and Cost in the Non-Health Care Economy**

|  |  | Cost | |
|---|---|---|---|
|  |  | Low | High |
| Risk | Low | (1)<br>Lost Spare Change | (2)<br>Fire/Flood |
|  | High | (3)<br>Oil Change | (4)<br>College |

With two risk levels and two cost levels, there are four different possible combinations, as shown in Table 21-1. The table also provides some concrete examples that show the kinds of incidents that each combination of risk and cost represents.

Cell 1 is low risk and low cost—think about the risk of losing some spare change. When that risk materializes, the amount of the loss is literally pocket change. No one buys (or sells) insurance against that risk because the losses are too small to be worth the bother.

Moving downward, Cell 3 is high risk but low cost. Think about the biannual maintenance on the furnace in your house or changing the oil in your car. And cars don't just need regular oil changes. As a car accumulates mileage, it also needs brake jobs, new tires, air filters, water pumps, timing belts, and lots of other things. Suppose that all of these repairs and preventive maintenance average $500 a year. Because the risk of having this work done is 100 percent, an insurer would have to charge a premium of $500 per year to cover the costs, plus an additional amount to cover its administrative overhead and profit. This arrangement would not really be insurance at all—it is just a form of prepayment of anticipated expenses, with the insurer holding the money. It is also a bad deal for consumers, who could obtain the services they need more cheaply and on their own timetable by purchasing them directly, without the hassle of going through their insurer. The result is that in the non-health care economy, no one sells insurance (or buys it) for anything that belongs in Cell 3.

Moving to the right, Cell 4 is high risk and high cost—like paying for college for your children or making mortgage payments. Most people save for college or take out student loans (thereby borrowing against future income). Mortgage payments are made out of current income. Just like Cells 1 and 3, in the non-health care economy, no one sells insurance (or buys it) for any of the type of things that are in Cell 4—even though college and mortgages can be very expensive.

Finally, the last possibility is Cell 2, which represents low-risk but high-cost situations, like a catastrophic house fire. Houses don't burn down that often, but when they do, few people can afford to replace them. This combination (low risk and high cost) makes it possible for insurers to protect people from the risk of an enormous financial loss in exchange for relatively modest premiums. A typical homeowners policy, which covers much more than fire-related damage, costs less than $1,000.[1]

As the examples in Table 21-1 imply, and as our discussion of each cell should make clear, in the non-health care economy, insurance is sold mainly to cover risks that belong in Cell 2, where there is a low (and often tiny) likelihood of a bad outcome, but with catastrophic consequences when the risk materializes. Conversely, when loss-causing events are highly likely (Cells 3 and 4), insurers can't offer inexpensive protection, so there isn't much (if any) demand for insurance. And, if the costs and risks are low enough (Cell 1), no one wants to buy or sell insurance against those situations either.

How does this framework apply to health care? Table 21-2 looks exactly like Table 21-1, but with different examples.

**Table 21-2. Risk and Cost in Health-Related Expenditures**

|  |  | Cost | |
| --- | --- | --- | --- |
|  |  | Low | High |
| Risk | Low | (1)<br>Band-Aids | (2)<br>Major Trauma/<br>Cancer |
|  | High | (3)<br>Childhood<br>Vaccines | (4)<br>Post-Retirement<br>Housing and Food |

Just as in Table 21-1, insurers don't add value for the kinds of problems that land in Cells 1, 3, and 4. For Cell 1, the cost of Band-Aids is sufficiently trivial that no one would buy insurance against that eventuality. Similarly, for Cell 3, if you have children, the likelihood of needing to pay for vaccines is 100 percent—at least, if you care about keeping your kid from dying of measles or whooping cough. And for Cell 4, the likelihood of needing housing and food in one's old age is quite high and the cost is large as well. These aren't the kinds of situations that normally give rise to a robust demand for insurance. And, except for the minority of seniors who require some form of long-term care, there is no market for post-retirement housing insurance.

Finally, as Cell 2 indicates, health insurance is a good way of protecting people against remote risks, such as the risk of being severely injured in a car crash and needing expensive medical treatments. As in Table 21-1, insurance works well for the type of problems that fall into Cell 2 because insurers can protect people from catastrophic outcomes while charging relatively modest premiums. When the risk is low but the ultimate cost is extremely high, voluntary markets emerge where consumers can transfer that financial risk to an insurer willing to accept it.

To sum up, health care coverage works well for low-probability, high-cost events (Cell 2), but like other types of insurance it has little to offer for other probability/cost combinations. Stated differently, insurance is a good way of paying for health care when each member of a sizable population faces a small risk of suffering a large loss. But insurance is a bad way of dealing with losses that do not fit this description, including inexpensive medical treatments and treatments for chronic illnesses and other maladies that people are certain to need. The way to deal with these costs is simply to pay for them. The money can come directly out of consumers' pockets or it can come from somewhere else, as it does when people who are too poor to pay for the needed services receive financial support—welfare or charity—from others. For everything other than low-probability, high-cost events, insurance doesn't work.

The type of insurance that works is often called catastrophic coverage. It protects people from large losses by applying after they meet substantial out-of-pocket minimums or deductibles. Catastrophic coverage is cheap because insurers expect people to use it infrequently. The type of insurance that doesn't work is called comprehensive coverage. It combines catastrophic coverage with a prepayment plan for medical expenses that fall into Cells 1, 3, and 4. This is the type of insurance that most people have and that Obamacare requires them to purchase.

Some policy provisions can make the difference between catastrophic coverage and comprehensive coverage hard to discern. For example, when selling coverage for catastrophic risks, an insurer may include coverage for certain inexpensive treatments—like vaccinations, hypertensive medications, or routine blood pressure monitoring—that are highly effective at preventing potentially serious maladies—like the flu, childhood diseases, heart attacks, or strokes. When items like these are covered, the package looks like it falls on the comprehensive side of the divide. But the reason for covering these treatments is that they make it less likely that subscribers will suffer illnesses that are expensive to treat and thereby keep the cost of catastrophic coverage down. Analytically, these provisions have the same function as discounts for nonsmokers or, in the case of automobile insurance, rebates to policyholders who avoid being involved in accidents for long periods. By encouraging behaviors that reduce the frequency of expensive claims, they generate savings in excess of their costs that insurers and policyholders can share.

## CROSS-SUBSIDIZATION: WELFARE IN DISGUISE

Left-leaning policymakers and policy wonks like comprehensive coverage because it redistributes resources in favor of people they want to help. This practice is usually called "cross-subsidization," but it would more accurately be described as welfare. How does cross-subsidization work?

Assume 10 people apply for health insurance. Eight are healthy. Two are sick. How much should each person pay? If the insurer is free to price the policies according to the expected cost that each applicant represents, the healthy people will pay less than the applicants who are sick. Lots of people don't like that idea because it makes it much more difficult for the infirm to obtain health insurance. This concern helps explain why Medicare was created.

But, if you aren't willing to create an entirely new program like Medicare, with the resulting on-budget expenses, what else can you do to fix this problem? The obvious solution is to force insurers to charge everyone the same premium. This is known as "community rating," and it is what Obamacare requires. Obamacare prohibits insurers from charging sick people more, from denying coverage on the basis of pre-existing conditions, and from charging older people more than three times as much as people who are younger. (The actual cost ratio between senior citizens and those under 65 is more like 6 to 1.)[2]

Community rating erases price differences or reduces them, but it also causes healthy applicants to be overcharged. Instead of paying premiums that reflect only the costs they are expected to generate, people who are young or healthy also pick up part of the tab for folks who are old or sick. This is cross-subsidization because the former are subsidizing the latter. By mandating community rating, the politicians, academics, and policy wonks who support Obamacare are using the insurance system to transfer resources from low-risk to high-risk groups in an off-budget fashion. This was a conscious decision, as we discuss further below.

Insurance markets don't tolerate cross-subsidization. Instead, competition forces premiums to reflect the costs that people are expected to generate. A carrier that wanted Person A to pay more so that Person B could pay less would quickly find that A went to a different company whose lower price reflected only A's expected cost. That's why young single males pay much more for auto insurance than middle-aged men who are married and have kids. An insurer who tried to make the latter pay more so that the former could save money would lose its middle-aged male customers in droves. That's also why homeowners who live in regions that are prone to earthquakes, floods, or wildfires are charged more than those whose areas are safer. It would be a bad business strategy to use premiums to force the latter to subsidize the former, particularly if the market for insurance coverage is remotely competitive. And, the more competitive the market, the more likely that premiums will reflects costs (and risks).

People are rarely bothered by the fact that insurance markets tie premiums to risks. Few seem to think that regulators should intervene and force carriers to charge everyone the same thing. Why should safe drivers pay more so that careless drivers can pay less? Why overcharge people who live in areas devoid of trees pay to subsidize people with houses in fire zones? In the wake of the hurricanes that recently devastated parts of Texas and Florida, many people who live inland are wondering why their tax dollars are used to subsidize insurance for people who choose to live near the coasts. Shouldn't the latters' taxes be increased to reflect the risk they incur by purchasing homes that are more likely to be flooded? As a general matter, people seem content to let prices vary across persons according to actual risks, which happens naturally when markets set insurance prices.

But many people think about health insurance differently. They think it is unfair and morally indefensible for high-risk people to pay more than low-risk people for the same coverage. Unfortunately, these proponents of cross-subsidization rarely acknowledge that their objective is to coerce low-risk people into giving wealth to others. Instead, they deliberately obscure the reality that the policies they support are a bad deal for most people.

Chris Conover discussed the impact community rating would have on young people, whom Obamacare overcharges so that older people can pay less.[3] Rates for people ages 18–24 had to increase by 45 percent above the actuarially fair price so that the rate for those ages 60–64 could be reduced by 13 percent. "Is this fair?" Conover wondered.

> Ask the typical 20–24 year-old—whose median weekly earnings are $461—whether it's fair to be asked to pay 50 percent higher premiums so that workers age 55–64—whose median weekly earnings are $887— can pay lower premiums. Think about that. The median earnings for older workers are $420 a week more than those of younger workers, or roughly $20,000 more a year. How is mandating a price break on health insurance for this far higher income group at the expense of the lower income group possibly fair?[4]

It isn't fair. It's immoral.

Jonathan Gruber, a health economist who helped design Obamacare, admitted that cross-subsidization is at the heart of the program. He also acknowledged that transparency about forced wealth transfers would have doomed the bill.

> If you had a law which . . . made it explicit that healthy people pay in [and] sick people get money it would not have passed. . . .
>
> Lack of transparency is a huge political advantage, and basically, call it the stupidity of the American voter or whatever, but basically that was really, really critical for getting the thing to pass.[5]

According to Gruber, if the American people had understood that Obamacare was really an off-the-books welfare program, Congress would not have passed it because even more Democrats would have voted against it.

Our view is simple. It is morally desirable to help poor people, people with chronic medical conditions, and others with the cost of health care. But it is a terrible idea to use the insurance system to accomplish this goal. Welfare programs are designed to redistribute wealth to those who have lost life's lottery; insurance is a financial instrument designed to *keep* people from losing that lottery. The two differ greatly and should not be confused or combined.

But they are routinely conflated and commingled, even by people who know better. Consider how three prominent health policy analysts argued against a recent Republican proposal to cap the rate of growth in Medicaid spending per capita. The proposal, which was modeled on a similar proposal made by President Bill Clinton in 1997, would convert Medicaid from an open-ended obligation of the U.S. Treasury to one in which Medicaid could still grow faster than GDP but slower than it had grown historically. The commentators argued that the cap would imperil Medicaid's ability to pay for nursing home care and described the nursing home benefit as "insurance for all of our mothers and fathers and, eventually, for ourselves." But their column then made it clear that Medicaid is not an insurance plan at all. Instead, it is a welfare program for the elderly poor:

> Medicaid is our nation's largest safety net for low-income people, accounting for one-sixth of all health care spending in the United States. . . . [N]early two-thirds of that spending is focused on older and disabled adults—primarily through spending on long-term care services such as nursing homes.
>
> Indeed, Medicaid pays nearly half of nursing home costs for those who need assistance because of medical conditions like Alzheimer's or stroke. In some states, overall spending on older and disabled adults amounts to as much as three-quarters of Medicaid spending. . . . [If Medicaid's budget were cut, m]any nursing homes would stop admitting Medicaid recipients . . . . Older and disabled Medicaid beneficiaries can't pay out-of-pocket for services and they do not typically have family members able to care for them. The nursing home is a last resort. Where will they go instead?[6]

The authors could and should have explained this problem without ever using the word "insurance." All they had to say is that many poor Americans need help paying for nursing homes and that, in the future, millions more will find themselves in this predicament. What is needed, they might well have concluded, is a safety net that protects old people against the consequences of being poor. That, however, is neither insurance nor even a plan for prepaying expected expenditures. It is welfare, plain and simple.

It should now be clear that both Medicare and Medicaid are hodge-podges of three different things: insurance, prepayment plans, and welfare. Both programs provide protection from low-probability catastrophic risks, and, to the extent they do, they provide insurance. But they also pay for many inexpensive treatments and services, like X-rays for strains and sprains and medications for aches and pains, while also covering things that people are certain to need, such as treatments for chronic illness. So they are prepayment plans too.

Both programs also transfer wealth. Medicaid does so overtly. It uses general tax revenues to pay for health care for the poor. Medicare is stealthier. It fosters the impression that beneficiaries pay for the services they receive by contributing tax dollars throughout their working lives and by paying Medicare premiums in their later years. In fact, the typical beneficiary takes out far, far more than he or she puts in, meaning that Medicare has an enormous welfare component. And, as we describe in further detail in Chapter 22, this welfare component is a reverse-Robin Hood scheme because it funnels resources from the less well off to the more well off.

The Medicare program is also grossly underfunded relative to its future obligations. And the fact that Medicare and Medicaid are entitlements means that spending grows on autopilot because Congress does not have to make annual appropriations to fund these programs.

Comprehensive private coverage is a hodgepodge too. Like Medicare and Medicaid, comprehensive private health insurance provides insurance against low-probability catastrophic risks. It also provides prepayment of expected medical expenses. That's why private health insurance covers well-baby care and many other readily predictable expenses.

Private health insurance may contain a welfare component too, although it's harder to see. Many employers charge different rates according to whether coverage is for a single individual, a couple, or a family, while ignoring other variables, such as age and family size, that also bear on expected costs. The decision to ignore these considerations can have real distributional consequences. They can force younger workers to subsidize older ones, small families to support larger ones, and infertile couples to help those who want comprehensive maternity coverage. Under plans like these, some amount of cross-subsidization is inevitable, although it is disciplined by the willingness of employees to participate, the willingness of employers to allow these wealth transfers, and any offsetting adjustments in wages.[7]

Government can also create cross-subsidies in private health insurance. Coverage mandates can have that effect. For example, all Obamacare policies have to cover a raft of preventive care treatments and wellness checkups without any cost sharing by insureds. Similarly, all Obamacare policies have to provide 10 "essential" benefits, including maternity and newborn care, mental health services, addiction treatment, preventive services, and pediatric services, such as well-child visits, vaccinations, and pediatric dental and vision care. The money to pay for those things had to come from somewhere. Some of it came from people who used those services, and the rest came from those who did not but were forced to buy policies that included the coverages anyway.

Direct regulation of health insurance premiums can result in cross-subsidization as well. As mentioned, Obamacare required young people to subsidize the elderly by capping the premium gradient (the ratio between highest and lowest premiums) at 3 to 1 when the real old-to-young cost ratio was closer to 6 to 1. In like fashion, when Obamacare eliminated the use of pre-existing conditions limitations, it created a large cross-subsidy that favored people who were predictably high cost.

## The Mandate to Insure

Insurance costs a lot because American health care is expensive. Cross-subsidies make premiums even higher for low-risk/low-cost enrollees, who are forced to transfer their wealth to others. As insurance prices rise, people naturally want to buy less of it, and they will not want to buy it at all if it costs more than the value they think it provides.

That's why Obamacare had an individual mandate coupled with a tax penalty imposed on people who opt out of the program. Cross-subsidies are hard to maintain when people can avoid being overcharged for insurance by refusing to buy it.

What does this mean for ordinary people, who don't spend all their time thinking about health policy? Consider what happened to Stacey and Eddie Albert—a nutritionist and a personal trainer, respectively. Before Obamacare, they had a bare-bones health insurance policy from Horizon Blue Cross Blue Shield of New Jersey for which they paid about $360 a month. The policy suited their needs and their budget, both were healthy, they rarely saw a doctor, and they had no children. But, when Obamacare came along, the price of coverage jumped to $650 per month. Some of that was because the Obamacare policy covered things that weren't covered under the old policy—like pediatric dental care and maternity services.[8] The Alberts didn't value those benefits and had gotten along perfectly well without them until Obamacare forced them to buy a bunch of coverages they didn't want. Their premiums were further inflated by overcharging them for the coverage they received so as to provide welfare for others.

The Alberts didn't use many medical services. In that respect, they are typical Americans, not exceptional ones. Although the United States now spends *an average* of more than $10,000 per person on medical services each year, most of this spending is concentrated on a small fraction of the population. For most Americans, the annual cost of health care is slightly below $1,000, an amount that most can afford to pay out of pocket.[9] If you sort the population by health care spending, the lowest-spending half accounts for a mere 3 percent of the nation's total annual health care bill [10]

Of course, spending is higher for Americans who are involved in accidents or suffer from chronic conditions, but many of them could manage their own expenses as well. The average cost per trauma victim is less than $3,000 per person who incurred an expense. The comparable annual figures for people with heart disease, cancer, mental disorders, and chronic obstructive pulmonary disease/asthma are $4,349, $5,631, $1,849, and $1,681, respectively.[11] Although no one enjoys spending sums like these on medical treatments, many consumers could cover them without breaking the bank.

But, as everyone knows, the problem is that spending on health care can vary greatly. All it takes is a bad case of trauma or an emergency surgery for appendicitis to move a person from the average category into the highest cost group—the 5 percent of Americans whose medical treatments account for 50 percent of total spending.[12] The mean annual expenditure for that group is about $43,000. Making the top 10 percent of spenders, who collectively account for 66 percent of medical expenses, is even easier. The mean outlay for that group is only $28,500. There's a lot of turnover in these high-cost groups too. Although nearly two-thirds of the members of the top 5 percent group suffer from long-term illnesses, every year about half of that share gets better and drops down to a lower bracket. Of course, this implies that lots of new people move into the high-cost group every year too.

Many people think that this distribution of costs makes it impossible for health insurance to work. This position betrays a fundamental misunderstanding of insurance economics. It is precisely the potential for incurred costs to vary by several orders of magnitude that creates a demand for insurance and allows catastrophic coverage to do its job—by placing a ceiling on the amount that a person must spend out of pocket on needed medical services in any policy period. When spending exceeds the ceiling, the insurance policy kicks in and protects the consumer from much or all of the burden of any additional medical treatments. And, because so few people incur catastrophic health care expenses, catastrophic coverage is affordable—as long as it isn't larded up with payments for predictable expenditures and cross-subsidies.

### KNOWN OR PREDICTABLE MEDICAL EXPENSES

Catastrophic coverage isn't a complete answer to everything that is wrong with the health care sector. We have addressed other problems that require attention in other chapters in Part 2. Here, we concentrate on the problem of dealing with known or predictable medical expenses.

Insurance can't do much to help people manage the consequences of illnesses that occurred *before* they were insured. When someone is highly likely to need expensive medical services year after year, there is no risk to insure. There is only a need to pay for the treatments. This is true, for example, of uninsured children born with significant, lifelong health problems. The medical services they require must be paid for somehow, and we should make it as easy and affordable as possible for people, including hopeful or expectant parents, to insure *before* health losses occur. But in cases where they don't, we shouldn't call whatever mechanism pays for their health care "insurance" because the need for the services is certain.

Insurance can't do much with the predictable costs of aging either. As people move from their thirties into their forties, fifties, and later decades, their expected medical costs rise inexorably. Because insurance premiums reflect expected costs, they rise with age too.

Even if the costs of aging were much less predictable, insurance still wouldn't be a good way of paying for them. Consider joint replacements. A 2015 study found that the average cost of total knee replacement surgery was about $31,000.[13] In that year, the average new car cost about $33,000, only $2,000 more.[14] People pay for their cars all by themselves; why can't they pay for new knee joints too? When it comes to financing the two, the main difference is that we're used to buying cars ourselves while we're used to using insurance to pay for medical treatments.

But paying for replacement knee joints with insurance has bad consequences. Prices rise because insurers add a substantial layer of expense. Insurance also stimulates demand and compounds the pricing problem by paying far more than consumers would if they were spending their own hard-earned money.

Consider the extent to which the average price for a total knee replacement varies, both within the same city and across states. In Dallas, Texas, the average charge for a total knee replacement in 2013 was about $40,000. However, one hospital in Dallas averaged $17,000, while another averaged $62,000. If patients paid for these procedures directly, the high-priced hospitals would go out of business, unless they could prove that they were vastly superior. Hospitals in New York City might not perform any knee replacements at all, unless they blockaded the bridges and tunnels to ensure their customers couldn't leave town. The average charge for a knee replacement in New York City in 2013 was just shy of $70,000. Cost-conscious New Yorkers could have the surgery done in Dallas and pocket the difference. Or they might pay a visit to Montgomery, Alabama, where the lowest-priced hospital charged only $11,000, and save even more.[15]

Cars need regular maintenance, but even when kept in good repair, they eventually wear out and are replaced. Human bodies deteriorate with age too, even when cared for well. Often, the options we choose for ourselves when we ail cost the same or less than those we select when dealing with our cars. So why do we pay for the latter directly while using insurance to pay for health care?

For most of us, the answer isn't that we have sufficient cash on hand to pay for cars but not for knee surgeries. When Americans buy new cars, we often take out loans that we pay off over time. In 2016, the average new car loan was for $30,000 and the average loan term was 68 months.[16] Presumably, the people who took out these loans had too little cash on hand to pay for knee replacements or cars, but only if they needed the former were they likely to pay with insurance.

The answer isn't that cars last longer than knee joints either. The opposite is true. Artificial knees typically are good for 20 years.[17] People would usually find knee surgery easier to afford than their first new car too, because joint replacements happen late in life, after the mortgage has been paid off and the kids are done with college.[18] New car buyers are usually much younger and have many more competing needs. In 2015, more than half of all new cars were sold to people 49 years of age or younger.[19] All things considered, knee replacement surgery seems to be more affordable than a new car—and it would be even easier to budget for if people bought it directly because it would cost much less than it does.

So why do people use insurance to pay for knee replacements and other medical procedures instead of borrowing money to pay for them? Why don't they save up in advance, the way people often do for their children's college expenses? For many reasons, none of them especially good. People think of new cars and college educations as gains and of medical treatments as losses, and they connect insurance to the latter, not the former. Tax breaks encourage people to use insurance to pay for medical treatments but not other things. The health care system teaches people that they're supposed to use insurance to pay for its products. And people who see others insuring against health care costs find it natural to do the same.

But it doesn't follow that insurance is a good way of dealing with medical expenses that are known or predictable. To the contrary, if you were trying to create a dynamic that would funnel ever-increasing amounts of money into the health care system, it would be hard to improve on Obamacare, which required everyone to have comprehensive insurance, backed up with huge amounts of federal funding to hide from everyone involved the true costs of running prepayment and welfare programs in the guise of an insurance program.

PRE-EXISTING CONDITIONS

What about individuals with pre-existing medical conditions? The plight of these unlucky individuals has preoccupied American health policy for decades, culminating with Obamacare's elimination of limitations on pre-existing conditions. What can we do about this problem if we move to a system of catastrophic coverage that does not cover known or predictable medical expenses?

The first point to understand is that much of the debate over pre-existing conditions is based on misleading statistics. Advocacy groups highlight the large number of Americans with chronic illnesses and imply that they are all at risk of being priced out of the insurance market.[20] This is complete nonsense. Insurers limit coverage of pre-existing conditions to ensure that new applicants are not gaming the system by purchasing coverage only when they think they will need it. Historically, people who maintained their coverage were not subject to limitations on newly developed conditions at renewal time, even if they experienced claims.[21] Indeed, the incentive to obtain and maintain insurance coverage derived partly from the fact that renewal at standard rates was usually guaranteed. (The same was ordinarily true for people who changed jobs, as long as they had coverage at the job they left.) Most insurers in the individual market voluntarily offered continuing coverage of this sort, and the 1996 Health Insurance Portability and Accountability Act roped in the few that did not.[22]

Greg Scandlen discusses the exaggeration of the frequency of coverage denials based on pre-existing conditions in his recent book, *Myth Busters: Why Health Reform Always Goes Awry*. He begins by observing that such denials occur only in the market where people who do not obtain coverage through their employers buy it directly. This market encompasses about 10.3 million people. He then points out that denials based on pre-existing conditions occur only when people buy insurance for the first time; denials do not happen when people who are already covered renew. That limits the at-risk group to about 1.8 million people per year. Finally, he notes that, in 2008, insurers accepted 87 percent of new applicants. The number denied coverage, 223,000, constituted "less than one tenth of one percent of the country's population."[23] Many of these unfortunates still had options too. They could join states' high-risk pools or obtain coverage through state-appointed insurers of last resort.

Obamacare itself showed that its architects exaggerated the severity of the problem of coverage denials based on pre-existing conditions. Although the legislation passed in 2010, the provision requiring insurers to accept all applicants would not take effect until 2014. Believing that they needed to address the problem of coverage denials more quickly, Obamacare's architects created a special program called the Pre-existing Conditions Insurance Plan (PCIP) that went into effect immediately. The U.S. Congressional Budget Office (CBO) projected that 200,000 people a year would enroll in PCIP.[24] Medicare's actuaries projected that 375,000 would.[25] In reality, *total* enrollment peaked just below 115,000,[26] just about enough to fill the University of Michigan's football stadium.[27] The neutral arbiters at the CBO and Medicare had pegged the *expected* annual demand at two to three times the *actual* total demand, reflecting the tendency to exaggerate the frequency of coverage denials for pre-existing conditions.

Prior to Obamacare, there were people with expensive illnesses who did not have health insurance, whether because they failed to purchase coverage when they should have, lacked the resources to do so, or lost their coverage along with their jobs. And, of course, not all of them may have felt the need to obtain coverage through the PCIP. So we should view these figures as a lower bound on the number of people who actually experience problems with obtaining coverage because of a pre-existing condition.

Assume for the sake of argument that we are talking about 500,000 people or even 1 million people per year. We note at the outset that this is at most 0.3 percent of the U.S. population. But, if we want to do something for these people, we should treat their problem just like we treat the problem of known or predictable medical expenses. We should subsidize them so they can obtain whatever level of coverage or treatment we collectively deem to be adequate. And we should do that in a transparent on-budget way, so that everyone voting for the legislation understands the associated trade-offs.

Obamacare supporters object that Congress and state legislatures won't provide sufficient funds to take care of the problem of pre-existing conditions if voters understand what is going on. That may or may not be true. But consider what it means that Obamacare supporters believe it to be true. If Congress and state legislatures won't provide the level of funding they want, it means that voters don't want what Obamacare supporters want. Obamacare supporters know this, and they therefore prefer to use (in Jonathan Gruber's words) a "lack of transparency" to deceive voters about what Obamacare really does. If Obamacare supporters believe the only way they can get what they want is to lie to their fellow citizens about what they are doing and why, that is a more damning indictment of their position than anything we can say about it.

Finally, even if our solution to the problem of pre-existing conditions isn't perfect, it is important to compare the stable and inexpensive catastrophic insurance market that will result from our proposals to the far more imperfect and dysfunctional insurance market that Obamacare has given us. Lots of people like the fact that Obamacare eliminated pre-existing condition terms, but they hate the individual mandate and the large subsidies that are required to make that decision remotely workable. We don't think this conflict can be finessed for much longer—and so we are offering a solution that will stick, while also reducing costs and making the system more responsive to its actual customers. Finally, our approach has the singular virtue of transparency about what it is trying to accomplish and how much it is costing us to do so.

### INCOMPETENT AND UNCONSCIOUS PATIENTS

One final issue is how we should deal with incompetent and unconscious patients, such as accident victims who are in no position to shop for low-priced health care. Skeptics seem to think that this problem is a compelling

argument against more market-oriented approaches to the financing and
delivery of health care.[28] But it is not a difficult problem, as Professor John
Cochrane explains:

> Yes, a guy in the ambulance on his way to the hospital with a heart attack
> is not in a good position to negotiate. But what fraction of health-care
> and its expense is caused by people with sudden, unexpected, debilitat-
> ing conditions requiring immediate treatment? How many patients are
> literally passed out? Answer: next to none. . . .
>
> Most of the expense and problem in our health care system involves
> treatment of chronic conditions or (what turns out to be) end-of-life
> care, and involve many difficult decisions involving course of treatment,
> extent of treatment, method of delivery, and so on. These people can
> shop. Our health care system actually does a pretty decent job with
> heart attacks.
>
> And even then . . . have they no families? If I'm on the way to the
> hospital, I call my wife. She is a heck of a negotiator.
>
> Moreover, health care is not a spot market, which people think
> about once, at fifty-five, when they get a heart attack. It is a long-term
> relationship. When your car breaks down at the side of the road, you're
> in a poor position to negotiate with the tow-truck driver. That is why
> you join AAA. If you, by virtue of being human, might someday need
> treatment for a heart attack, might you not purchase health insurance, or
> at least shop ahead of time for a long-term relationship to your doctor,
> who will help to arrange hospital care?
>
> And what choices really need to be made here? Why are we even
> talking about "negotiation?" Look at any functional, competitive busi-
> ness. As a matter of fact, roadside car repair and gas stations on inter-
> states are remarkably honest, even though most of their customers meet
> them once. In a competitive, transparent market, a hospital that routinely
> overcharged cash customers with heart attacks would be creamed by
> Yelp.com reviews, to say nothing of lawsuits from angry patients. Life
> is not a one-shot game. Competition leads to clear posted prices, and
> businesses anxious to gain a reputation for honest and efficient service.[29]

Like the old Yiddish joke about the man who kills his parents and
then throws himself on the mercy of the court because he is an orphan,
those who allow third-party payment to create widespread, rampant price
gouging oppose letting consumers control health care dollars because, god

forbid, someone might get gouged. If there is a problem with overcharging the unconscious and incompetent, it is because our politically controlled third-party payer system encourages health care providers to overcharge *everyone*. Politicians, medical professionals, hospitals, insurance companies, and many others making money off our health care system are protecting those high prices from the cost-reducing effects of competition.

## A STURDIER THREE-LEGGED STOOL

Jonathan Gruber, the prominent health economist whose remarks on transparency were quoted above, observed that Obamacare relied on a "three-legged stool" to reform health insurance markets: "new rules that prevent insurers from denying coverage or raising premiums based on pre-existing conditions, requirements that everyone buy insurance, and subsidies to make that insurance affordable."[30] That approach doubled down on a failed strategy. It used health insurance to pay for most health care expenditures, insulated patients from the direct costs of their decisions, and hid the enormous costs that resulted. Obamacare's architects positioned their three-legged stool atop a massive health care bubble.

Moving forward also requires a three-legged stool—but not the one found in Obamacare. The first leg is catastrophic coverage for remote risks with the potential to inflict large losses. The second leg is having people pay out of pocket for medical treatments that are expected and predictable. And the third leg is an explicit on-budget welfare system that provides financial support to people who are poor or otherwise deemed deserving of public support.

# CHAPTER 22: MORALITY AND HEALTH CARE

## Medicare: Standing Robin Hood on His Head

Most of the chapters in this book are chock-full of statistics and economically oriented policy analyses. This one is different. It addresses moral matters that are hard to quantify but nonetheless important. The basic question is whether government health care programs like Medicare, Medicaid, and the VHA have compelling moral justifications. We think not. To the contrary, they are subject to obvious moral complaints. Medicare is an intergenerational Ponzi scheme that moves dollars from younger people who are relatively poor to older people who are relatively rich, while making health care more dangerous and expensive for everyone and wasting one-third of the dollars it doles out. How can a moral case be made for a program like that? Medicaid helps the poor, but it does so inefficiently and is needlessly paternalistic. Poor people would fare better if the program was replaced with cash grants. The VHA suffers similar deficiencies. Veterans should receive cash so they can buy medical services anywhere.

Americans love Robin Hood, the legendary English bandit who took from the rich and gave to the poor. And, like him, we are givers. The vast majority of us donate to charities every year. Total giving exceeds

$200 billion a year, with most of the dollars coming from individuals and much of it being earmarked for people in need.[1]

The impulse to help others is one of the moral pillars of civilization. But it also makes Medicare seem odd, because Medicare is a reverse Robin Hood scheme. Medicare's dominant tendency is to move dollars from the poor to the rich. Young people, including those who are raising families, saddled with educational debts, and struggling to make ends meet, are taxed to buy medical services for seniors, who tend to be much wealthier. That is the opposite of charity.[2]

The wealth disparity between young and old is large. In 2013, the median net worth of a family headed by a person ages 35–44 was $46,700. Families whose heads were ages 65–74 had a median worth of $232,100, almost five times as much.[3] Young people are much more likely than the elderly to live in poverty too. In 2015, 20 percent of America's children lived in poverty, as did 12 percent of adults ages 19–64. The comparable figure for Americans 65 years and up was only 9 percent.[4]

The elderly's wealth and income advantages are easy to explain. Old people have had their entire working lives to accumulate wealth and build careers, and many of them have done so. They've paid off their mortgages and their cars, and many built retirement savings or stock portfolios. Young people have yet to live through their working years. Consequently, they tend to have less wealth, lower earnings, and more debt.

That Medicare forces people who are relatively poor to support people who are relatively rich is abhorrent. Every moral theory we know of posits that wealth transfers should run in the opposite direction. It's easy to see why. When poor young people, especially those with children, acquire houses, cars, education, medical services, and many other things, the welfare gains are enormous because the benefits are large and pay out over many years. But, when the equivalent number of dollars are spent on seniors, the utility gains are small because the improvements in the quality of life are frequently minor and life expectancy is short. This is especially true of intensive medical treatments delivered in the last months of life that cost tens of thousands of dollars.

If children are the future, we shouldn't force young people to pay for old people's health care. We should reverse our spending priorities.

The ratio of federal benefits to the old versus the young is roughly 3 to 1. A ratio of 1 to 3 would make more sense.

## MEDICARE: AN INTERGENERATIONAL PONZI SCHEME

Years ago, one of us asked a health policy expert who supported Medicare to defend the morality of moving money from poorer people to those who are richer. The answer went something like this: *Everyone gets old. Medicare is an inter-generational pact that ensures that health care will be available when we're aged and infirm.* There are so many things wrong with this answer that it's hard to know where to begin.

Consider the premise: "Everyone gets old." That's not true. We all know people who died before they turned 65, the eligibility threshold for Medicare. Of every 100,000 baby boomers born between 1949 and 1951, only 67,555 lived to age 65.[5] African-American baby boomers born during the same years fared even more poorly. Only 48,649 per 100,000 lived to Medicare's eligibility age. The unfortunates who died early never received any Medicare benefits. But many did pay Medicare taxes, so they both died young and were taxed to help others whose lives were longer. There are also many people like Tom Petty, the rock star, who die shortly after turning 65. For them, Medicare is also a bad deal.

Medicare isn't a "pact" either. Tens of millions of people who are paying Medicare taxes today were born after 1965, the year Medicare was created. No one asked them whether they'd rather buy health care for other people or use the money in some other way, such as saving it for their own retirements. Nor, obviously, has anyone asked the permission of the hundreds of millions of yet-to-be-born Americans who will have to pay Medicare taxes in the future, if the program is to survive. Medicare isn't a "pact." It is governmentally imposed coercion, and it is intellectually dishonest to obscure this truth by babbling on about a "pact" that doesn't exist.

The argument that Medicare is an intergenerational pact also assumes that Medicare will last forever. That is far from guaranteed, if only because the demographics are against it. When Medicare was created, there were 4.5 working people for every eligible beneficiary.[6] Over time, the ratio has steadily declined. In 2016, there were only 3.1 workers per beneficiary.

In 2030, there will be only 2.4.[7] As the ratio of workers to beneficiaries falls, taxes per worker will have to rise.

Will tomorrow's workers keep paying those taxes? Or will they rise up and demand that Congress repeal Medicare? No one can be certain. But if you're confident that they will let themselves be fleeced, you might read *Boomsday*, a novel by Christopher Buckley. He foresees an uprising against Medicare by young workers who stage protests at golf courses and nursing homes. Nor is Buckley alone in predicting a revolt. Phillip Longman, a demographer and investigative journalist, expressed the same concern, writing, "The 75 million members of the Baby Boom generation . . . have good reason to fear desertion by their successors."[8] If you think that's far-fetched, remember how unlikely it seemed that Donald Trump would win the 2016 election. Strange things can happen, and the baby boom generation has imposed an impossible burden on younger Americans.

The truth is that Medicare is a Ponzi scheme in which money from new participants is used to pay earlier participants. The program will last only as long as the government supports it. How much longer that will be is anyone's guess, but it seems likely that support for the program among taxpaying workers will steadily erode. Even if Medicare survives, Congress may address its rising cost by raising the eligibility age, increasing premiums and copays, capping benefits, excluding services from coverage, or taking other steps that force retirees to shoulder more costs. Aging baby boomers may soon discover that, after paying Medicare taxes throughout their careers, they are the big losers in an intergenerational Ponzi scheme.

In case the defects already pointed out aren't sufficiently fatal, the claim that Medicare is an intergenerational pact has one more glaring flaw. Its central thrust is that it is fair to tax today's young people because they will eventually benefit from taxes that tomorrow's young people will be made to pay. That is utterly wrong. Would you say that it is fair for older kids to steal younger kids' lunch money because the younger kids will soon grow up and steal from the new kids who come in behind them? Of course not. The fact that a person may benefit from a forced transfer of wealth in the future does not justify forcibly taking wealth from that person today. For the same reason, no one should think it morally desirable to coercively move wealth from young people to old people today simply because dollars will be coercively taken from future generations tomorrow. Everyone should recognize that coercive transfers are presumptively immoral and that their immorality is increased when the victims are poor and the beneficiaries are rich. The possibility that today's plunderees will be tomorrow's plunderers shows only that an immoral practice can continue far longer than it should—and that redistributionist schemes will have no shortage of apologists.

### MEDICARE: NEITHER PRUDENT NOR JUST

The Harvard philosopher Norman Daniels, who has devoted much of his academic career to the subject of justice between generations, rejects most of the points we just made. In *Am I My Parents' Keeper?*, he offers a Prudential Lifespan Account of justice between age groups, according to which public institutions like Medicare and Social Security help people improve their lives by budgeting resources prudently over time. These institutions are also equitable, he contends, because when they are applied consistently, everyone benefits from them at the appropriate stage of life. Thus, of Social Security he writes:

> [I]f the Social Security system remains stable, young workers will be entitled to claim benefits when they age and retire. There is an inter-generational compact that has the effect of transferring resources from an individual's working years to his retirement years, insuring that basic needs can be met over the whole lifespan.[9]

And of Medicare he states:

> What is crucial about the health-care system is that we pass through it as we grow older. The system transfers resources from stages of our lives in which we have relatively little need for them into stages in which we do. We pay for health care we do not use in our middle years, but we receive health care we do not pay for in . . . old age. . . . The inflated premium in *our* adult years is needed to pay for *our* needs in other stages of *our* lives. . . . We all benefit from an institution that reallocates health-care resources from stages of our lives in which we have many resources and few needs into those stages in which we have fewer resources and greater needs.[10]

On Daniels' view, then, what justifies the Social Security and Medicare programs is not that they redistribute wealth *across* persons. It is that they help individuals move wealth from fat years to lean years. The programs are redistributive *within* persons across different stages of life.

This argument suffers from a host of deficiencies, some of which Daniels acknowledges. For example, it works only if one assumes that Social Security and Medicare will last indefinitely, which seems unlikely. But, even if the argument were sound, it would not justify Medicare. It would warrant only a legal requirement or other inducement that causes people to save money for the predictable medical needs of old age.

To see this, imagine that, over the course of a lifetime, all Americans earn enough money to pay for all of their medical needs. But there is a problem: most of the dollars come in during their working years, and many people save too little to pay for medical treatments they will need after they retire. Would Medicare be the only way to solve this problem? No. Any program that encouraged or required people to save more during their working years would do the trick.

There could be another problem, though. Even if we succeeded in getting people to save more during their working years, we might fear that, after retiring, many would spend their accumulated wealth on travel, gambling, or other entertainments instead of designating the money for health care. Even if this were true, though, we still would not need Medicare. We would only have to encourage people to use the money for medical treatments or require them to do so by limiting the uses to which the saved dollars could be put.

To put the point succinctly: if the problem is that people save too little or spend what they do save unwisely, the solution is not Medicare. Medicare neither encourages savings nor discourages profligacy in retirement. It does the opposite. Medicare discourages workers from saving during their income-generating years by assuring them that the government will give them heavily subsidized health care when they retire. And it encourages profligacy in old age by telling seniors that, no matter how they spend their retirement dollars, their access to medical services won't be imperiled. Medicare is a Rube Goldberg–style mechanism that takes care of the elderly by politicizing the health care economy, driving up health care costs for everyone, wasting hundreds of billions of dollars a year, moving money from the poor to the rich, degrading the quality of care, and discouraging individuals from acting responsibly. And that's even without considering the overwhelming financial challenges to the long-term viability of the program.

## PROOF OF CONCEPT

Some readers may be thinking that it is fine in theory to suggest that people should save during their working years for the medical treatments they will need in old age, but the idea will never work in practice. How can anyone be expected to save that much? And what about the poor and less fortunate? Can we seriously think that, when they become seniors, they should pay for their own care too?

Doubters may reconsider when they learn what Singapore does. Singapore, an Asian city-state with a population of roughly 5.6 million, requires residents to put a defined share of their earnings into tax-free "Medisave" accounts, from which funds can be withdrawn only to pay for health care. To prevent Singaporeans from depleting their Medisave accounts too early, the spending rules require them to pay out of pocket for most of the ordinary medical treatments they need. To encourage thrift, the law also allows Singaporeans to bequeath any funds left in their accounts at death to their heirs. Singapore provides for its poorest citizens by topping up their Medisave accounts, operating a safety net of public hospitals that provide standardized care at bargain-basement prices and, on rare occasions, by dipping into a fund and helping to pay some of the bills.[11] But treatments are not doled out for free. All Singaporeans must contribute something to the cost of their care.

Singapore's Medisave is much better than our Medicare. It prevents people from overspending during their fruitful years, encourages prudent purchasing of medical services when illness strikes, and reinforces the ethic of personal responsibility for health and health care.[12] Medicare does none of these things. If anything, Medicare discourages saving and encourages irresponsibility by telling people that, when they are old, the government will give them health care for free. Medisave is also less coercive than Medicare. Singaporeans keep both the money they set aside and the interest it earns. They do not regard their forced savings program as a tax because the money is still theirs.

Medisave also has the singular advantage of insulating the health care payment system from government control.[13] As Professor David A. Reisman, an economist who lives in Singapore, explains:

> [Singapore's] personal-account, defined-contribution system shelters social security from the rise in dependency [on the government]. There is no pooling, no sharing, no cross-subsidisation [sic] and no redistribution. There is no crediting-in of payments for university students or the unemployed. Retirement balances are sealed off from the electoral cycle and the vote motive. Save-as-you-earn, [Medisave] does not presuppose that pension plans should be augmented out of tax revenues or that there should be an intergenerational promise. For that reason, there is no looming exhaustion of reserves and no pension-driven pressure for a budget deficit. There is no imminent threat that payouts will have to be pruned back because current and future generations will not tolerate the higher tax rates of PAYGO [pay-as-you-go] in an ageing society where the worker-to-pensioner ratio is decreasing.[14]

In contrast, Medicare is an unfunded, pay-as-you-go system, whose survival depends on a never-ending inflow of new tax dollars and deficit spending. Its future, including its eligibility threshold and the coverage it provides, is subject to the whims of voters and manipulation by scheming politicians. Medisave, by contrast, is fully funded at all times, privately owned and controlled, and resistant to governmental interference. By switching to a program designed along the lines of Medisave, Americans would eliminate both the political corruption of medicine and the medical corruption of politics.

Finally, and perhaps most important, Singapore lets patients decide how their health care dollars are spent. Unlike the Medicare program, which puts health care dollars under the control of bureaucrats, Singapore's mandated savings program leaves consumers in charge. They decide which services to use and how much to pay for them. This approach encourages providers to compete for business by improving quality of care, cutting their fees, and offering guarantees. First-party payment also makes life much more difficult for fraudsters.

In sum, a Singaporean-style savings program would be far more compatible with the ideals of small government, individual freedom, and personal responsibility than Medicare. But Singapore is a small city-state with only 5.6 million people. And its system of government is, to put it mildly, quite different from our own. Could a similar program take root in the United States, across 50 states and 325 million people?

We think so. Tens of millions of Americans already participate in voluntary retirement plans. Most of these individuals do so via their employers, who withhold contributions from their wages. Others contribute on their own. For these people, a transition to a mandated or tax-incentivized savings program would be nearly invisible. Americans are also accustomed to paying Social Security and Medicare taxes. In 2014, 166 million workers had dollars deducted from their wages in the form of payroll taxes to support these programs.[15] Converting these dollars from taxes into savings plan contributions should generate enthusiasm—not resistance—among workers. Finally, 35 million Americans have tax-favored, health-care-targeted flexible spending accounts (FSAs), and 30 million are expected to have similar health savings accounts (HSAs) by 2018.[16] People with these accounts would obviously be comfortable with a program that rewarded them for saving for old age.

## MEDICAID: WRONGLY PATERNALISTIC

Medicaid isn't a Ponzi scheme. It's a welfare program for the poor, albeit one with a strange design. Poverty is a money problem. Poor people have too little of it, and the solution is to give them more. Medicaid doesn't do that. Not a single dollar winds up in any poor person's hands. Instead, Medicaid pays health care providers to treat poor people for free.

The health care industry likes this arrangement, which ensures that its members receive every one of the nearly $600 billion that Medicaid pays out each year. But is this the best way to help the poor? We think not.

To see why, ask yourself a question. Across the United States, the average amount spent per Medicaid enrollee per year is about $6,500.[17] Suppose that poor people were offered a choice: receive $6,500 in cash and use it to buy an insurance package equivalent to Medicaid or receive $6,500 in cash and use it some other way. If you think that some, many, or most poor people would spend the money some other way, you're with the majority and you should agree that forcing them to take Medicaid in lieu of cash isn't the welfare-maximizing approach.

We are not the first to contend that Medicaid could help the poor more by giving them cash. Many economists and commentators with libertarian leanings have made this point. But centrist health policy thinkers don't agree. After observing that "every developed country, including the United States, subsidize[s] health insurance for the poor," Harold Pollack, Bill Gardner, and Timothy Jost explain:

> Part of the reason is that those countries have broader moral and public-health criteria for thinking about health insurance and poor people's lives. Universal health care expresses a commitment to the well-being of fellow citizens. Everyone should have access to a decent minimum of care; caring for others in distress is a primary expression of human solidarity.[18]

These are lofty sentiments, but they do not survive scrutiny.

Consider the assertion, "Universal health care expresses a commitment to the well-being of fellow citizens." That's not really what it does. It expresses a commitment to something—access to medical services—that can affect people's well-being (for better or for worse) and that, in the opinion of mainstream health policy thinkers, matters more than other goods and services that affect people's well-being and could be bought with the same dollars. This more accurate way of framing the commitment makes two things clear. First, health care does not equal well-being but is only one of many means by which well-being might be maintained or improved. Second, Medicaid policy is fundamentally paternalistic. If the program were actually devoted to the well-being of fellow citizens, it would hand out cash and let people spend it on goods and services that, from *their* perspective, have the most potential to help. Instead, Medicaid pays only for medical treatments. In effect, Pollack, Gardner, and Jost are saying that they know how poor people should spend money better than poor people do themselves. They want poor people to have what *they* think the poor need, not what poor people themselves might want.

There is a good reason why paternalism has a bad name, apart from dealing with minors and the mentally incompetent. By giving benefits in-kind rather than in cash, the state expresses the opinion that recipients cannot be trusted

> . . . to make what [the state] regards as wise choices about how to spend their money. This, despite the fact that both economic theory and a growing body of empirical evidence suggest that individuals are better off with the freedom of choice that a cash grant brings. In kind grant programs like SNAP (food stamps) persist in their present form not because they are effective but because they are the product of a classic Bootleggers-and-Baptists coalition: well-meaning members of the public like the idea that welfare recipients have to use their vouchers on food rather than alcohol and cigarettes, and the farm lobby likes that beneficiaries are forced to buy its own products. Poor people, meanwhile, are deprived of the opportunity to save [what] a cash grant would give them, and they are forced to waste time and effort trading what SNAP allows them to buy for what they really want.[19]

A bootleggers-and-Baptists coalition supports Medicaid too. Well-meaning health policy types such as Pollack, Gardner, and Jost like the idea that poor people have to buy medical services—and so do health care providers. Their touted "commitment to the well-being of fellow citizens" really just amounts to leaving poor people less well-off than they could be, while wasting hundreds of billions of dollars on fraud and health care services of little or no value.

Pollack, Gardner, and Jost also offer a second justification. They argue that Medicaid works, citing a study that, they report, "found that [a] previous expansion of state Medicaid programs significantly reduced all-cause mortality."[20] That claim can be disputed—recall the study of Oregon's Medicaid expansion, which found negligible health effects—but the argument fails even if they are right. What Pollack, Gardner, and Jost need to provide, but do not, is a study that compares the impact of two different programs: one that doles out Medicaid and one that gives out cash. Without a comparative study, there is no way to establish that poor people benefit more from in-kind awards of access to health care than from cash grants.

Let there be no mistake: cash grants help poor people immensely. The Earned Income Tax Credit and the Child Tax Credit transfer more than $100 billion to the working poor every year.[21] These outlays generate documented reductions in poverty and health improvements, especially among women and children.[22] These effects are not surprising. Recipients spend the money they receive on necessities like food, housing, clothing, transportation, furniture, and school supplies. "The overall pattern suggests that recipients allocate their refunds carefully, meeting essential needs that they may have difficulty addressing with regular income."[23] We know of no basis upon which Pollack, Gardner, and Jost could reasonably posit that poor people intrinsically derive greater value from government-subsidized medical services than from cash grants of equal size. Indeed, there are strong reasons to believe the opposite—starting with the revealed preferences of the poor when they are spending their own money.

What's true of Medicaid also applies to Medicare. Instead of paying for seniors' health care, the federal government could give them money and let them decide how to spend it. Its refusal to do this makes sense from a bootleggers-and-Baptists perspective, but not from a moral one. The vast majority of seniors are competent and make important choices for themselves. They decide whether to sell their homes and move closer to their grandchildren or into retirement centers, whether to draw money out of their retirement accounts, and whether and where to take vacations. There is little reason to fear that they would spend Medicare dollars unwisely if given control of them. However, there is reason to think that many of them would buy things other than medical services with the money, which is why the bootleggers won't let the federal government give them control.

Some people, elderly, poor, or otherwise, lack the competence needed to handle their own affairs. These people require special arrangements, which typically include judicial proceedings and the appointment of legal guardians. But, even for these people, there is no moral argument for bestowing benefits in-kind rather than in cash. Once a guardian is appointed, a competent decisionmaker exists and the need for governmental paternalism disappears. The government's proper role is to monitor the guardian's performance, for example, by policing mismanagement of assets and self-dealing.

## MEDICAID: INEFFICIENT

We said above that we see no basis for thinking that poor people intrinsically benefit more from health care coverage than from cash grants of equal size. In fact, the opposite is more likely true. Poor people probably derive greater value from things they buy with cash than from the medical services that Medicaid provides at the public's expense.

The reason is simple. When people spend their own money, they purchase things whose subjective value exceeds the dollars they have to give up. Rather than spend $10 on an item that bestows only $5 worth of value, a person would hold onto the cash. But, when a third party pays for an item or service, a beneficiary will rationally accept it even if the cost exceeds the subjective benefit by far. Who cares if a medical service that costs $10 conveys only $5 worth of value when the government foots the bill? And who cares if the service actually costs $100 or even $1,000? By accepting the service, the recipient would still be $5 better off. The cost to taxpayers is irrelevant.

Medicaid, Medicare, and private health insurance all tempt beneficiaries to use medical services imprudently. That's a big part of the reason why America is awash in unnecessary treatments. That's also why switching from Medicaid to cash grants would make poor people better off. Rather than undergo medical treatments with little potential to help, they would buy high-value goods and services of other types.

The study that occasioned the commentary by Pollack, Gardner, and Jost suggested that low-value consumption is a real problem in Medicaid. Looking yet again at Oregon's health insurance experiment (see Chapter 15), a team of researchers from the Massachusetts Institute of Technology, Harvard, and Dartmouth attempted to measure the value recipients derived from services covered by Medicaid. The authors concluded: "All of our estimates indicate a welfare benefit from Medicaid to recipients that is below the government's cost of providing Medicaid."[24] In plain English, if we took the money the government is spending on

Medicaid, gave it to Medicaid enrollees, and offered them the right to buy into Medicaid, the people who purportedly benefit from this program wouldn't buy it. Think about that. The people receiving Medicaid don't think the benefits are worth what the government is spending.

Indeed, we think it is likely that Medicaid recipients derive less than the 40 cents of value the researchers estimated recipients derive from one dollar of Medicaid spending. The basic reason for this conclusion is straight-forward. Prior to enrolling in Medicaid, the people who won Oregon's lottery paid only 20–40 cents on the dollar for the medical services they received. The rest of the cost of their care was either borne by others or absorbed as charity care. Medicaid primarily benefited those other payers and charitable providers by freeing them from having to pitch in.[25] Other studies have also found that "Medicaid significantly reduces the provision of uncompensated care by hospitals."[26] No wonder the bootleggers like Medicaid—it exists for them, not the poor.

Pollack, Gardner, and Jost do not dispute our conclusion that Medicaid is perceived as a bad deal even by those who benefit from it. "Given the choice between a Medicaid benefit that costs $4,000 and $4,000 in simple cash," they write, "many or most low-income people might well prefer to take the cash." But they defend Medicaid against this scathing critique by arguing that poor people's willingness to pay for medical services is irrelevant:

> Voters want to provide for the health of their neighbors and to protect [their] neighbors from the financial ruin that often follows serious illness. When my neighbor requires $50,000 for a life-saving kidney transplant, that need has special urgency, as do other basic necessities such as nutri-tion and shelter. The moral interest of the community does not hinge on my neighbor's willingness to pay. We respond to critical needs because we understand the consequences of failing to meet them, not just for the individual in question but for all those whose lives are connected to hers.[27]

Once again, this argument invokes lofty-sounding sentiments but does not survive scrutiny. To begin with, it is unclear why Pollack, Gardner, and Jost talk about voters' desires. If it is morally right to protect people from the financial consequences of illnesses, then it is hard to see why voters' preferences should matter. But, if voters' preferences do matter, they don't offer Pollack, Gardner, and Jost much solace. As Obamacare architect Jonathan Gruber confessed (Chapter 21), the entire premise of that law is that voters do *not* want what Pollack, Gardner, and Jost think they do. Voters had to be fooled because Obamacare would not have been passed if its true potential to transfer wealth to sick people had been understood. Opinion polls further show that most Americans support reductions in Medicaid spending[28] and that most also believe that the federal government should play either a minor role in making America's health care system work well or no role at all.[29] And any argument based on voters' preferences has to deal with the outcome of the 2016 election, which gave control of the federal government to people who are not fond of Medicaid. By resting their defense of Medicaid on voters' desires, Pollack, Gardner, and Jost have built their cathedral on a foundation made of sand.

One should also ask why "the financial ruin that often follows serious illness" ought to be treated differently from financial calamities with other causes. Millions of people have suffered financially after losing their jobs or on account of stock market declines. Millions of others, most of whom are women and children, have been impoverished by divorces, financial abuses committed by lovers or spouses, or the deaths of breadwinners who had little or no life insurance. Floods, earthquakes, and other natural disasters have taken their toll on millions more. And perhaps the leading cause of poverty is the misfortune of having been born poor, a fact for which no one bears any personal responsibility. Because extreme financial difficulties can occur for many reasons, an argument is needed to explain why sick people are singled out for special treatment. Pollack, Gardner, and Jost do not provide one.

The need to explain why financial difficulties stemming from illnesses are special becomes even more urgent when one remembers that Medicaid spends as much money as all other forms of public assistance combined. In 2016, combined federal and state spending on Medicaid totaled about $575 billion.[30] Federal spending on Medicaid alone ($369 billion) exceeded all other federal welfare outlays in 2016.[31] Instead of paying for medical services for a selected group, the hundreds of billions spent on Medicaid could have been used to provide a financial cushion for all of America's poor.

The assertion that Medicaid protects people who become ill from financial ruin is also overstated. Medicaid absorbs only their medical expenses. But many sick people experience financial ruin for other reasons, even when their health care costs are covered. Consider victims who suffer from post-traumatic stress disorder, paralysis, fibromyalgia, back pain, or other maladies that are cheap to treat but that can prevent people from working. Medicaid covers the relatively minor costs of pills and wheelchairs for these people but otherwise leaves them in poverty.

Having mentioned that Medicaid provides long-term care coverage for seniors, we can also point out that many Medicaid beneficiaries bear little resemblance to the kidney transplant recipient that Pollack, Gardner, and Jost use to make their point. Medicaid is, disproportionately and increasingly, a retirement program that protects people from the predictable consequences of aging, not from the financial costs of severe illnesses that strike people at random.[32] Why we are doling out retirement funds inefficiently through Medicaid rather than giving people cash via Social Security or the Earned Income Tax Credit is anybody's guess.

Thus, even though Medicaid moves money in the right direction (from richer to poorer), there is no clear moral justification for this program either. Medicaid absorbs an enormous fraction of the dollars that are available to provide poverty relief. And, like Medicare, it treats people disrespectfully, by denying them the opportunity to make their own choices. Medicaid also doles out money inefficiently by paying for medical services that benefit providers substantially more than beneficiaries. Poor people would do much better if Medicaid simply handed out cash. Even those who use the money to buy health care or nursing home services would be better off because they would be in the driver's seat.

## WHAT ABOUT POOR DECISIONS?

Many health policy scholars worry that people would make poor decisions if they were required to pay for medical treatments with their own money. In support, they cite an important study known as the RAND Health Insurance Experiment (HIE). The HIE concluded that people who face greater cost sharing cut back on their use of health care, including treatments that physicians believe are medically necessary.[33] The desire to ensure that everyone receives all medically appropriate treatments has led some commentators to conclude that everyone must be supplied with comprehensive health insurance that imposes minimal out-of-pocket costs.

A typical example of the genre is provided by Professor Allison K. Hoffman of the University of Pennsylvania School of Law, who wrote a long article and a short column on the topic.[34] Citing the HIE, Hoffman says that "people generally do a poor job of differentiating between effective and ineffective medical care," and that "poor and sick people . . . fare better when they have access to free or low-cost care."[35] She then observes that, since Obamacare took effect, "people have been using increased levels of preventive care and are complying more with drugs and treatment recommended by their doctors."[36] From there, it is only a short step to the conclusion that we should avoid any and all strategies that force consumers to use their own money to pay for health care. After all, what kind of monster would be interested in policies that might place people's health and lives at risk?

The deep problem with Hoffman's approach is that it focuses on health care instead of health. The HIE did *not* find that people who cut back on medical treatments were less healthy than those who got everything the doctor ordered for free. To the contrary, it found that, even though people who were treated for free used more medical treatments, their health was effectively the same as that of people who had to pay.

The HIE is one of the most important studies ever conducted of the effect of insurance on health care and health. (The studies of Oregon's Medicaid Experiment, which we discuss in Chapter 15, are its chief rivals.) The HIE included more than 7,700 people belonging to 2,750 families from across the United States. Families were randomly assigned to five different health insurance plans. Some plans offered free medical care, while others required participants to share costs. Among the latter plans, some imposed higher cost-sharing levels than others. Out-of-pocket costs were capped to protect poorer families. Families participated in the HIE for three to five years.

Predictably enough, participants who shared in the cost of medical treatments used less health care than people who received services for free: "cost sharing reduced the use of nearly all health services. . . . [Participants] with cost sharing made one to two fewer physician visits annually and had 20 percent fewer hospitalizations than those with free care. Declines were similar for other types of services as well, including dental visits, prescriptions, and mental health treatment."[37] Usage reductions correlated with the level of cost sharing too. Participants "with 25 percent coinsurance spent 20 percent less than participants with free care, and those with 95 percent coinsurance spent about 30 percent less."[38] The HIE makes it clear that demand for health care is actually fairly elastic and that insurance encourages the consumption of health care by making treatments cheaper for patients at the point of service.

Although participants in cost-sharing plans used fewer medical treatments, the HIE found that, "in general, the reduction in services induced by cost sharing had no adverse effect on participants' health."[39] The only statistically significant differences were improved vision owing to eyeglasses and lower blood pressure. The first of these findings is trivial. Since retailers have moved into optometry, eye exams and eyeglasses have become cheap enough for people to pay for themselves. The second finding is more troubling but could well be the result of data mining. If you study enough dependent variables, you're likely to stumble across at least a few statistically significant findings.

In sum, Hoffman is on solid ground in contending that, when health care is free, patients are more likely to comply with doctors' recommendations and to use more preventive treatments. That's because, when health care is free, everyone uses more of everything. But giving away health care for free has enormous downsides too. It encourages people to use treatments that are ineffective, harmful, and wasteful, and to rely on intensive medical treatments to cure what ails them instead of doing other things that would be cheaper and more efficacious, like exercising, dieting, sleeping more, and cutting back on smoking. The lavish public spending that is needed to make medical treatments free also diverts enormous amounts of money from other public health priorities that deliver more bang for the buck, like sanitation, housing, education, school lunches, and pollution abatement. A person who wanted to maximize the use of medical treatments would make health care free at the point of delivery; a person who wanted to make people healthy would not.

The definition of "effective" medical care also involves further complexities. At first glance, the matter might seem like a question to be decided by doctors using data and their clinical judgment—either a treatment is effective or it isn't. But effectiveness isn't the only thing that matters. Cost matters too. There are significant problems with ignoring costs when deciding whether people should use medical treatments.

Imagine that you once had a rich uncle (Sam) who gave you a new top-of-the-line Lexus to drive. Uncle Sam is now broke, and you have to buy your own car. Another top-of-the-line Lexus would be an "effective" car for you. It would get you from place to place, in luxury and with the utmost safety. But a much cheaper car—even a used car—would get you where you need to go—albeit with considerably less luxury and probably a little less safety. Which car should you choose from the vast array of options?

The answer depends, at least in part, on the price of each car, the amount you can afford to spend, and your desires and priorities. If your budget is tight, you might reasonably decide to buy something cheaper than a top-of-the-line Lexus because, for you, that car isn't cost effective. Or you might purchase the Lexus and make room for it in your budget by cutting other expenses. By itself, effectiveness-as-transportation doesn't tell you what you should do.

Suppose you decide to buy a less expensive car. The fact that you used to drive a Lexus when it was free doesn't imply that a Lexus provides a valid baseline against which to measure your future transportation choices, particularly now that you have to foot the bill. Nor should we listen to the complaints of those who believe you are making a bad choice by purchasing something other than a Lexus. (Of course, it is no doubt a coincidence that those who make this argument are quite often in the business of making and selling Lexuses.)

The key is that the HIE didn't ask whether participants in cost-sharing plans made cost-effective choices—decisions that maximized their expected health status given the positive cost of health care and their other needs and priorities. It also didn't ask whether participants in the free plans made cost-effective choices. It just found that participants in cost-sharing plans used fewer services that doctors ranked as effective. Given the HIE's failure to find significant health effects, the natural inference to draw is that participants in cost-sharing plans found other uses for their dollars that they rightly thought were better for them.

To be sure, good consumer choices are preferable to bad ones. Ideally, patients would use only cost-effective medical treatments, whether spending their own money or dollars provided by their insurers. But it is first-party payment (and not third-party payment) that encourages patients to learn whether treatments confer benefits that exceed their costs. And only first-party payment encourages patients to seek out alternatives that are better and cheaper.

Some medical treatments are so cost effective that everyone should have them, including people who are so poor or so short sighted they might not buy them on their own. Vaccinations against childhood diseases fall into this category. Solving this problem doesn't require third-party payment. Instead, we should identify the few treatments that fit this description and design means of delivering them. Mass inoculations already take place at schools, workplaces, and other locations. Vaccines are available at little or no cost at retail outlets too. If we want to improve population health, that's the best way to go about doing so.

## The Veterans Health Administration: A Moral Jumble

Several of the moral criticisms we have leveled against Medicare and Medicaid apply with equal or greater force to the VHA, a $65 billion program that provides medical services for almost nine million veterans each year.[40] This program, too, is paternalistic. Instead of giving America's veterans access to health care, we could give them cash and let them choose how to use it. The VHA is also inefficient. If veterans were given money instead of access to health care, many would spend the dollars in other ways that enhance their welfare more.

The VHA has also experienced scandalous quality problems.[41] In 2014, it emerged that veterans needing care often experienced long waits, that many died before being seen, and that VHA administrators had deceived their superiors by maintaining secret lists of patients who were in the queue.[42] In 2017, investigations of VHA medical centers conducted by *USA Today* and the GAO found that "the [VHA] has for years concealed medical mistakes and misconduct by health care workers."[43] It failed to open investigations promptly when errors were reported, failed to document investigations properly, failed to file mandatory reports on providers who committed malpractice to the National Practitioner Data Bank, entered into hundreds of secret settlements of malpractice claims, and hired doctors with histories of harming patients.[44] Given this dismal record and the VHA's proven willingness to lie to Congress, why should anyone trust the VHA with the care of our nation's veterans?

The discussion of moral issues relating to the VHA can be streamlined by asking one question: Why does a separate health care system for veterans exist? Even if one believes, as we do, that veterans who put their lives at risk are entitled to preferential treatment, there is no obvious need for a separate health care system to deliver that treatment. Most American veterans—about 13 million of them—use the same health care providers as everyone else. The veterans who are eligible for treatment in VHA facilities are those with service-related disabilities or who are poor. They constitute a minority of America's former uniformed military personnel.

Do the differences between VHA-eligible veterans and other service personnel provide a moral justification for the existence of a separate health care system? It does not seem so to us. Start with veterans who are poor. Rather than have a separate medical system for them, the federal government could put them on Medicaid or enroll them in Medicare. This would enable them to obtain health care via the private sector, just like other people who participate in these programs. Many poor veterans would see this as a plus, especially those who live a considerable distance from the nearest VHA facility.

Insofar as poor veterans are concerned, history provides the only reason for having a separate VHA system: neither Medicaid nor Medicare existed when the VHA was created. But, now that these programs do exist, the need for a separate system for veterans with low incomes has disappeared. And, if (as we recommend) Medicaid and Medicare were both converted to cash-grant programs, poor veterans would have the same access to medical services as everyone else—better access, if (as we would suggest) their grants were significantly topped up in recognition of their past service.

Turning from poor veterans to those with service-related disabilities, the need for a federally run system for the latter is not obvious either. The Veterans Access, Choice, and Accountability Act of 2014 (the Choice Act) suggests as much. When waiting times at VHA facilities exceed 30 days or the nearest VHA facility is more than 40 miles away, the Choice Act entitles veterans to see civilian providers who accept Medicare or participate in TRICARE, another federal program for veterans and their families. The plain implication would seem to be that all veterans, including those with service-related disabilities, can be treated adequately outside the VHA.

This makes sense. Although veterans are special and those with service-related disabilities may have special needs, hospitals, physicians, therapists, and other civilian providers can deliver all of the medical treatments that are available through the VHA. And, if injured veterans benefit by being in the company of others with service-related disabilities, civilian providers can help with that too. They need only attract veterans in numbers by developing practices that cater to them or by hiring them onto their staffs. In fact, nothing would prevent a private sector hospital company from operating a string of VHA-style facilities, and one would surely do so if veterans wanted a separate health care system and had the means to pay for it.

The Choice Act actually makes clear the difficulty of justifying the existence of the VHA. Why offer the option of using civilian providers only when the delay or distance requirement is met? Why not give veterans this option in all contexts? Many veterans might reasonably think it better to use private providers than to wait even 10 days for appointments or to venture even 10 miles to VHA facilities. Nothing requires civilian patients to encounter such obstacles before seeing providers whose hours and locations are convenient. Many veterans might also envy the freedom that civilians have to use the providers who are best at handling their medical needs. By subjecting veterans who want to use non-VHA providers to the indicated limits, the Choice Act denies them the opportunity of taking advantage of the most appealing options while also protecting the VHA from private sector competition that would pressure it to improve. One is inevitably led to the conclusion that the limitations on the Choice Act are there to protect the VHA—and the jobs that VHA facilities provide in congressional districts—rather than to ensure that veterans receive the high-quality care they deserve at convenient locations.

Some writers have defended the VHA by pointing out that, for a time and in certain ways, VHA hospitals provided better care than private facilities.[45] In a 2005 article, we also touted the superiority of VHA hospitals, while noting that the impetus to serve veterans better came from Congress in response to decades of high-profile scandals involving quality of care at VHA facilities.[46] VHA personnel certainly didn't seem inclined to take the necessary steps to prevent these problems from exploding into full-blown scandals—raising questions about whether that system should be trusted with the care of veterans at all.

Even so, the argument that VHA facilities are sometimes better than civilian facilities misses the point. Oldsmobiles may have been better cars than Renaults, but the U.S. auto market drove both brands to extinction because both were inferior. The same goes for the civilian medical sector and the VHA. Both could be and should be much better than they are, and both would be better if patients bought medical services directly instead of relying so heavily on third-party payers.

# CONCLUSION

For the last half century, the chief object of American health policy has been to ensure that consumers pay the smallest possible fraction of the cost of medical care at the point at which treatments are delivered. Obamacare, the State Children's Health Insurance Program, Medicare, Medicaid, the U.S. Veterans Health Administration (VHA), and tax-advantaged private insurance arrangements—along with the long list of coverage mandates that go with them—all reduce direct financial responsibility for medical services to a minimum. As explained in Chapter 15, the evil genius of third-party payment is that it encourages consumption and drives up costs by making medical services cheap for patients at the point of sale.

The public officials, insurers, and health care providers who benefit from all this spending defend third-party payment arrangements by arguing that health care is too complicated and too expensive for consumers to manage on their own, and by contending that people who are directly responsible for health care costs will use medical services less often than they should. Better that government bureaucrats spend tax dollars and that private insurers spend premium dollars, they argue, than that consumers pay for medical services themselves. They don't want consumers to consider the possibility that market mechanisms might remediate excessive costs and complications as successfully in health care as they have in other sectors. This is to be expected. Widespread reliance on third-party payment arrangements benefits insurers and health care providers, so they want nothing to interfere with it.

Advocates of tax breaks for dollars spent on medical services and insurance claim to be doing consumers favors too. They want us to believe that they are making medical treatments and insurance coverage more affordable, when they are actually making both more expensive by stimulating demand and by encouraging people to rely on insurance more often and more heavily than they should. The deduction from the federal income tax that applies to interest on home mortgages drives up home prices by encouraging people to buy instead of renting and by encouraging buyers to pay more. That's why realtors, whose income depends on home sales, are this tax break's biggest fans. Likewise, insurers and health care providers love tax exemptions for insurance and medical treatments. By encouraging consumption, these tax breaks bring hundreds of billions of dollars to their doors.

This modern faith in pervasive third-party payment—one might even call it a fetish or an obsession—reached its apotheosis in Obamacare, the goal of which was to provide almost everyone with coverage for almost everything. Elderly people would have Medicare. Poor people would have Medicaid. And everyone else would have private insurance, provided by employers or bought on exchanges, with expansive coverage mandates and substantial subsidies and penalties deployed to encourage compliance. If the goal was to maximize spending, Obamacare made perfect sense. One thing we know for certain about comprehensive health insurance coverage and political control of the health care economy is that both add massively to costs.

Those of us who believe that American health care should be better and cheaper think that Obamacare was crazy. To fix the myriad problems with our health care system—including excessive cost and consumption, quality problems, and the loss of an estimated $1 trillion a year to fraud, waste, and abuse—we need to identify their root causes and address them. An abundance of evidence, including everything from peer-reviewed academic studies of the impact of Medicare and tax breaks on costs to news reports about surprise bills, retail outlets, and frauds, makes it clear that the politicized third-party payment system is the main culprit. Instead of expanding the reach of that system, as Obamacare did, we should face facts and start paying for health care the same way we pay for everything else. When hundreds of millions of people spend their own money on health care, they will behave differently, and health care providers will too. Consumers will look for services that offer better value for the dollar, and doctors, hospitals, drug companies, and other medical outlets will try to provide them. Prices will fall and both the availability and the quality of medical treatments will improve.

Many health care providers won't like this new world in which they must compete for business. They benefit from existing arrangements, which pay them whatever they ask and send them more dollars year after year. We should stop indulging them, and we should stop listening to their apologists and lobbyists too. Markets do a good job of supplying food, clothing, housing, transportation, and other essentials. They can help us meet our needs for medical treatments.

One of the most wonderful things about markets is that they automatically reward sellers who treat consumers well and automatically punish those who don't. Both the carrot and the stick are important. For American health care to improve, providers that deliver high-quality services at reasonable prices must be rewarded and inferior providers must fail. There must be turnover and opportunities for new entrants. A near-death experience made the American automobile industry more efficient and pro-consumer, and decades later, innovators like Tesla are still forcing existing manufacturers to do better by deploying new technologies and business models. If and when the businesses that operate in the American health care sector are subjected to intense competition, they will respond the same way. And if they don't, they will fall by the wayside and new businesses will emerge that will offer Americans cheaper and better health care.

Change won't come easily. Old-line health care companies have rigged the game in their favor. They benefit from a guaranteed flow of dollars and massive subsidies. They control market entry. And they have convinced the American public that they should not have to operate like other businesses. They possess great political power too and will use it to ruthlessly stifle competition. That's why the changes that are needed won't be imposed from above. If they occur at all, it will be in response to the demands of self-paying consumers who use their dollars to support innovative providers and break local cartels.

We are optimistic because the army of self-paying consumers is bound to grow and will become more influential over time. Unless Congress raises taxes significantly or inflates the deficit massively, Medicare, Medicaid, and Obamacare will all have to change. All will have to shift increasing fractions of the cost of health care to their beneficiaries, as may smaller programs like the VHA. As rising costs drive up premiums, deductibles, and copays, private insurance will seem like less of a bargain too. Millions of consumers will react to these changes by looking for a better alternative. If it is allowed to do so, the retail sector will give them what they want— better medical treatments at less cost—and draw business away from traditional providers. As new purchasing patterns and norms develop and as public support for old-style financing arrangements wanes, traditional providers will adapt or fail. Either way, pressure from below will make American health care better and less expensive.

What roles will private insurance and government agencies play in a system based primarily on first-party payment? The former will help people deal with catastrophes, and the latter will provide financial support to people who are too poor to meet their needs. But, by and large, both insurers and public agencies will get out of the business of buying health care for consumers. In the new, retail-dominated health care marketplace, consumers will be in the driver's seat and there will be no good reason for insurers or government bureaucrats to displace them.

As a nation, we currently spend 18 percent of GDP on health care. If given full control of their dollars, few American households would voluntarily spend that large a fraction of their gross income on health care. The government and private payers should stop dragging us in a direction we do not want to go.

The First Rule of Holes is that, when you find yourself in one, stop digging. Americans are in an enormous hole, but we are still digging. Our system functions as though it is expensive by design. It moves dollars into the medical sector as quickly as the Treasury can print them. But, instead of recognizing that excessive reliance on third-party payment arrangements and political control of the health care economy are the main drivers of spiraling costs and mediocre quality, we keep demanding more of both. To make American health care better and cheaper, consumers should use their own money to purchase medical treatments directly—the same way they buy everything else.

# NOTES

## Epigraphs

[1]See also "From the Bookshelves: 'Critical,'" Tom Daschle interview by Jackie Judd, *The Healthcast* (podcast), Kaiser Family Foundation, March 20, 2008, at 2:16, https://web.archive.org/web/20091113171751/http://podcast.kff.org/podcast/2008/032008_kn_daschle_audio.mp3. Michael F. Cannon, "Can Congress Manage the Health Care Sector?," *Cato at Liberty* (blog), May 1, 2008, https://www.cato.org/blog/can-congress-manage-health-care-sector.

[2]Phil Gramm, 142 Cong. Rec. S9923 (September 5, 1996).

[3]Naomi Lin, "Bill Clinton Calls Obamacare 'the Craziest Thing in the World,' Later Tries to Walk It Back," *CNN Politics*, October 5, 2016, http://www.cnn.com/2016/10/04/politics/bill-clinton-obamacare-craziest-thing/index.html.

## Introduction

[1]Megan Headley, "Why Are Medical Errors Still a Leading Cause of Death?," *Patient Safety & Quality Healthcare*, April 5, 2017, https://www.psqh.com/analysis/why-are-medical-errors-still-a-leading-cause-of-death/.

[2]Chad Terhune, "Putting a Lid on Waste: Needless Medical Tests Not Only Cost $200B—They Can Do Harm," *Kaiser Health News*, May 24, 2017, http://khn.org/news/putting-a-lid-on-waste-needless-medical-tests-not-only-cost-200b-they-can-do-harm/.

[3]Lisa Du and Wei Lu, "U.S. Health-Care System Ranks as One of the Least-Efficient: America Is Number 50 out of 55 Countries That Were Assessed,"

*Bloomberg.com*, September 28, 2016, https://www.bloomberg.com/news/articles/2016-09-29/u-s-health-care-system-ranks-as-one-of-the-least-efficient.

[4]Centers for Medicare and Medicaid Services, "CMS Releases 2015 National Health Expenditures," news release, December 2, 2016, https://www.cms.gov/Newsroom/MediaReleaseDatabase/Press-releases/2016-Press-releases-items/2016-12-02.html.

[5]Emily Ekins, "Large Majorities Support Key Obamacare Provisions, Unless They Cost Something," *Cato at Liberty* (blog), April 25, 2017, https://www.cato.org/blog/large-majorities-support-key-obamacare-provisions-unless-they-cost-something.

[6]Carolyn Y. Johnson, "Trump on Drug Prices: Pharma Companies Are 'Getting Away with Murder,'" *Washington Post*, January 11, 2017, https://www.washingtonpost.com/news/wonk/wp/2017/01/11/trump-on-drug-prices-pharma-companies-are-getting-away-with-murder/?utm_term=.eef4204841db.

[7]Emily Kopp, "White House Task Force Echoes Pharma Proposals," *Kaiser Health News*, June 16, 2017, http://khn.org/news/exclusive-white-house-task-force-echoes-pharma-proposals/.

[8]Sydney Lupkin, "Drugmakers Dramatically Boosted Lobbying Spending in Trump's First Quarter," *Kaiser Health News*, April 21, 2017, http://khn.org/news/drugmakers-dramatically-boosted-lobbying-spending-in-trumps-first-quarter/.

[9]Ibid.

[10]Ibid.

[11]Jay Hancock, Sydney Lupkin, and Elizabeth Lucas, "With Drug Costs in Crosshairs, Health Firms Gave Generously to Trump's Inauguration," *Kaiser Health News*, April 19, 2017, http://khn.org/news/with-drug-costs-in-crosshairs-health-firms-gave-generously-to-trumps-inauguration/.

[12]Theodore R. Marmor and Jonathan Oberlander, "Medicare at Fifty," in *The Oxford Handbook of U.S. Health Law*, eds. I. Glenn Cohen, Allison K. Hoffman, and William M. Sage (New York: Oxford University Press, 2017).

[13]Charles Silver, "Healthcare Insurance: America's Collective Action Nightmare," *The Health Care Blog*, March 7, 2017, http://thehealthcareblog.com/blog/2017/03/07/healthcare-insurance-americas-collective-action-nightmare/.

[14]Christy Ford Chapin, "How Did Health Care Get to Be Such a Mess?," *New York Times*, June 19, 2017, https://www.nytimes.com/2017/06/19/opinion/healthinsuranceamericanmedicalassociation.html?emc=eta1&_r=0.

[15]On the lack of cost controls in Medicare, see Uwe E. Reinhardt, "How the Medical Establishment Got the Treasury's Keys," *New York Times*, February 28, 2014, http://economix.blogs.nytimes.com/2014/02/28/how-the-medical-establishment-got-the-treasurys-keys/?_php=true&_type=blogs&src=recg&_r=0; and Ezekiel Emanuel, *Reinventing American Health Care: How the Affordable Care Act Will Improve Our Terribly Complex, Blatantly Unjust, Outrageously*

*Expensive, Grossly Inefficient, Error Prone System* (New York: PublicAffairs, 2014), p. 21. For more on the guaranteed hospital profit, see Herman Miles Somers and Anne Ramsay Somers, *Medicare and the Hospitals: Issues and Prospects* (Washington: Brookings Institution, 1967). On moving money to health care businesses, see Rick Mayes, "The Origins, Development, and Passage of Medicare's Revolutionary Prospective Payment System," *Journal of the History of Medicine and Allied Sciences* 62, no. 1 (2007): 21–55, https://academic.oup.com/jhmas/article-abstract/62/1/21/724956. A discussion of the hikes in physicians' fees and hospital charges that came on the heels of Medicare's enactment can be found in Theodore R. Marmor, *The Politics of Medicare* (New York: Transaction Publishers, 1970), pp. 85–90.

[16]U.S. Department of Justice, "Departments of Justice and Health and Human Services Announce over $27.8 Billion in Returns from Joint Efforts to Combat Health Care Fraud," news release, March 19, 2015, https://www.justice.gov/opa/pr/departments-justice-and-health-and-human-services-announce-over-278-billion-returns-joint.

[17]"The $272 Billion Swindle: Why Thieves Love America's Health Care System," *The Economist,* May 31, 2014, https://www.economist.com/news/united-states/21603078-why-thieves-love-americas-health-care-system-272-billion-swindle.

[18]Kim Janssen, "Cost of Name-Brand Prescription Drugs Doubled over Last 5 Years: Report," *Chicago Tribune,* March 15, 2016, http://www.chicagotribune.com/business/ct-prescription-drug-prices-0316-biz-20160315-story.html

[19]Sarah Kliff, "The Problem Is the Prices: Opaque and Sky High Bills Are Breaking Americans—And Our Health Care System," *Vox,* October 16, 2017, https://www.vox.com/policy-and-politics/2017/10/16/16357790/health-care-prices-problem.

[20]Associated Press, "Woman Gives Birth in Car, Hospital Charges Full Delivery Fee," *News10.com,* November 2, 2016, http://news10.com/2016/11/02/womangivesbirthincarhospitalchargesfulldeliveryfee/.

[21]Letitia Stein and Alexandra Zayas, "Florida Trauma Centers Charge Outrageous Fees the Moment You Come Through the Door," *Tampa Bay Times,* March 7, 2014, http://www.tampabay.com/news/health/florida-trauma-centers-charge-outrageous-fees-the-moment-you-come-through/2169148.

[22]Ibid.

[23]Sarah Kliff, "The Problem Is the Prices: Opaque and Sky High Bills Are Breaking Americans—and Our Health Care System," *Vox.com,* October 16, 2017, https://www.vox.com/policy-and-politics/2017/10/16/16357790/health-care-prices-problem.

[24]Kimberly Mitchell, "Like Magic? ('Every System Is Perfectly Designed . . .')," *IHI Improvement Blog,* Institute for Healthcare Improvement, August 21, 2015, http://www.ihi.org/communities/blogs/_layouts/15/ihi/community/blog/itemview.aspx?List=7d1126ec-8f63-4a3b-9926-c44ea3036813&ID=159.

²⁵See Veronique de Rugy, "U.S. Health Care Spending More than Twice the Average for Developed Countries," Mercatus Center, George Mason University, September 17, 2013, http://mercatus.org/publication/us-health-care-spending-more-twice-average-developed-countries. To read more on the missing "bang for your buck," see Anna Edney, "U.S. Health System among Least Efficient before Obamacare," *Bloomberg News*, September 18, 2014, http://www.bloomberg.com/news/print/2014-09-18/u-s-health-system-among-least-efficient-before-obamacare.html. For more on secretive hospitals, see Elizabeth Cohen and John Bonifield, "Secret Deaths: CNN Finds High Surgical Death Rate for Children at Florida Hospital," *CNN.com*, June 2, 2015, http://www.cnn.com/2015/06/01/health/st-marys-medical-center/. For information on the amount of money the feds recouped from wrongdoers, see the Department of Health and Human Services and the Department of Justice, *Annual Report of the Departments of Health and Human Services and Justice, Health Care Fraud and Abuse Control Program FY 2014*, March 19, 2015, https://oig.hhs.gov/publications/docs/hcfac/FY2014-hcfac.pdf; to learn about how much money criminals are thought to steal from Medicare, see Thomas Sullivan, "Big Data, CMS and OIG Discuss 'The Use of Data to Stop Medicare Fraud' before House Ways and Means Subcommittee," *Policy and Medicine*, April 8, 2015, http://www.policymed.com/2015/04/cms-and-oig-discuss-the-use-of-data-to-stop-medicare-fraud-before-house-ways-and-means-subcommittee.html.

²⁶For discussion of variation in complication and death rates after surgery, see Marshall Allen and Olga Pierce, "Surgery Risks: Why Choosing the Right Surgeon Matters," *ProPublica*, July 13, 2015, https://www.propublica.org/article/surgery-risks-patient-safety-surgeon-matters. For a critique of *ProPublica*'s methodology and a reply, see Mark W. Friedberg, Peter J. Pronovost, David M. Shahian, et al., "A Methodological Critique of the ProPublica Surgeon Scorecard," *RAND Health Quarterly* 5, no. 4 (2016), http://www.rand.org/content/dam/rand/pubs/perspectives/PE100/PE170/RAND_PE170.pdf; Stephen Engelberg and Olga Pierce, "Our Rebuttal to RAND's Critique of Surgeon Scorecard," *ProPublica*, October 7, 2015, https://www.propublica.org/article/our-rebuttal-to-rands-critique-of-surgeon-scorecard?utm_source=et&utm_medium=email&utm_campaign=dailynewsletter&utm_content=&utm_name=.

²⁷Infection rates vary greatly across hospitals. See Joel Keehn, "12 Hospitals You Might Want to Avoid for Infections," *Consumer Reports*, December 7, 2015, https://www.consumerreports.org/cro/health/12-hospitals-to-avoid.

²⁸On variation in survival rates across hospitals for patients receiving the same procedures, see John Commins, "Choose Hospitals on Performance Data, Consumers Urged," *Health Leaders Media*, October 20, 2015,

http://healthleadersmedia.com/print/QUA321847/ChooseHospitalsonPerformance DataConsumersUrged.

[29]Brian Krans, "Campaign Launched to Fight Back Against Massive, Surprise 'Out of Network' Medical Bills," *HealthlineNews*, November 3, 2015, http:// www.healthline.com/healthnews/campaignlaunchedtofightbackagainstmassive surpriseoutofnetworkmedicalbills110315#1.

[30]For further discussion and resources on central line-associated bloodstream infections, see Chapter 13, "Bad Business." For employer and employee tax exclusions, see Matthew Rae, Gary Claxton, Nirmita Panchal, and Larry Levitt, "Tax Subsidies for Private Health Insurance," The Henry J. Kaiser Family Foundation, October 27, 2014, http://files.kff.org/attachment/tax-subsidies-for-private-health-insurance-issue-brief.

[31]Ryan Basen, "AMA Does Not Want PA Autonomy," *MedPage Today*, June 15, 2017, https://www.medpagetoday.com/meetingcoverage/ama/66039.

[32]Peter Whoriskey and Dan Keating, "How a Secretive Panel Uses Data That Distort Doctors' Pay," *Washington Post*, July 20, 2013, http://www.washingtonpost .com/business/economy/how-a-secretive-panel-uses-data-that-distorts-doctors-pay/2013/07/20/ee134e3a-eda8-11e2-9008-61e94a7ea20d_story.html.

[33]Peter Whoriskey and Dan Keating, "Medicare Pricing Drives High Healthcare Costs," *Washington Post*, December 31, 2013, http://www.washingtonpost .com/business/economy/medicare-pricing-drives-high-health-care-costs/2013/12/31/24befa46-7248-11e3-8b3f-b1666705ca3b_story.html.

[34]Goodreads.com, "Mahatma Gandhi," https://www.goodreads.com/quotes/84976-there-goes-my-people-i-must-follow-them-for-i. The quote is probably apocryphal. Suzy Platt, ed., *Respectfully Quoted: A Dictionary of Quotations* (New York: Barnes & Noble, 1993), p. 194.

[35]Samuel Greengard, "Understanding Knee Replacement Costs: What's on the Bill?," *Healthline*, February 23, 2015, http://www.healthline.com/health/total-knee-replacement-surgery/understanding-costs#1.

[36]The website of the Surgery Center of Oklahoma, http://www.surgery centerok.com/.

[37]Mark Hendrickson, "The Real Class Warfare in America Today," *Forbes.com*, May 2, 2014, http://www.forbes.com/sites/markhendrickson/2014/05/02/the-real-class-warfare-in-america-today/.

PART 1

[1]Margot Sanger-Katz, "Even Insured Can Face Crushing Medical Debt, Study Finds," *New York Times*, January 5, 2016, http://nyti.ms/1O82fb2.

## CHAPTER 1

[1]J. Weston Phippen, "Who Wants to Punch Martin Shkreli in the Face (for Charity)?," *Atlantic*, September 28, 2016, https://www.theatlantic.com/news/archive/2016/09/martin-shkreli-punch-face/502010/.

[2]Devin Leonard and Annmarie Hordern, "Who Bought the Most Expensive Album Ever Made?," *Bloomberg.com*, December 9, 2015, http://www.bloomberg.com/features/2015-martin-shkreli-wu-tang-clan-album/.

[3]Ben Popken, "Industry Insiders Estimate EpiPen Costs No More than $30," *NBCNews.com*, September 6, 2016, http://www.nbcnews.com/business/consumer/industryinsidersestimateepipencostsnomore30n642091.

[4]Robert Langreth and Rebecca Spalding, "Shkreli Was Right: Everyone's Hiking Drug Prices," *Bloomberg*, February 2, 2016, https://www.bloomberg.com/news/articles/2016-02-02/shkreli-not-alone-in-drug-price-spikes-as-skin-gel-soars-1-860.

[5]Ibid.

[6]Robert Langreth, "Drug Prices Defy Gravity, Doubling for Dozens of Products," *Bloomberg Business*, April 30, 2014, https://www.bloomberg.com/news/articles/2014-04-30/drug-prices-defy-gravity-doubling-for-dozens-of-products.

[7]Robert Pearl, "New Checks and Balances for Big Pharma," *The Health Care Blog*, May 12, 2017, http://thehealthcareblog.com/blog/2017/05/12/thelouisianapurchase/.

[8]Remarks by Andy Slavitt, "The Need to Partner on Drug Innovation, Access and Cost," delivered at the Biopharma Congress in Washington, D.C., *The CMS Blog*, November 3, 2016, https://blog.cms.gov/2016/11/04/remarks-by-andy-slavitt-the-need-to-partner-on-drug-innovation-access-and-cost/.

[9]Stephen W. Schondelmeyer and Leigh Purvis, "Trends in Retail Prices of Brand Name Prescription Drugs Widely Used by Older Americans, 2006 to 2015," *Rx Watch Pricing Report,* AARP Public Policy Institute, December 2016, http://www.aarp.org/content/dam/aarp/ppi/2016-12/trends-in-retail-prices-dec-2016.pdf.

[10]Aimee Picchi, "Prognosis for RX in 2017: More Painful Drug-Price Hikes," *CBSNews.com*, December 30, 2016, http://www.cbsnews.com/news/drug-prices-to-rise-12-percent-in-2017/.

[11]Alfred Engelberg, "Memo to the President: The Pharmaceutical Monopoly Adjustment Act of 2017," *Health Affairs Blog*, September 13, 2016, http://healthaffairs.org/blog/2016/09/13/memo-to-the-president-the-pharmaceutical-monopoly-adjustment-act-of-2017/.

[12]Aaron S. Kesselheim, Jerry Avorn and Ameet Sarpatwari, "The High Cost of Prescription Drugs in the United States: Origins and Prospects for Reform,"

*JAMA* 316, no. 8 (2016): 858–71, https://jamanetwork.com/journals/jama/article-abstract/2545691.

[13]Evan Sernoffsky, "California Voters Reject Drug-Price Measure Prop 61," *SFGate.com*, November 9, 2016, http://www.sfgate.com/bayarea/article/California-voters-reject-drug-price-measure-Prop-10604256.php; Maureen Cruise, "Vote Yes on Prop 61, the California Drug Price Relief Act," *LA Progressive*, November 2, 2016, https://www.laprogressive.com/california-prop-61/. See also Deena Beasley, "Support for California Drug Spending Limits Stokes Industry Fears," *Business Insider*, October 5, 2016, http://www.businessinsider.com/r-support-for-california-drug-spending-limits-stokes-industry-fears-2016-10; David Lazarus, "Drug Companies Spend Millions to Keep Charging High Prices," *Los Angeles Times*, August 26, 2016, http://www.latimes.com/business/lazarus/la-fi-lazarus-drug-prices-20160826-snap-story.html.

[14]Brian Keppler, "Congress Has a Little Drug Problem," *The Health Care Blog*, March 16, 2016, http://thehealthcareblog.com/blog/2016/03/16/congress-has-a-drug-problem/. See also OpenSecrets.org, "Top Industries," https://www.opensecrets.org/lobby/top.php?indexType=i.

[15]Engelberg, "Memo to the President."

[16]Ike Swetlitz, "As Epipen Prices Skyrocket, Consumers and EMTs Resort to Syringes for Severe Allergies," *PBS Newshour*, July 6, 2016, http://www.pbs.org/newshour/rundown/as-epipen-prices-skyrocket-consumers-and-emts-resort-to-syringes-for-life-threatening-allergies/; Carmen Heredia Rodriguez, "The Need to Replace EpiPens Regularly Adds to Concerns about Cost," *PBS Newshour*, October 2, 2016, http://www.pbs.org/newshour/rundown/epipens-replace-cost/.

[17]Sanofi US, "UPDATED: Sanofi US Issues Voluntary Nationwide Recall of All Auvi-Q Due to Potential Inaccurate Dosage Delivery," news release posted on U.S. Food and Drug Administration website, October 30, 2015, https://www.fda.gov/Safety/Recalls/ucm469980.htm.

[18]Ariana Eunjung Cha, "Senator's Daughter Who Raised Price of EpiPen Got Paid $19 Million Salary, Perks in 2015," *Washington Post*, August 24, 2015, https://www.washingtonpost.com/news/to-your-health/wp/2016/08/24/senators-daughter-who-raised-price-of-epipen-got-paid-19-million-salary-perks-in-2015/.

[19]Mark Maremont and Theo Francis, "Mylan Chairman Received Nearly $100 Million Last Year," *Wall Street Journal*, May 2, 2017, https://www.wsj.com/articles/mylan-chairman-received-nearly-100-million-last-year-1493717400.

[20]Charles Ornstein, "A Drug Quintupled in Price. Now, Drug Industry Players Are Feuding over the Windfall," *ProPublica*, May 31, 2017, https://www.propublica.org/article/drug-quintupled-in-price-now-drug-industry-players-feuding-over-windfall?utm_source=pardot&utm_medium=email&utm_campaign=dailynewsletter#.

[21]Shefali Luthra, "Getting Patients Hooked on an Opioid Overdose Antidote, Then Raising the Price," *Kaiser Health News*, January 30, 2017, http://khn.org/news/getting-patients-hooked-on-an-opioid-overdose-antidote-then-raising-the-price/.

[22]David Belk, "Brand Name Medication Prices," *True Cost of Healthcare*, 2015, http://truecostofhealthcare.net/wp-content/uploads/2015/05/Brand-Name-Medication-Prices-2.pdf.

[23]Joseph Walker, "Drugmakers' Pricing Power Remains Strong," *Wall Street Journal*, July 14, 2016, http://www.wsj.com/articles/drugmakerspricingpower remainsstrong1468488601.

[24]Cynthia Koons, "Pfizer Raised Prices on 133 Drugs This Year, and It's Not Alone," *Bloomberg*, October 2, 2015, http://www.bloomberg.com/news/articles/20151002/pfizerraisedpriceson133drugsthisyearanditsnotalone.

[25]Aristotle, *Politics*, bk. 1, sec. 1259a.

[26]For a synopsis of the options for gaining monopoly control that the law makes available to pharma companies, see Engelberg, "Memo to the President."

[27]Special Committee on Aging, United States Senate, *Sudden Price Spikes in Off-Patent Prescription Drugs: The Monopoly Business Model That Harms Patients, Taxpayers, and the U.S. Health Care System*, December 2016, https://www.aging .senate.gov/imo/media/doc/Drug%20Pricing%20Report.pdf.

[28]Marcia Angell, "Why Do Drug Companies Charge So Much? Because They Can," *Washington Post*, September 25, 2015, https://www.washingtonpost .com/opinions/why-do-drug-companies-charge-so-much-because-they-can/2015/09/25/967d3df4-6266-11e5-b38e-06883aacba64_story.html?tid= a_inl.

[29]Victor Luckerson, "Everything to Know about the Arrested Drug Price-Hiking CEO," *Time.com*, December 17, 2015, http://time.com/4153512/martin-shkreli-pharmaceuticals-arrested-turing-daraprim/.

[30]David Crow, "Drugmaker Raises Price of Acne Cream to $10,000 a Tube," *CNBC.com*, September 21, 2016, http://www.cnbc.com/2016/09/21/drugmakerraisespriceofacnecreamto10000atube.html.

[31]Jackie Wattles, "Drugmaker Fined $100M for Hiking Price 85,000%," *CNN.com*, January 18, 2017, http://money.cnn.com/2017/01/18/news/drug pricingmallinckrodtftcfine/index.html.

[32]U.S. Government Accountability Office, *Generic Drugs under Medicare Part D: Generic Drug Prices Declined Overall, but Some Had Extraordinary Price Increases*, August 2016, http://www.gao.gov/assets/680/679022.pdf.

[33]Trefis Team, "Why Are Generic Drug Prices Shooting Up?," *Forbes.com*, February 27, 2015, http://www.forbes.com/sites/greatspeculations/2015/02/27/why-are-generic-drug-prices-shooting-up/#26f1ccab377e.

[34]Melody Petersen, "Here's Why Drug Prices Rise Even When There's Plenty of Competition," *Los Angeles Times*, September 1, 2016, http://www.latimes.com/business/la-fi-mylan-price-hikes-20160830-snap-story.html.

[35]Ibid.

[36]Mary Hiers, "Cost of Viagra at CVS, Walgreens, and Walmart," *AccessRX*, April 25, 2012, http://www.accessrx.com/blog/erectile-dysfunction/viagra/cost-viagra-cvs-walgreens-walmart/.

[37]WebMD, "Erectile Dysfunction: Medicines to Treat ED," http://www.webmd.com/erectile-dysfunction/guide/cialis-levitra-staxyn-viagra-treat-ed.

[38]AccessRX Staff, "The Climbing Cost of Cialis—Price Has Increased 105% in Six Years," *AccessRX*, January 8, 2010, http://www.accessrx.com/blog/erectile-dysfunction/cost-of-cialis-price-up-105-percent/#ixzz2jbv3lrsu.

[39]Don Amerman, "Low Price Levitra Erectile Dysfunction Medication Order Online at AccessRx," *AccessRX,* November 12, 2012, https://www.accessrx.com/blog/erectile-dysfunction/levitra/low-price-levitra-erectile-dysfunction-medication-order-online-at-accessrx-m1102/.

[40]Ibid.

[41]Lydia Ramsey, "The Prices for Life-Saving Diabetes Medications Have Increased Again," *Business Insider,* May 15, 2017, http://www.businessinsider.com/insulin-prices-increased-in-2017-2017-5.

[42]Lydia Ramsey, "A 93-Year-Old Drug That Can Cost More Than a Mortgage Payment Tells Us Everything That's Wrong with American Healthcare," *Business Insider,* September 16, 2016, http://www.businessinsider.com/insulin-prices-increase-2016-9.

[43]U.S. Government Accountability Office, *Generic Drugs under Medicare Part D.*

[44]Ibid.

[45]Ed Silverman, "Mylan Raised Prices for Some Drugs by Huge Amounts," *STAT,* June 10, 2016, https://www.statnews.com/pharmalot/2016/06/10/mylan-drug-prices-increase/.

[46]Gloria Riviera, Katie Yu, and Lauren Effron, "With Generic Prescription Drug Prices Surging, Families Are Feeling the Squeeze," *ABCNews.com*, May 28, 2015, http://abcnews.go.com/Health/generic-prescription-drug-prices-surging-families-feeling-squeeze/story?id=31374562.

[47]Stephen Feller, "Criminal Charges Expected for Generic Drug Price-Fixing by End of Year," UPI, November 3, 2016, http://www.upi.com/Business_News/2016/11/03/Criminal-charges-expected-for-generic-drug-price-fixing-by-end-of-year/2761478224768/.

[48]Eric Kroh, "Generic Drug Price-Fixing Suits Just Tip of the Iceberg," *Law360.com,* January 6, 2017, https://www.law360.com/articles/877707/generic-drug-price-fixing-suits-just-tip-of-the-iceberg.

[49]Eric Kroh, "20 States Sue Generic-Drug Companies over Collusion," *Law360.com*, December 15, 2016, https://www.law360.com/articles/873185/20-states-sue-generic-drug-companies-over-collusion; Kevin McCoy, "Lawsuit: Steak Dinners, Girls Nights Out Keyed Generic Drug Price-Fixing," *USAToday*, December 15, 2016, http://usat.ly/2hLOfyv.

[50]See Tim Worstall, "Markets Work: Martin Shkreli, Daraprim and Turing Pharma Edition," *Forbes.com*, October 23, 2015, http://www.forbes.com/sites/timworstall/2015/10/23/marketstheyworkmartinshkrelidaraprimandturing pharmaedition/print/.

[51]Priti Radhakrishnan, "Pharma's Secret Weapon to Keep Drug Prices High," *STAT*, June 14, 2016, https://www.statnews.com/2016/06/14/secondary-patent-gilead-sovaldi-harvoni/.

[52]Tahir Amin and Aaron S. Kesselheim, "Second Patenting of Branded Pharmaceuticals: A Case Study of How Patents on Two HIV Drugs Could Be Extended for Decades," *Health Affairs* 31, no. 10 (2012): 2286–94.

[53]Robin Feldman and Connie Wang, "May Your Drug Price Be Ever Green," October 29, 2017. Available at SSRN: https://ssrn.com/abstract=3061567.

[54]Ibid.

[55]Song Hee Hong, Marvin D. Shepherd, David Scoones, and Thomas T. H. Wan, "Product-Line Extensions and Pricing Strategies of Brand-Name Drugs Facing Patent Expiration," *Journal of Managed Care Pharmacy* 11, no. 9 (2005): 746–54.

[56]Ibid.

[57]U.S. Federal Trade Commission v. Actavis, Inc., 133 S. Ct. 1630 (2012).

[58]U.S. Federal Trade Commission, *Pay-for-Delay: How Drug Company Pay-Offs Cost Consumers Billions*, 2010, https://www.ftc.gov/reports/pay-delay-how-drug-company-pay-offs-cost-consumers-billions-federal-trade-commission-staff.

[59]Community Catalyst and US PIRG, *Top Twenty Pay-for-Delay Drugs: How Drug Industry Payoffs Delay Generics, Inflate Prices and Hurt Consumers*, July 2013, http://www.uspirg.org/sites/pirg/files/reports/Top_Twenty_Pay_For_Delay_Drugs_USPIRG.pdf. See also U.S. Federal Trade Commission, Bureau of Competition, "Overview of Agreements Filed in FY 2013," December 22, 2014, https://www.ftc.gov/news-events/press-releases/2014/12/ftc-staff-issues-fy-2013-report-branded-drug-firms-patent.

[60]Arthur Allen, "A Giant Pain in the Wallet: How Drug Companies Are Making Crucial, Common Drugs up to 100 Times More Expensive," *Slate.com*, March 29, 2011, http://www.slate.com/articles/health_and_science/medical_examiner/2011/03/a_giant_pain_in_the_wallet.html.

[61]Many articles name URL Pharma as the company that obtained FDA approval for colchicine. See, for example, Aaron S. Kesselheim and Daniel H. Solomon, "Incentives for Drug Development—the Curious Case of Colchicine,"

*New England Journal of Medicine* 362, no. 22 (2010): 2045–47, http://www.nejm
.org/doi/full/10.1056/NEJMp1003126. The *Federal Register* identifies Mutual
Pharmaceutical, Inc., a subsidiary of URL Pharma, as the company so we use
that name here. FDA, *Single-Ingredient Oral Colchicine Products; Enforcement Action
Dates*, October 1, 2010, https://www.federalregister.gov/documents/2010/10/01/
2010-24684/single-ingredient-oral-colchicine-products-enforcement-action-dates.

[62]U.S. Department of Health and Human Services and U.S. Food and Drug
Administration, "FDA Orders Halt to Marketing of Unapproved Single-Ingredient
Oral Colchicine," news release, September 30, 2010, http://www.fda.gov/
NewsEvents/Newsroom/PressAnnouncements/2010/ucm227796.htm.

[63]Allan S. Brett, "Spotlight on Colchicine: The Colcrys Controversy,"
*NEJM Journal Watch*, June 10, 2010, http://www.jwatch.org/jw2010061
00000001/2010/06/10/spotlight-colchicine-colcrys-controversy.

[64]Kurt Ullman, "Colcrys Approval Triggers Questions," *Rheumatologist*,
May 1, 2010, http://www.the-rheumatologist.org/details/article/865591/Colcrys_
Approval_Triggers_Questions.html.

[65]Orphan Drug Act, Title 21, 316.3 (12).

[66]Aaron S. Kesselheim, Jessica M. Franklin, Seoyoung C. Kim, John D. Seeger,
and Daniel H. Solomon, "Reductions in Use of Colchicine after FDA Enforcement
of Market Exclusivity in a Commercially Insured Population," *Journal of General
Internal Medicine* 30, no. 11 (2015): 1633–38, doi:10.1007/s11606-015-3285-7.

[67]Lisa Schenker, "FDA Approves Northbrook Company's $89,000 Muscular
Dystrophy Drug," *Chicago Tribune*, February 9, 2017, http://www.chicagotribune
.com/business/ct-muscular-dystrophy-drug-fda-approval-0210-biz-20170209-
story.html.

[68]Sarah Jane Tribble and Sydney Lupkin, "Sky-High Prices for Orphan Drugs
Slam American Families and Insurers," *Kaiser Health News*, January 17, 2017.

[69]Ed Silverman, "FDA Designated a Record Number of Orphan Drugs Last
Year," *STAT*, February 11, 2016, https://www.statnews.com/pharmalot/2016/02/
11/fda-designates-record-number-of-orphan-drugs/.

[70]Michael G. Daniel, Timothy M. Pawlik, Amanda N. Fader, Nestor F. Esnaola,
and Martin A. Makary, "The Orphan Drug Act: Restoring the Mission to Rare
Diseases," *American Journal of Clinical Oncology* 39, no. 2 (2016): 210–13, https://jhu
.pure.elsevier.com/en/publications/the-orphan-drug-act-restoring-the-mission-
to-rare-diseases-4.

[71]Ibid.

[72]Ed Silverman, "Law for Rare Disease Drugs Needs Revamping,"
Researchers Say," *STAT*, November 30, 2015, https://www.statnews.com/
pharmalot/2015/11/30/orphan-drug-act-rare-diseases/; Daniel et al., "The
Orphan Drug Act."

[73]Harris Meyer, "Does the FDA Enable Drugmakers to Jack Up Prices on Cheap Old Drugs?," *Modern Healthcare Vital Signs (blog),* October 17, 2016, http://www.modernhealthcare.com/article/20161017/BLOG/161019928.

[74]Joanne Armstrong, "Unintended Consequences—The Cost of Preventing Preterm Births after FDA Approval of a Branded Version of 17OHP," *New England Journal of Medicine* 364, no. 18 (2011): 1689–91, http://www.nejm.org/doi/full/10.1056/NEJMp1102796.

[75]Allen, "A Giant Pain in the Wallet."

[76]Ed Silverman, "A New Drug and the High Cost of Premature Births," *Pharmalive.com,* March 10, 2011, http://www.pharmalive.com/new-drug-high-cost-premature-births; Yesha Patel and Martha M. Rumore, "Hydroxyprogesterone Caproate Injection (Makena) One Year Later," *Pharmacy and Therapeutics* 37, no. 7 (July 2012), http://www.ncbi.nlm.nih.gov/pmc/articles/PMC3411212/; Pharmalot, "KV Pharmaceuticals under Federal Scrutiny for Price Gouging," *Seeking Alpha,* March 19, 2011, http://www.firstwordpharma.com/node/354087.

[77]Jim Doyle, "KV Pharmaceutical Files for Bankruptcy," *St. Louis Post-Dispatch,* August 7, 2012, http://www.stltoday.com/business/local/kv-pharmaceutical-files-for-bankruptcy/article_4a26c62c-dfde-11e1-9ffb-0019bb30f31a.html.

[78]Courtney Hutchison, "KV Pharma Cuts Price of Costly Premature Birth Prevention Drug," *ABCNews,* April 1, 2011, http://abcnews.go.com/Health/Womens Health/kv-pharma-cuts-price-makena-costly-drug-prevents/story?id=13274910.

[79]Charles L. Hooper, "Never Mind: FDA Changes Own Rules in Midstream," *Library of Economics and Liberty,* November 5, 2012, http://www.econlib.org/library/Columns/y2012/Hooperdrugs.html.

[80]U.S. Department of Health and Human Services and U.S. Food and Drug Administration, "FDA Takes Action Against KV Pharmaceutical Company: Company Making, Marketing and Distributing Adulterated and Unapproved Drugs," news release, March 2, 2009, http://www.firstwordpharma.com/node/354087.

[81]U.S. Department of Justice, Office of Public Affairs, "Former Drug Company Executive Pleads Guilty in Oversized Drug Tablets Case: St. Louis Judge Imposes Sentence of $1 Million Fine, $900,000 Forfeiture, 30 Days in Jail," news release, March 10, 2011, http://www.justice.gov/opa/pr/2011/March/11-civ-306.html; Joseph Whittington and Andrew M. Harris, "Ex-KV Pharmaceutical CEO Pleads Guilty, Gets 30-Day Sentence," *Bloomberg Business,* March 10, 2011, http://www.bloomberg.com/news/articles/2011-03-10/ex-kv-pharmaceutical-ceo-hermelin-pleads-guilty-to-drug-label-law-breach.

[82]Jim Doyle, "KV Pharmaceutical Agrees to $17 Million Settlement," *St. Louis Post-Dispatch,* December 6, 2011, http://www.stltoday.com/business/local/kv-pharmaceutical-agrees-to-million-settlement-with-doj/article_3c947aee-2054-11e1-8c50-001a4bcf6878.html#ixzz1l2nvv3Uz.

[83]Nicholas Fogelson, "Boycott Makena: March of Dimes Responds to KV Pharmaceuticals," *Academic OB/GYN* (blog), March 24, 2011, http://academicobgyn.com/2011/03/24/boycott-makena-march-of-dimes-responds-to-kv-pharmaceuticals/.

[84]Jennifer Howse, "March of Dimes Demands Prompt and Decisive Action from Ther-Rx," March of Dimes website, March 23, 2011, http://www.marchofdimes.org/news/march-of-dimes-demands-prompt-and-decisive-action-from-ther-rx.aspx.

[85]Ryan M. Mott, "Colchicine, Guaifenesin, and the Constitutionality of FDA Market Exclusivity for Approval Pioneers," unpublished paper, University of Michigan Law School, March 19, 2012, http://works.bepress.com/ryan_mott/1, citing Tammy M. Muccio, "Guaifenesin and FDA Approval of Marketed Unapproved Drugs: Protecting the Public or Protecting Profits?," *Harvard Law School* 2 (May 3, 2007), http://leda.law.harvard.edu/leda/data/834/Muccio_07.pdf.

[86]Sinead M. Murphy, Araya Puwanant, Robert C. Griggs, and the Consortium for Clinical Investigations of Neurological Channelopathies (CINCH) and Inherited Neuropathies Consortium (INC) Consortia of the Rare Disease Clinical Research Network, "Unintended Effects of Orphan Product Designation for Rare Neurological Diseases," *Annals of Neurology* 72, no. 4 (2012): 481–90, https://www.ncbi.nlm.nih.gov/pmc/articles/PMC3490440/.

[87]Ibid.

[88]Elisabeth Rosenthal, "The Soaring Cost of a Simple Breath," *New York Times*, October 12, 2013, http://www.nytimes.com/2013/10/13/us/the-soaring-cost-of-a-simple-breath.html?pagewanted=all.

[89]Ibid.

[90]Partners Healthcare Asthma Center, "Ozone, CFC's and Your Asthma," in *The Best of Breath of Fresh Air: 1995–2000,* http://www.asthma.partners.org/newfiles/BoFAChapter10.html.

[91]Nick Baumann, "Why You're Paying More to Breathe," *Mother Jones*, July/August 2011, http://www.motherjones.com/environment/2011/07/cost-increase-asthma-inhalers-expensive.

[92]Ibid.

[93]Rosenthal, "The Soaring Cost of a Simple Breath."

[94]ProCon.org, "State-by-State Guide to Physician-Assisted Suicide," February 21, 2017, https://euthanasia.procon.org/view.resource.php?resourceID=000132.

[95]Roxanne Nelson, "When Dying Becomes Unaffordable," *Medscape*, November 9, 2017, https://www.medscape.com/viewarticle/888271.

[96]Langreth, "Drug Prices Defy Gravity, Doubling for Dozens of Products."

CHAPTER 2

[1]Bruce Japsen, "At $1,000 a Pill, Hepatitis C Drug Sovaldi Rattles Medicaid Programs," *Forbes.com*, April 28, 2014, http://www.forbes.com/sites/brucejapsen/2014/04/28/pricey-hepatitis-pill-sovaldi-rattles-medicaid-programs/.

[2]Kristen Fischer, "New Hep C Drug Sovaldi Ignites Fierce Pricing Debate," *Healthline*, April 11, 2014, http://www.healthline.com/health-news/new-hepatitis-c-drug-stirs-controversy-041114.

[3]U.S. Department of Health and Human Services, Centers for Medicare and Medicaid Services, *National Health Expenditure Projections 2012–2022*, http://www.cms.gov/Research-Statistics-Data-and-Systems/Statistics-Trends-and-Reports/NationalHealthExpendData/downloads/proj2012.pdf.

[4]Priti Radhakrishnan, "Pharma's Secret Weapon to Keep Drug Prices High," *STAT*, June 14, 2016, https://www.statnews.com/2016/06/14/secondary-patent-gilead-sovaldi-harvoni/.

[5]John Carroll, "Merck Goes Toe-to-Toe with Gilead's Hep C Goliath, Flags Discount with Blockbuster OK," *FierceBiotech*, January 28, 2016, http://www.fiercebiotech.com/regulatory/merck-goes-toe-to-toe-gilead-s-hep-c-goliath-flags-discount-blockbuster-ok.

[6]Ed Silverman, "Gilead Hep C Drug Prices Blamed for England's Health Service Rationing Treatment," *STAT*, July 28, 2016, https://www.statnews.com/pharmalot/2016/07/28/gilead-hepatitis-drug-prices/.

[7]U.S. Senate Committee on Finance, "Wyden–Grassley Sovaldi Investigation Finds Revenue-Driven Pricing Strategy behind $84,000 Heptatitis Drug," December 1, 2015, http://www.finance.senate.gov/newsroom/ranking/release/?id=3f693c730fc24a4cba92562723ba5255.

[8]Silverman, "Gilead Hep C Drug Prices."

[9]Ed Silverman, "Colorado Is Latest State to Be Sued for Restricting Access to Hepatitis C Drugs," *STAT*, September 26, 2016, https://www.statnews.com/pharmalot/2016/09/22/colorado-sued-for-restricting-hepatitis-c-medicine/.

[10]Stephanie M. Lee, "$1,000 Hepatitis C Pill a Tough Miracle to Swallow," *SFGate*, May 8, 2014, http://www.sfgate.com/health/article/1-000-hepatitis-C-pill-a-tough-miracle-to-swallow-5455230.php.

[11]Ed Silverman, "Less Than 1 Percent of State Prisoners with Hepatitis C Get Treated Due to Drug Costs," *STAT*, October 5, 2016, https://www.statnews.com/pharmalot/2016/10/05/prisons-hepatitis-drug-prices-gilead/.

[12]Associated Press, "Pricey Drugs Overwhelm Medicare Safeguard," *STAT*, July 25, 2016, https://www.statnews.com/2016/07/25/medicare-drug-prices-harvoni-solvaldi/.

[13]Charles Ornstein, "Medicare Spending for Hepatitis C Cures Surges," *ProPublica*, October 16, 2015, https://www.propublica.org/article/medicare-spending-for-hepatitis-c-cures-surges.

[14]Associated Press, "Pricey Drugs Overwhelm Medicare Safeguard."

[15]Shannon First, "Reining in Medicare Rx Costs: What Will Work?," *MedPage Today*, November 4, 2016, http://www.healthleadersmedia.com/health-plans/reining-medicare-rx-costs-what-will-work-0.

[16]Chuck Grassley, "Grassley Presses the Administration on Reasons for Alarming Increase in Medicare Catastrophic Drug Spending," news release, July 27, 2017, https://www.grassley.senate.gov/news/news-releases/grassley-presses-administration-reasons-alarming-increase-medicare-catastrophic.

[17]Caroline Humer, "Express Scripts Drops Gilead Hep C Drugs for Cheaper AbbVie Rival," *Reuters*, December 22, 2014, http://www.reuters.com/article/us-express-scripts-abbvie-hepatitisc-idUSKBN0K007620141222.

[18]U.S. Senate Committee on Finance, *The Price of Sovaldi and Its Impact on the U.S. Health Care System*, (Washington: Government Printing Office, December 2015), https://www.finance.senate.gov/imo/media/doc/1%20The%20Price%20of%20Sovaldi%20and%20Its%20Impact%20on%20the%20U.S.%20Health%20Care%20System%20(Full%20Report).pdf.

[19]Avik Roy, "The Sovaldi Tax: Gilead Can't Justify the Price It's Asking for Hepatitis C Therapy," *The Apothecary* (blog), *Forbes.com*, June 7, 2014, http://www.forbes.com/sites/theapothecary/2014/06/17/the-sovaldi-tax-gilead-cant-justify-the-price-its-asking-americans-to-pay/.

[20]Letter from Sen. Bernard Sanders to the Honorable Robert A. McDonald, Secretary, U.S. Dept. of Veterans Affairs, May 12, 2015, https://www.sanders.senate.gov/download/051215-letter/?inline=file.

[21]Roy, "The Sovaldi Tax."

[22]Robert Langreth, "Gilead CEO Becomes Billionaire on $84,000 Hepatitis Drug," *Bloomberg Business*, March 3, 2014, http://www.bloomberg.com/news/2014-03-03/gilead-ceo-becomes-billionaire-on-84-000-hepatitis-drug.html.

[23]Merrill Goozner, "Why Sovaldi Shouldn't Cost $84,000," *Modern Healthcare*, March 3, 2014, http://www.modernhealthcare.com/article/20140503/MAGAZINE/305039983.

[24]See also National Institute of Allergy and Infectious Diseases, "Investigational Oral Regimen for Hepatitis C Shows Promise in NIH Trial," *NIH News*, August 27, 2013, http://www.nih.gov/news/newsreleases/2013/Pages/hepCtrial.aspx.

[25]Aaron S. Kesselheim, Yongtian Tina Tan, and Jerry Avorn, "The Roles of Academia, Rare Diseases, and Repurposing in the Development of the Most Transformative Drugs," *Health Affairs* 34, no. 2 (2015): 286–93.

[26]Robert Weisman, "Doctors Challenge Vertex over High Price of Cystic Fibrosis Drug," *Boston Globe*, July 20, 2015, http://www.bostonglobe.com/business/2015/07/20/researcher-and-group-doctors-challenge-vertex-price-new-cystic-fibrosis-drug/d5PZMlj6T6uzq0usm2xLEL/story.html. See also Ed Silverman, "How High? The Backlash over Rising Prescription Drug Prices Gains Steam," *Pharmalot* (blog), *Wall Street Journal,* July 21, 2015, http://blogs.wsj.com/pharmalot/2015/07/21/how-high-the-backlash-over-rising-prescription-drug-prices-gains-steam/.

[27]Silverman, "How High?"

[28]Alfred Engelberg, "Memo to the President: The Pharmaceutical Monopoly Adjustment Act of 2017," *Health Affairs Blog,* September 13, 2016, http://healthaffairs.org/blog/2016/09/13/memo-to-the-president-the-pharmaceutical-monopoly-adjustment-act-of-2017/.

[29]Ibid.

[30]Ibid.

[31]Stan Finkelstein and Peter Temin, *Reasonable RX: Solving the Drug Price Crisis* (Upper Saddle River, NJ: FT Press, 2008), chap. 4.

[32]Joe Nocera, "The $300,000 Drug," *New York Times*, July 18, 2014, http://www.nytimes.com/2014/07/19/opinion/joe-nocera-cystic-fibrosis-drug-price.html?_r=0.

[33]Robert Pear, "Medicare, Reversing Itself, Will Pay More for an Expensive New Cancer Drug," *New York Times*, August 8, 2015, http://www.nytimes.com/2015/08/09/us/medicare-reversing-itself-will-pay-more-for-an-expensive-new-cancer-drug.html?emc=edit_th_20150809&nl=todaysheadlines&nlid=15782921.

[34]Richard Knox, "Cancer Drug Mark-Ups: Year of Gleevec Cost $159 to Make but Sells for $106K," *CommonHealth*, September 25, 2015, http://www.wbur.org/commonhealth/2015/09/25/cancer-drug-cost.

[35]Reuters, "These New Cancer Drugs Are Helping Patients Live Years Longer," *Fortune*, May 19, 2016, http://fortune.com/2016/05/19/cancer-drugs-keytruda-opdivo/.

[36]Tracy Staton, "Payers Beware: Bristol-Myers Prices PD-1 Cancer Med at $143,000 in Japan," *FiercePharma*, September 4, 2014, http://www.fiercepharma.com/sales-and-marketing/payers-beware-bristol-myers-prices-pd-1-cancer-med-at-143-000-japan; Tracy Staton, "With $120K Price Tag, Yervoy Hailed as Potential Blockbuster," *FiercePharma*, March 28, 2011, http://www.fiercepharma.com/pharma/120k-price-tag-yervoy-hailed-as-potential-blockbuster.

[37]Eric Palmer, "Roche Looks to Earn Even More from Perjeta with EU Nod," *FiercePharma*, December 14, 2012, http://www.fiercepharma.com/financials/roche-looks-to-earn-even-more-from-perjeta-eu-nod.

[38]Aimee Picchi, "The Cost of Biogen's New Drug: $750,000 per Patient," *CBSNews.com*, December 29, 2016, http://www.cbsnews.com/news/the-cost-of-biogens-new-drug-spinraza-750000-per-patient/.

[39]Keith Speights, "The 7 Most Expensive Prescription Drugs in the World," *The Motley Fool*, April 18, 2017, https://www.fool.com/investing/2017/04/18/the-7-most-expensive-prescription-drugs-in-the-wor.aspx.

[40]Ibid.

[41]Ibid.

[42]Ibid.

[43]Liz Szabo, "Dozens of New Cancer Drugs Do Little to Improve Survival, Frustrating Patients," *Kaiser Health News*, February 13, 2107, http://khn.org/news/dozensofnewcancerdrugsdolittletoimprovesurvivalfrustratingpatients/.

[44]Ibid.

[45]Ben Hirschler, "Academics Call Time on $100,000 Cancer Drugs," *Reuters.com*, February 9, 2017, http://www.reuters.com/article/health-cancer-pharmaceuticals-prices-idUSL1N1FU1EC.

[46]Liz Szabo, "Cascade of Costs Could Push New Gene Therapy above $1 Million per Patient," *Kaiser Health News*, October 17, 2017, https://khn.org/news/cascade-of-costs-could-push-new-gene-therapy-above-1-million-per-patient/.

[47]Ibid.

[48]AHIP Center for Policy and Research, *High-Priced Drugs: Estimates of Annual Per-Patient Expenditures for 150 Specialty Medications*, April 8, 2016, https://www.ahip.org/report-high-priced-drugs-expenditures/.

[49]Stephen Barlas, "Are Specialty Drug Prices Destroying Insurers and Hurting Consumers? A Number of Efforts Are Under Way to Reduce Price Pressure," *Pharmacy and Therapeutics* 39, no. 8 (2014): 563–66, http://www.ncbi.nlm.nih.gov/pmc/articles/PMC4123806/.

[50]AHIP Center, *High-Priced Drugs*.

[51]Carolyn Y. Johnson, "Specialty Drugs Now Cost More than the Median Household Income," *Washington Post*, November 20, 2015, https://www.washingtonpost.com/news/wonk/wp/2015/11/20/specialty-drugs-now-cost-more-than-most-household-incomes/?utm_term=.df93c2adc145.

[52]William Shrank, Alan Lotvin, Surya Singh, and Troyen Brennan, "In the Debate about Cost and Efficacy, PCSK9 Inhibitors May Be the Biggest Challenge Yet," *Health Affairs Blog*, February 17, 2015, http://healthaffairs.org/blog/2015/02/17/in-the-debate-about-cost-and-efficacy-pcsk9-inhibitors-may-be-the-biggest-challenge-yet/; Gina Kolata, "New Alternatives to Statins Add to a Quandary on Cholesterol," *New York Times*, August 29, 2015, http://www.nytimes.com/2015/08/30/health/new-alternatives-to-statins-add-to-a-quandary-on-cholesterol.html?emc=edit_th_20150830&nl=todaysheadlines&nlid=15782921&_r=0.

[53]Peggy Peck, "PCSK9 Inhibitors: Now That We Have Them, What Do We Do?," *MedPage Today*, September 8, 2015, http://www.medpagetoday.com/Cardiology/Dyslipidemia/53451?xid=nl_mpt_DHE_2015-09-09&eun=g452253d0r.

[54]Ibid.

[55]Andrew Pollack, "Express Scripts Says It Will Cover 2 New Cholesterol Drugs," *New York Times*, October 6, 2015, http://nyti.ms/1RsFiCq.

[56]Ibid.

[57]Ibid.

[58]Institute for Clinical and Economic Review, "ICER Draft Report on Effectiveness, Value, and Pricing Benchmarks for PCSK9 Inhibitors for High Cholesterol Posted for Public Comment," news release, September 8, 2015, http://www.icer-review.org/pcsk9-draft-report-release/.

[59]Shannon Firth, "D.C. Week: Libido Pill OK'd; Healthcare Draws Attention in 2016 Race," *Medpage Today*, August 22, 2015, http://www.medpagetoday.com/Washington-Watch/Washington-Watch/53195; Andrew Pollack, "F.D.A. Approves Addyi, a Libido Pill for Women," *New York Times*, August 18, 2015, https://www.nytimes.com/2015/08/19/business/fda-approval-addyi-female-viagra.html; David Kroll, "FDA Approves Addyi (Flibanserin), 'A Milestone Moment' in Women's Health," *Forbes*, August 18, 2015, http://www.forbes.com/sites/davidkroll/2015/08/18/fda-approves-addyi-flibanserin-a-milestone-moment-in-womens-health/.

[60]Pollack, "F.D.A. Approves Addyi."

[61]Kroll, "FDA Approves Addyi (Flibanserin)."

[62]Caroline Chen, Cynthia Koons, and Anna Edney, "Valeant Buys Female Libido-Drug Maker Sprout for $1 Billion," *Bloomberg.com*, August 20, 2015, https://www.bloomberg.com/news/articles/2015-08-20/valeant-pharma-to-buy-female-libido-drug-maker-for-1-billion.

[63]GoodRX, "Addyi," https://www.goodrx.com/addyi.

[64]Gretchen Morgenson, "To Stop Price Spikes on Prescription Drugs, a Widening Radar," *New York Times*, December 23, 2016, http://nyti.ms/2hgUcSA.

[65]Charles Ornstein, "The Obscure Drug with a Growing Medicare Tab," *New York Times*, August 4, 2014, http://nyti.ms/1olTDzt.

[66]Charles Ornstein, "A Drug Quintupled in Price. Now, Drug Industry Players Are Feuding over the Windfall," *ProPublica*, May 31, 2107, https://www.propublica.org/article/drug-quintupled-in-price-now-drug-industry-players-feuding-over-windfall?utm_source=pardot&utm_medium=email&utm_campaign=dailynewsletter#.

[67]Andrew Pollack, "Drug Maker's Donations to CoPay Charity Face Scrutiny," *New York Times*, December 18, 2013, http://www.nytimes.com/2013/12/19/business/shake-up-at-big-co-pay-fund-raises-scrutiny-on-similar-charities.html.

[68]Benjamin Elgin and Robert Langreth, "How Big Pharma Uses Charity Programs to Cover for Drug Price Hikes: A Billion-Dollar System in Which Charitable Giving Is Profitable," *Bloomberg.com*, May 19, 2016, https://www.bloomberg.com/news/articles/2016-05-19/the-real-reason-big-pharma-wants-to-help-pay-for-your-prescription.

[69]Ibid.

[70]Office of Inspector General, U.S. Department of Health and Human Services, "Supplement Special Advisory Bulletin: Independent Charity Patient Assistance Programs," 79 *Federal Register* 104 (May 16, 2014): 31120–23, http://oig.hhs.gov/fraud/docs/alertsandbulletins/2014/independent-charity-bulletin.pdf.

[71]Corrected Expert Report of Joel W. Hay, PhD, ¶ 119, April 22, 2016, submitted in United States of America, ex rel. Beverly Brown v. Celgene Corp., Civil Action No. CV10-03165 GHK, https://www.lexis.com/research/retrieve?_m=fd361b888752f2fba6924da901ac0034&csvc=le&cform=byCitation&_fmtstr=CITE&docnum=1&_startdoc=1&wchp=dGLbVzt-zSkAA&_md5=3c697f98066c6bdf57c869f189efe2c4.

[72]Ibid.

[73]Bloomberg News, "PAN Foundation Responds to Bloomberg Article: Dan Klein," *Bloomberg,* August 3, 2016, https://www.bloomberg.com/news/articles/2016-08-03/pan-foundation-responds-to-bloomberg-article-dan-klein.

[74]John R. Graham, "EpiPen: A Case Study in Health Insurance Failure," *NCPA Health Policy Blog*, September 13, 2016, http://healthblog.ncpa.org/epipen-a-case-study-in-health-insurance-failure/.

## Chapter 3

[1]Robert Draper, "The Toxic Pharmacist," *New York Times*, June 8, 2003, http://www.nytimes.com/2003/06/08/magazine/the-toxic-pharmacist.html?src=pm&pagewanted=3; Josh Freed, "Thousands of Diluted Drug Doses," Associated Press, April 19, 2002, http://www.cbsnews.com/news/thousands-of-diluted-drug-doses/.

[2]Ibid.

[3]Danny McDonald, "Pharmacist in NECC Meningitis Outbreak Case Acquitted of Murder," *Boston Globe*, October 25, 2017, https://www.bostonglobe.com/metro/2017/10/25/chin/sSmR8lC4AZloK4HidEmGWI/story.html.

[4]Susan Morse, "Feds Nab 10 More in $100 Million Tricare Fraud," *Healthcare IT News*, October 21, 2016, http://www.healthcareitnews.com/news/feds-nab-10-more-100-million-tricare-fraud; Kevin Krause, "Dallas Firm That Marketed Compounded Pain Creams Busted in Massive Health Care Fraud, Kickback Case," *DallasNews.com*, February 24, 2016, https://www.dallasnews.com/news/

crime/2016/02/24/drug-compounders-marketing-firm-busted-for-alleged-massive-health-care-fraud-involving-doctor-kickbacks.

[5]Krause, "Dallas Firm Busted."

[6]Ibid.

[7]Paula McMahon, "Feds Charge 16 in Massive $175M Prescription Cream Fraud Based in South Florida," *Sun-Sentinel*, September 1, 2016, http://www.sun-sentinel.com/local/palm-beach/fl-compound-cream-fraud-20160901-story.html; Carolina Bolado, "Alleged Ringleader Pleads Guilty in $175M Health Fraud," *Law360*, January 19, 2017, https://www.law360.com/articles/882839/alleged-ringleader-pleads-guilty-in-175m-health-fraud.

[8]Times Staff, "New Port Richey Pharmacy at Center of Federal Insurance Fraud Indictment," *Tampa Bay Times*, August 10, 2016, http://www.tampabay.com/news/publicsafety/crime/new-port-richey-pharmacy-at-center-of-federal-indictment/2288992; Frances McMorris, "New Port Richey Pharmacy Owner Pleads Guilty in Massive Fraud Scheme," *Tampa Bay Business Journal*, November 6, 2017, https://www.bizjournals.com/tampabay/news/2017/11/06/new-port-richey-pharmacy-owner-pleads-guilty-in.html.

[9]McMorris, "New Port Richey Pharmacy Owner Pleads Guilty."

[10]Ibid.

[11]Nathan Hale, "3 Sentenced in Fla. for $175 Health Care Fraud Scheme," *Law360*, March 24, 2017, https://www.law360.com/articles/905509/3-sentenced-in-fla-for-175m-health-care-fraud-scheme.

[12]Ryan Moore, "Feds: Hub City Doctor, Christmas Tree Farm Named in Federal Pharmacy Investigation," WDAM-TV, February 15, 2017, http://www.wdam.com/story/34516678/feds-hub-city-doctor-christmas-tree-farm-named-in-federal-pharmacy-investigation.

[13]United States v. Real Property Located at 19 Crane Park, Hattiesburg, Lamar County, Mississippi, Improvements, and Fixtures Thereon, et al., No. 3:16cv27 TSL-RHW (S.D. Miss., February 10, 2017).

[14]Ibid.

[15]Ibid.

[16]Lici Beveridge, "Details Emerge in Alleged Compounding Pharmacy Scheme," *Hattiesburg American*, February 15, 2017, http://www.hattiesburgamerican.com/story/news/crime/2017/02/15/details-emerge-alleged-compounding-pharmacy-scheme/97940600/.

[17]Tom McLaughlin, "Feds Seize Homes in Gulf Breeze, WaterColor, Sandpiper Cove as Part of TRICARE Fraud Case," *Northwest Florida Daily News*, June 8, 2016, http://www.nwfdailynews.com/news/20160608/feds-seize-homes-in-gulf-breeze-watercolor-sandpiper-cove-as-part-of-tricare-fraud-case; Lici Beveridge, "Complaint Outlines Depth of Alleged Pharmacy

Fraud," *Clarion Ledger*, February 19, 2017, http://www.clarionledger.com/ story/news/local/2017/02/19/complaint-outlines-depth-alleged-pharmacy-fraud/98114652/.

[18]Ryan Moore, "2 Criminally Charged in 2016 Pharmacy Raids," WDAM, July 13, 2017, http://www.wdam.com/story/35880218/2-criminally-charged-in-2016-pharmacy-raids.

[19]Amended Complaint, U.S. v. Par Pharmaceuticals, No. 06 C 06131, (N.D. Ill., July 7, 2011), http://i.bnet.com/blogs/par-complaint1.pdf.

[20]Ibid.

[21]Ibid.

[22]Ibid.

[23]Ibid.

[24]Ibid.

[25]Ibid.

[26]Ibid.

[27]U.S. Department of Justice, United States Attorney for the Northern District of Illinois, "CVS Caremark Corp. to Pay $36.7 Million to U.S., 23 States, and D.C. to Settle Medicaid Prescription Drug Fraud Allegations," news release, March 18, 2008, https://www.justice.gov/archive/opa/pr/2008/March/08_crt_214.html.

[28]Jim Edwards, "Hard to Swallow: Walgreens Wrote 'One Liners' to Sell Illegal Price Hikes to Patients," *CBS Money Watch*, September 9, 2011, http://www.bnet.com/blog/drug-business/hard-to-swallow-walgreens-wrote-8220one-liners-8221-to-sell-illegal-price-hikes-to-patients/9629.

[29]Ibid.

[30]Ibid.

[31]Amended Complaint, U.S. v. Par Pharmaceuticals, No. 06 C 06131, (N.D. Ill., July 7, 2011), http://i.bnet.com/blogs/par-complaint1.pdf.

[32]Ibid.

[33]U.S. Department of Justice, Office of Public Affairs, "Nation's Largest Nursing Home Pharmacy and Drug Manufacturer to Pay $112 Million to Settle False Claims Act Cases," news release, November 3, 2009, http://www.justice.gov/opa/pr/nation-s-largest-nursing-home-pharmacy-and-drug-manufacturer-pay-112-million-settle-false.

[34]John Kennedy, "Par Pharmaceutical Beats FCA Prescription-Switch Claims," *Law 360*, August 18, 2017, https://www.law360.com/articles/955531/par-pharmaceutical-beats-fca-prescription-switch-claims.

[35]Dawn M. Gencarelli, "Average Wholesale Price for Prescription Drugs: Is There a More Appropriate Pricing Mechanism?," National Health Policy Forum Issue Brief no.775, George Washington University, June 7, 2002.

[36] Chris George, "Seven States Consider Lawsuit Against Drug Companies for Fraud," *Wyoming Tribune-Eagle*, April 25, 2001, p. A1 (list of drugs by DOJ that are overpriced).

[37] First Amended Complaint, Citizens for Consumer Justice, et al., v. Abbott Laboratories, Inc., et al., No. 01-12257 PBS, (D. Mass. March 18, 2002), at 35, ¶¶ 150–51.

[38] Amended Master Consolidated Class Action Complaint, In re Pharmaceutical Industry Average Wholesale Price Litigation, M.D.L. No. 1456, 01-12257-PBS, July 25, 2003, at 338, https://www.courtlistener.com/opinion/2309518/in-re-pharmaceutical-industry-average-wholesale-price-litigation/.

[39] Abby Alpert, Mark Duggan, and Judith Hellerstein, "Perverse Reverse Price Competition: Average Wholesale Prices and Medicaid Pharmaceutical Spending," *Journal of Public Economics* 108 (2013): 44–62.

[40] Prepared Statement of William J. Scanlon, Director, Health Care Issues, United States General Accounting Office, before the Subcommittee on Health and the Subcommittee on Oversight and Investigations of the Committee on Energy and Commerce, House of Representatives, 107th Cong., 1st Sess., *Medicare Drug Reimbursements: A Broken System for Patients and Taxpayers* (Washington: Government Printing Office, September 21, 2001), https://www.gpo.gov/fdsys/pkg/CHRG-107hhrg75756/html/CHRG-107hhrg75756.htm.

[41] Sentencing Memorandum of the United States, U.S. v. TAP Pharmaceutical Products, Inc., Criminal Action No. 01-CR-10354-WGY, U.S. District Court for the District of Massachusetts, Eastern Division, December 4, 2001, http://www.prescriptionaccesslitigation.org/pdf/20020123-Sentencing-Memo.pdf.

[42] U.S. Department of Justice, "Astrazeneca Pharmaceuticals LP Pleads Guilty to Healthcare Crime; Company Agrees to Pay $355 Million to Settle Charges," news release, June 20, 2003, https://www.justice.gov/archive/opa/pr/2003/June/03_civ_371.htm.

[43] Joshua Partlow and Marc Kaufman, "U.S., Drug Company Settle Scam Charges," *Washington Post*, June 21, 2003, p. E1.

[44] Ibid.

[45] "Health Care Fraud Report," *BNA* 7, no. 6 (March 19, 2003): 215.

[46] GlaxoSmithKline, "Statement Concerning AWP Complaint Filed by New York's Attorney General," February 13, 2003, on file with authors.

[47] John E. Calfee and Michael S. Greve, "The New Pharmaceutical Litigation: What Is It and Where Is It Going?," American Enterprise Institute press briefing, June 18, 2002.

[48] Ibid.

[49] Testimony of George F. Grob, Deputy Inspector General for Health and Human Services, before the Committee on Energy and Commerce, House of Representatives, 107th Cong., 1st Sess., *Medicare Drug Reimbursements: A Broken*

*System for Patients and Taxpayers*, (Washington: Government Printing Office, September 21, 2001), https://www.gpo.gov/fdsys/pkg/CHRG-107hhrg75756/html/CHRG-107hhrg75756.htm (stating that the Office of the Inspector General has been investigating drug prices since the mid-1980s).

[50]Defendants' Memorandum of Law in Support of Their Motion to Dismiss the Commonwealth's Amended Complaint, p. 14, filed in Commonwealth of Kentucky, Ex Rel. Albert Chandler, III, Attorney General v. Warrick Pharmaceuticals Corporation, Schering-Plough Corporation, Schering Corporation, and Dey, Inc., Civil Action No. 03-CI-1135 (Kentucky—Franklin Circuit Court, Division II), February 6, 2004, https://awp.doj.wi.gov/sites/default/files/states-documents/Kentucky/MotionsBriefs/KY_Abbott_Warrick-Dey_Brief_Supporting_Motion_Dismiss_Amended_complaint-02-06-2004.pdf.

[51]U.S. Department of Health and Human Services, Office of the Inspector General, ACN 06-40216, "Changes to the Medicaid Prescription Drug Program Could Save Millions," 1984; U.S. Department of Health and Human Services, Office of the Inspector General, A-06-89-00037, "Use of Average Wholesale Prices in Reimbursing Pharmacies in Medicaid and the Medicare Catastrophic Coverage Act Prescription Drug Program," 1989.

[52]U.S. Department of Health and Human Services, Office of the Inspector General, OEI-03-94-00390, "Medicare Payments for Nebulizer Drugs," February 1996, http://oig.hhs.gov/oei/reports/oei-03-94-00390.pdf.; U.S. Department of Health and Human Services, Office of the Inspector General, OEI-03-04-00393, "Suppliers' Acquisition Costs for Albuterol Sulfate," June 1996, http://oig.hhs.gov/oei/reports/oei-03-94-00393.pdf; U.S. Department of Health and Human Services, Office of the Inspector General, OEI-03-94-00392, "A Comparison of Albuterol Sulfate Prices," June 1996, https://oig.hhs.gov/oei/reports/oei-03-94-00392.pdf; U.S. Department of Health and Human Services, Office of the Inspector General, OEI-03-94-00391, "Questionable Medicare Payments for Nebulizer Drugs," March 1997, https://oig.hhs.gov/oei/reports/oei-03-94-00391.pdf.

[53]U.S. Department of Health and Human Services, Office of the Inspector General, OEI-03-97-00290, "Excessive Medicare Payments for Prescription Drugs," December 1997, https://oig.hhs.gov/oei/reports/oei-03-97-00290.pdf.

[54]U.S. Department of Health and Human Services, Office of the Inspector General, OEI-03-00-00311, "Medicare Reimbursement of Albuterol," June 2000, https://oig.hhs.gov/oei/reports/oei-03-00-00311.pdf.

[55]Statement of William J. Scanlon Director, Health Care Issues, U.S. Government Accountability Office, GAO-01-1142T, "Medicare Part B Drugs: Program Payments Should Reflect Market Prices," September 21, 2001, http://www.gao.gov/assets/110/108994.pdf.

[56]"Concerns about Average Wholesale Price-Based Reimbursement Raised Again," *Oncology*, November 1, 2001, http://www.physicianspractice.com/practice-management/concerns-about-average-wholesale-price-based-reimbursement-raised-again.

[57]See Gardiner Harris, "Plan Would Slash What Medicare Pays for Cancer Drugs," *New York Times*, July 27, 2004, (estimating that Medicare will save $16 billion over a decade by eliminating AWP-based payment for cancer drugs); U.S. Department of Health and Human Services, Office of Inspector General, *The 2002 Red Book* (Washington: Government Account Office, 2002), pp. 14 and 69, https://oig.hhs.gov/publications/docs/redbook/2002%20Red%20Book.pdf ($1.6 billion estimate). Testimony of George F. Grob, Deputy Inspector General for Health and Human Services, before the Committee on Energy and Commerce, House of Representatives, 107th Cong., 1st Sess., *Medicare Drug Reimbursements: A Broken System for Patients and Taxpayers* (Washington: Government Printing Office, September 21, 2001), https://www.gpo.gov/fdsys/pkg/CHRG-107hhrg75756/html/CHRG-107hhrg75756.htm (estimating overpayments are $1 billion–$2 billion).

[58]Letter from Pete Stark, Ranking Member, Subcommittee on Health, U.S. House of Representatives, to Alan F. Holmer, President, Pharmaceutical Research and Manufacturers of America, September 28, 2000, reprinted in *Congressional Record*, 20114-20116, September 20, 2000, https://books.google.com/books?id=b4xdPiDceH8C&lpg=PA20114&ots=0SkgfSXjuq&dq=which%20congressman%20prevent%20medicare%20from%20abandoning%20awps&pg=PA20115#v=onepage&q=which%20congressman%20prevent%20medicare%20from%20abandoning%20awps&f=false.

[59]Hearing on President's Fiscal Year 1998 Budget Proposal for Medicare, Medicaid, and Welfare Before the Senate Committee on Finance, 105th Cong. 265 (1997) (written response of Secretary Donna Shalala to questions of Senator Hatch) (App. 52).

[60]H. Rep. No. 105-149, at 1354, Balanced Budget Act of 1997, Committee on the Budget, House of Representatives, 105th Cong., 1st Sess., https://www.congress.gov/congressional-report/105th-congress/house-report/149.

[61]This history is set out in Defendants' Memorandum of Law in Support of Their Motion to Dismiss the Commonwealth's Amended Complaint, pp. 17–19, filed in Commonwealth of Kentucky, ex rel. Albert Chandler, III, Attorney General vs. Warrick Pharmaceuticals Corporation, Schering-Plough Corporation, Schering Corporation, and Dey, Inc., Civil Action No. 03-CI-1135 (Kentucky–Franklin Circuit Court, Division II), February 6, 2004, available at https://awp.doj.wi.gov/sites/default/files/states-documents/Kentucky/MotionsBriefs/KY_Abbott_Warrick-Dey_Brief_Supporting_Motion_Dismiss_Amended_complaint-02-06-2004.pdf.

[62]Robert Pearl, "America's Broken Health Care System: The Role of Drug, Device Manufacturers," *Forbes.com*, April 24, 2014, http://www.forbes.com/sites/robertpearl/2014/04/24/americas-broken-health-care-system-the-role-of-drug-device-manufacturers/.

[63]Peter Whoriskey and Dan Keating, "An Effective Eye Drug Is Available for $50. But Many Doctors Choose a $2,000 Alternative," *Washington Post*, December 7, 2013, http://www.washingtonpost.com/business/economy/an-effective-eye-drug-is-available-for-50-but-many-doctors-choose-a-2000-alternative/2013/12/07/1a96628e-55e7-11e3-8304-caf30787c0a9_story.html.

[64]Ibid.

[65]Ibid.

[66]Centers for Medicare and Medicaid Services, *Medicare Drug Spending Dashboard*, https://www.cms.gov/Research-Statistics-Data-and-Systems/Statistics-Trends-and-Reports/Dashboard/2015-Medicare-Drug-Spending/medicare-drug-spending-dashboard-2015-data.html.

[67]Whoriskey and Keating, "An Effective Eye Drug."

[68]Ibid.

## CHAPTER 4

[1]Peter Waldman, David Armstrong, and Sydney Freedberg, "Deaths Linked to Cardiac Stents Rise as Overuse Seen," *Bloomberg Business*, September 25, 2013, http://www.bloomberg.com/news/articles/2013-09-26/deaths-linked-to-cardiac-stents-rise-as-overuse-seen.

[2]Ibid.

[3]Mary Ann Roser, "State Medical Board Accuses Well-Known Cardiologist of Unnecessary Heart Procedures and Patient's Death," *Statesman.com*, November 21, 2010, http://www.statesman.com/news/news/local/state-medical-board-accuses-well-known-cardiolog-1/nRTHX/.

[4]Ibid.

[5]Ibid.

[6]Waldman, Armstrong, and Freedberg, "Deaths Linked to Cardiac Stents Rise."

[7]Ibid.

[8]David Fleshler, "Broward Health to Pay $69.5 Million on Federal Charges," *Sun-Sentinel*, September 15, 2015, http://www.sun-sentinel.com/local/broward/fl-hospital-settlement-20150915-story.html; Jeff Overley, "Ga. Hospital Inks $35M FCA Deal Over Doc Pay, Billing," *Law360.com*, September 4, 2015, http://www.law360.com/articles/699791/ga-hospital-inks-35m-fca-deal-over-doc-pay-bill.

[9]Waldman, Armstrong, and Freedberg, "Deaths Linked to Cardiac Stents Rise."

[10]Kathleen Stergiopoulos and David L. Brown, "Initial Coronary Stent Implantation with Medical Therapy vs. Medical Therapy Alone for Stable Coronary Artery Disease: Meta-Analysis of Randomized Controlled Trials," *Archives of Internal Medicine* 172, no. 4 (2012): 312–19, https://jamanetwork.com/journals/jamainternalmedicine/fullarticle/1108733.

[11]Kathleen Stergiopoulos, William E. Boden, Pamela Hartigan, et al., "Percutaneous Coronary Intervention Outcomes in Patients with Stable Obstructive Coronary Artery Disease and Myocardial Ischemia: A Collaborative Meta-Analysis of Contemporary Randomized Clinical Trials," *JAMA Internal Medicine* 174, no. 2 (2014): 232–40, https://jamanetwork.com/journals/jamainternalmedicine/fullarticle/1783047.

[12]Peggy Peck, "COURAGE at 15: Still No Edge for Stenting," *MedPage Today*, November 11, 2015, http://www.medpagetoday.com/cardiology/pci/54659.

[13]Peter Waldman, "Doctors Use Euphemism for $2.4 Billion in Needless Stents," *Bloomberg*, October 29, 2013, http://www.bloomberg.com/news/articles/2013-10-30/doctors-use-euphemism-for-2-4-billion-in-needless-stents.

[14]U.S. Senate, "Senator Everett McKinley Dirksen Dies," September 7, 1969, https://www.senate.gov/artandhistory/history/minute/Senator_Everett_Mckinley_Dirksen_Dies.htm.

[15]Nicole Lou, "Criteria Reduce Inappropriate PCI," *MedPage Today*, November 10, 2015, http://www.medpagetoday.com/Cardiology/PCI/54625.

[16]Nicole Lou, "Registry: Too Many Heart Caths before Noncardiac Surgery," *MedPage Today*, March 28, 2016, http://www.medpagetoday.com/Cardiology/PCI/56981?xid=nl_mpt_DHE_2016%AD03%AD29&eun=g452253d0r.

[17]Waldman, Armstrong, and Freedberg, "Deaths Linked to Cardiac Stents Rise."

[18]Shelley Wood, "DeMaio Resolves Unnecessary Stenting Charges with Board," *Medscape HeartWire*, November 28, 2011, http://www.medscape.com/viewarticle/754271.

[19]Ibid.

[20]Ibid.

[21]Shawn J. Soper, "Doctor Sentenced to 8 Years in Stent Case," *Dispatch/Maryland Coast Dispatch*, November 25, 2011, http://mdcoastdispatch.com/2011/11/23/doctor-sentenced-to-8-years-in-stent-case/; Bob Herman, "Retired Cardiologist Convicted, Faces up to 35 Years in Prison for Unnecessary Stents, Fraudulent Billing," *Becker's Hospital Review*, July 27, 2011, http://www.beckershospitalreview.com/hospital-key-specialties/retired-cardiologist-convicted-faces-up-to-35-years-in-prison-for-unnecessary-stents-fraudulent-billing.html; Molly Gamble, "Trial Begins for Maryland Cardiologist

Accused of Implanting 200 Unnecessary Stents," *Becker's Hospital Review*, July 13, 2011, http://www.beckershospitalreview.com/hospital-management-administration/trial-begins-for-marylands-dr-john-mclean-over-stent-implants .html; Tricia Bishop, "Salisbury Stent Doctor Sentenced to Federal Prison," *Baltimore Sun*, November 10, 2011, http://articles.baltimoresun.com/2011-11-10/health/bs-md-mclean-sentenced-20111108_1_stent-patients-unnecessary-coronary-stents-federal-prison.

[22]One case was tried, to a mixed conclusion. Glenn Weinberg, a Baltimore businessman, claimed to have lost millions of dollars in income because he had to scale back his career after Dr. Midei implanted three unnecessary stents. At trial, Weinberg won on liability, but the jurors deadlocked on the issue of damages, and a mistrial was declared. Jessica Anderson, "Juror Says Midei Panel Split over Damages," *Baltimore Sun*, November 7, 2013, http://articles .baltimoresun.com/2013-11-07/news/bs-md-midei-folo-20131107_1_mark-midei-stents-maryland-live; Jessica Anderson and Scott Calvert, "Jury Weighing Damages in $150 Million Stent Suit," *Baltimore Sun*, November 1, 2013, http://articles.baltimoresun.com/2013-11-01/news/bs-md-co-midei-damages-closings-20131101_1_midei-and-st-mark-midei-maryland-live; Jessica Anderson, "Midei Breached Medical Care Standards with Stents, Jury Finds," *Baltimore Sun*, October 23, 2013, http://articles.baltimoresun.com/2013-10-23/news/bs-md-midei-verdict-20131023_1_other-former-midei-patients-mark-midei-stents.

[23]Ian Duncan, "$37 Million Settlement Deal Reached in Midei Stent Case," *Baltimore Sun*, April 7, 2014, http://articles.baltimoresun.com/2014-04-07/news/bs-md-stent-settlement-20140407_1_midei-glenn-weinberg-unnecessary-heart-stent-procedures.

[24]Ibid. One of us (DAH) was an expert for MidAtlantic Cardiovascular Associates in a case brought by a group of cardiac surgeons (Cardiac Surgery Associates) after unsuccessful merger negotiations. For further background, see Joyce Frieden, "Dispute Splits Cardiologists, Cardiac Surgeons," *Internal Medicine News*, March 15, 2004, https://www.thefreelibrary.com/Dispute+splits+cardiologists, +cardiac+surgeons.-a0115499688.

[25]Associated Press, "Md. Hospital to Pay $22M in Unnecessary Stent Case," *Bloomberg Businessweek*, November 9, 2010, http://www.businessweek.com/ap/financialnews/D9JCSLD80.htm; Margaret Dick Tocknell, "St. Joseph Medical Center Settles Stent Cases," *HealthLeaders Media*, May 7, 2013, http://www.health leadersmedia.com/content/LED-291861/St-Joseph-Medical-Center-Settles-Stent-Cases.

[26]Drug-eluting stents are coated with a medication that helps prevent future cardiac events.

[27]Larry Husten,"Mark Midei Can't Get a Job Taking Blood Pressure at a Walmart," *Forbes*, April 8, 2012, https://www.forbes.com/sites/larryhusten/2012/04/08/mark-midei-cant-get-a-job-taking-blood-pressure-at-a-walmart/#2dcbe-3a26c17; Larry Husten, "Senate Report on Mark Midei and Abbott: 30 Stents in 1 Day, Pig Roasts, and More," *CardioBrief*, December 6, 2010, http://cardiobrief.org/2010/12/06/senate-report-on-mark-midei-and-abbott-30-stents-in-1-day-pig-roasts-and-more/; Maryland State Board of Physicians, "Final Decision and Order," July 13, 2011, http://www.mbp.state.md.us/BPQAPP/orders/d3004207.131.pdf.

[28]Ibid.

[29]Molly Gamble, "Former Cardiologist at St. Joseph's Hospital in Kentucky Pleads Guilty to Overstenting," *Becker's Hospital Review*, June 6, 2013, http://www.beckershospitalreview.com/legal-regulatory-issues/former-cardiologist-at-st-josephs-hospital-in-kentucky-pleads-guilty-to-overstenting.html.

[30]Bill Estep, "Hundreds of Patients Allege Needless Heart Procedures Done at Saint Joseph-London," *Lexington Herald-Leader*, September 6, 2012, http://www.kentucky.com/2012/09/06/2326087_hundreds-of-patients-allege-needless.html?rh=1#storylink=cpy; Andrew Wolfson "Hundreds Sue Hospital Over Heart Procedures," *Courier-Journal* (Kentucky), February 16, 2013, http://www.courier-journal.com/story/news/2014/05/28/hundreds-sue-hospital-over-heart-procedures/9683369/.

[31]Terry Dickson, "Waycross Hospital Pays $840,000 in Lawsuit over Unqualified Physician," *Florida Times-Union*, January 20, 2012, http://jacksonville.com/news/crime/2012-01-19/story/waycross-hospital-pays-840000-lawsuit-over-unqualified-physician; United States' Complaint, U.S. ex rel. Lana Rogers v. Najam Azmat, M.D., and Satilla Health Services, Inc., d/b/a Satilla Regional Medical Center, No. CV507-92 (S.D. Ga. July 7, 2010), http://www.vernialaw.com/FCA%20Documents/Pleadings/US%20ex%20rel%20Rogers%20v%20Azmat%20SDGA.pdf; Sydney P. Freedberg, "Mother Dies Amid Abuses in $110 Billion U.S. Stent Assembly Line," *Bloomberg.com*, October 9, 2013, http://www.bloomberg.com/news/articles/2013-10-10/mother-dies-Amid-abuses-in-110-billion-u-s-stent-assembly-line; Jan Skutch, "Doctor Sentenced in Garden City Pill-Mill Scam," *Savannah Morning News*, August 9, 2014, http://savannahnow.com/news/2014-08-08/doctor-sentenced-federal-court.

[32]United States' Complaint, U.S. ex rel. Lana Rogers v. Najam Azmat, M.D., and Satilla Health Services, Inc., d/b/a Satilla Regional Medical Center, No. CV507-92 (S.D. Ga. July 7, 2010), http://www.vernialaw.com/FCA%20Documents/Pleadings/US%20ex%20rel%20Rogers%20v%20Azmat%20SDGA.pdf.

[33]Freedberg, "Mother Dies Amid Abuses."

[34]R. G. Dunlap, "Doctor Followed an Unsettled Path to Lexington," *Louisville Courier-Journal*, December 18, 2011, http://archive.courier-journal.com/article/20111218/NEWS01/101240008/Doctor-followed-an-unsettled-path-Lexington.

[35]Ibid.

[36]Ibid.

[37]Ibid.

[38]Ibid.

[39]Ibid.

[40]Ibid.

[41]Ibid.

[42]Ibid.

[43]Ibid.

[44]Joe Carlson, "Beating the System: Physician Faces Charges after Years of Allegations, Lawsuits in Multiple States," *Modern Healthcare*, March 16, 2013, http://www.modernhealthcare.com/article/20130316/MAGAZINE/303169974; Joe Carlson, "Georgia Suspends Medical License of Jailed Surgeon 'Dr. Hazmat,'" *Modern Healthcare*, April 2, 2013, http://www.modernhealthcare.com/article/20130402/NEWS/304029948.

[45]Ibid.

[46]Ibid.

[47]Ibid.

[48]Ajay J. Kirtane, Hemal Gada, Sripal Bangalore, Dean J. Kereiakes, and Gregg W. Stone, "TCT-845 Percutaneous Coronary Intervention Is Associated with Lower Mortality Compared with Optimal Medical Therapy in Patients with Stable Ischemic Heart Disease and Objective Evidence of Ischemia or Abnormal Fractional Flow Reserve: A Meta-Analysis of Randomized Controlled Trials," *Journal of the American College of Cardiology* 62, no. 18 (2013): B255s, https://core.ac.uk/download/pdf/82727836.pdf.

[49]Shelley Wood, "Stents, ICDs, Inappropriate? Then, under New Audit Program, CMS Won't Pay," *Medscape*, December 3, 2011, http://www.medscape.com/viewarticle/791095.

[50]Ibid.

[51]Ibid.

[52]Stephen Klaidman, *Coronary: A True Story of Medicine Gone Awry* (New York: Scribner, 2007).

[53]Ibid.

[54]Ibid.

[55]Ibid.

[56]Ibid.

[57]Anupam B. Jena, Vinay Prasad, Dana P. Goldman, and John Romley, "Mortality and Treatment Patterns among Patients Hospitalized with Acute Cardiovascular Conditions during Dates of National Cardiology Meetings," *JAMA Internal Medicine* 175, no. 2 (2015): 237–44, https://jamanetwork.com/journals/jamainternalmedicine/fullarticle/2038979.

[58]Ibid.

[59]Rasha Al-Lamee, David Thompson, Hakim-Moulay Dehbi, et al. "Percutaneous Coronary Intervention in Stable Angina (ORBITA): A Double-Blind, Randomised Controlled Trial" (published online November 2), *Lancet* (2017), http://www.thelancet.com/journals/lancet/article/PIIS0140-6736(17)32714-9/fulltext?elsca1=tlxpr.

[60]David L. Brown and Rita F. Redberg, "Last Nail in the Coffin for PCI in Stable Angina" (published online November 2), *Lancet* (2017), http://www.thelancet.com/journals/lancet/article/PIIS0140-6736(17)32757-5/fulltext.

[61]Gina Kolata, "'Unbelievable': Heart Stents Fail to Ease Chest Pain," *New York Times*, November 2, 2017, https://www.nytimes.com/2017/11/02/health/heart-disease-stents.html.

[62]Brown and Redberg, "Last Nail in the Coffin."

[63]Gina Kolata, "Why 'Useless' Surgery Is Still Popular," *New York Times*, August 3, 2016, https://www.nytimes.com/2016/08/04/upshot/the-right-to-know-that-an-operation-is-next-to-useless.html.

[64]See Shannon Brownlee, "Newtered: Gingrich's Congress Emasculated the One Agency Capable of Controlling Health Care Costs and Improving Quality," *Washington Monthly*, October 2007, 2015, http://www.washingtonmonthly.com/features/2007/0710.brownlee.html. On questionable spinal fusion surgeries, including surgeries performed by doctors who received payments from a device manufacturer, see John Carreyrou and Tom McGinty, "Top Spine Surgeons Reap Royalties, Medicare Bounty," *Wall Street Journal*, December 20, 2010, http://www.wsj.com/articles/SB10001424052748703395204576024023361023138.

[65]See, e.g., Jeff Overley "'Extreme' Dental Billing Abounds in Calif., OIG Says," *Law360*, May 18, 2015, http://www.law360.com/articles/657144/extreme-dental-billing-abounds-in-calif-oig-says; Lacie Glover, "Dental Billing Fraud Is More Common Than You Think," *FoxNews.com*, January 9, 2015, http://www.foxnews.com/health/2015/01/09/dental-billing-fraud-is-more-common-than-think/; "Report: Indiana Dentists Were Paid Too Much for Services," *Herald Bulletin*, November 6, 2014, http://www.heraldbulletin.com/news/local_news/report-indiana-dentists-were-paid-too-much-for-services/article_32de315d-9d71-58ec-b82c-425d7adeeb9c.html.

[66]Steven Reinberg, "Many Older Americans May Get Unneeded Breast, Prostate Cancer Screenings," *HealthDay News*, January 21, 2016, https://consumer.healthday.com/senior-citizen-information-31/senior-citizen-news-778/many-older-americans-may-get-unneeded-breast-prostate-cancer-screenings-707268.html.

[67]John Fauber, "Study: Two-Thirds of New Cancer Drugs Not Found to Extend Life," *Milwaukee-Wisconsin Journal Sentinel*, October 19, 2015,

http://www.jsonline.com/news/health/study-two-thirds-of-new-cancer-drugs-dont-extend-life-b99599343z1-334332891.html.

[68]Dong W. Chang and Martin F. Shapiro, "Association between Intensive Care Unit Utilization during Hospitalization and Costs, Use of Invasive Procedures, and Mortality," *JAMA Internal Medicine* 76, no. 10 (2016): 1492-99.

[69]Louis L. Nguyen, Ann D. Smith, Rebecca E. Scully, et al. "Provider-Induced Demand in the Treatment of Carotid Artery Stenosis: Variation in Treatment Decisions between Private Sector Fee-for-Service vs. Salary-Based Military Physicians," *JAMA Surgery* 152, no. 6 (2017): 565–72, https://jamanetwork.com/journals/jamasurgery/article-abstract/2606979.

[70]David Epstein, "When Evidence Says No, but Doctors Say Yes," *ProPublica*, February 22, 2017, https://www.propublica.org/article/when-evidence-says-no-but-doctors-say-yes.

[71]Interventional cardiologist Samin Sharma reportedly earned $4.8 million in 2012. Larry Husten, "What Ails Mt. Sinai Hospital Ails the Entire US Healthcare System," *Forbes.com*, March 6, 2014, http://www.forbes.com/sites/larryhusten/2014/03/06/what-ails-mt-sinai-hospital-ails-the-entire-us-healthcare-system/. See also Larry Husten, "Million Dollar Bonuses for Five Ohio State University Electrophysiologists," *Forbes.com*, April 16, 2012, http://www.forbes.com/sites/larryhusten/2012/04/16/million-dollar-bonuses-for-five-ohio-state-university-electrophysiologists.

[72]For a recent example of a settlement of a federal investigation alleging that a hospital paid unlawful kickbacks to a cardiology practice, see Ayla Ellison, "NY Hospital to Pay $18.8M to Settle Kickback Allegations," *Becker's Hospital Review*, May 15, 2015.

[73]Sanjaya Kumar and David B. Nash, *Demand Better! Revive Our Broken Healthcare System*, 1st edition (Bozeman, MT: Second River Healthcare Press, 2011).

## Chapter 5

[1]The Second City Network, "Completely Honest Ob/Gyn," YouTube video, 2:21. Posted by "The Second City," October 30, 2011, http://www.youtube.com/watch?v=xG6K5hbPJKs.

[2]Childbirth Connection, "Why Is the National U.S. Cesarean Section Rate So High?" National Partnership for Women and Families, August 2016, http://www.nationalpartnership.org/research-library/maternal-health/why-is-the-c-section-rate-so-high.pdf.

[3]See M. Joffe, J. Chapple, C. Paterson, and R. W. Beard, "What Is the Optimal Caesarean Section Rate? An Outcome Based Study of Existing Variation," *Journal of Epidemiology and Community Health* 48, no. 4 (1994): 406–11.

[4]Jeffrey Clemens and Joshua D. Gottlieb, "Do Physicians' Financial Incentives Affect Medical Treatment and Patient Health?," *American Economic Review* 104, no. 4 (2014): 1320–49.

[5]Center for Medical Consumers, "Cuts in Doctor-Payments Cut Unproven ADT Use," November 12, 2010, https://medconsumers.wordpress.com/2010/11/12/cuts-in-doctor-payments-cut-unproven-adt-use/.

[6]Vahakn B. Shahinian, Yong-Fao Kuo, Scott M. Gilbert, et al, "Reimbursement Policy and Androgen-Deprivation Therapy for Prostate Cancer," *New England Journal of Medicine* 363, no. 19 (2010): 1822–32, doi:10.1056/NEJMsa 0910784, http://www.nejm.org/doi/full/10.1056/NEJMsa0910784.

[7]Peter Waldman, "Prostate Patients Suffer as Money Overwhelms Best Therapy," *Bloomberg.com,* November 6, 2012, http://www.bloomberg.com/news/2012-11-06/prostate-patients-suffer-as-money-overwhelms-optimal-therapy.html.

[8]Ibid.

[9]John Carreyou and Maurice Tamman, "A Device to Kill Cancer, Lift Revenue," *Wall Street Journal,* December 7, 2010, http://www.wsj.com/articles/SB10001424052748703904804575631222900534954.

[10]Melody Petersen, "AstraZeneca Pleads Guilty in Cancer Medicine Scheme," *New York Times*, June 21, 2003, http://www.nytimes.com/2003/06/21/business/astrazeneca-pleads-guilty-in-cancer-medicine-scheme.html. See Chapter 3 for more details.

[11]Waldman, "Prostate Patients Suffer."

[12]Charles Bankhead, "New Ventures May Help Make Up for Lost Reimbursement," *Urology Times*, December 1, 2004, http://urologytimes.modern medicine.com/urology-times/news/clinical/practice-management/new-ventures-may-help-make-lost-reimbursement?id=&sk=&date=&pageID=2#sthash.3tYajwTk.dpuf.

[13]Ibid.

[14]Ibid.

[15]Ibid.

[16]Ibid.

[17]Jean M. Mitchell, "Urologists' Use of Intensity-Modulated Radiation Therapy for Prostate Cancer," *New England Journal of Medicine* 369, no. 17 (2013): 1629–37, http://www.nejm.org/doi/full/10.1056/NEJMsa1201141. See also Zosia Chustecka, "Financial Incentives Driving Prostate Cancer Testing and IMRT?," *Medscape*, April 18, 2012, http://www.medscape.com/viewarticle/761871.

[18]Gene Emery, "Costly Prostate Treatment Common When Docs Own the Machine," *Reuters,* October 23, 2013, http://www.reuters.com/article/2013/10/23/us-prostate-therapy-idUSBRE99M1C920131023.

[19]Waldman, "Prostate Patients Suffer."

[20]"Some Doctors Rake in Big Profits by Pushing Prostate Cancer Treatments," *Newsmax,* November 6, 2012, https://www.newsmax.com/Health/Health-News/ Some-Doctors-May-Put-Profit-Ahead-of-Prostate-Cancer-Patients-prostate- cancer-treatment-intensity-modulated-radiation-therapy-IMRT-and-prostate- cancer/2012/11/06/id/484403/. See also Jay Hancock, "After Urologists Get Machine, Cancer Treatments Soared," *Baltimore Sun,* January 17, 2012, http:// articles.baltimoresun.com/2012-01-17/health/bs-bz-hancock-chesapeake- urology-20120114_1_imrt-prostate-cancer-cancer-treatments.

[21]Waldman, "Prostate Patients Suffer."

[22]Ibid.

[23]Ibid.

[24]Ibid.

[25]Jean M. Mitchell, "Urologists' Self-Referral for Pathology of Biopsy Spec- imens Linked to Increased Use and Lower Prostate Cancer Detection," *Health Affairs* 31, no. 4, (2012): 741–49.

[26]Mark Hoithaus, "Pathology, IMRT Studies Heat Up Self-Referral Debate," *Urology Times* 40, no. 6 (2012): 1, http://urologytimes.modernmedicine.com/ urology-times/news/modernmedicine/modern-medicine-news/pathology- imrt-studies-heat-self-referral-deb?id=&sk=&date=&&pageID=1#sthash .Ptd8g35g.dpuf. See also "Urologists Denounce *New England Journal of Medicine* Article Regarding Prostate Cancer Treatment," *Imaging Technology News,* October 24, 2013, https://www.itnonline.com/content/urologists-denounce-new-england- journal-medicine-article-regarding-prostate-cancer-treatment.

[27]Hoithaus, "Pathology, IMRT Studies."

[28]Ibid. Dr. Kapoor laid out his methodological critique in a letter to the editors of *Health Affairs.* See Deepak A. Kapoor and David Penson, "Letter to the Editor in response to Jean Mitchell's study, Urologists' Self-Referral for Pathology of Biopsy Specimens Linked to Increased Use and Lower Prostate Cancer Detec- tion," *Health Affairs* 31, no. 4 (2012): 741–49, http://lugpa.org/evidence-not- finances-drives-urologists-care-a-critique-of-jean-mitchells-article/.

[29]Mireille Jacobson, Craig C. Earle, Mary Price, and Joseph P. Newhouse, "How Medicare's Payment Cuts for Cancer Chemotherapy Drugs Changed Patterns of Treatment," *Health Affairs* 29, no. 7 (2010): 1391–99, http://content .healthaffairs.org/content/29/7/1391.full.

[30]Reed Abelson, "Doctors Recouped Cuts in Medicare Pay, Study Finds," *New York Times,* June 16, 2010, http://www.nytimes.com/2010/06/ 17/health/17drug.html.

[31]Ibid.

[32]Virgil Dickson, "CMS Cancels Part B Demo, Industry and Advocates Rejoice," *Modern Healthcare,* December 16, 2016, http://www.modernhealthcare .com/article/20161217/magazine/312179879.

[33]Richard A. Hirth, Marc N. Turenne, John R. C. Wheeler, et al., "The Initial Impact of Medicare's New Prospective Payment System for Kidney Dialysis," *American Journal of Kidney Diseases* 62, no. 4 (2013): 662–69.

[34]Ibid.

[35]Andrew Pollak, "Lawsuit Says Drugs Were Wasted to Buoy Profit," *New York Times*, July 25, 2011, http://www.nytimes.com/2011/07/26/health/26dialysis.html.

[36]Ibid.

[37]Ibid.

[38]Ibid.

[39]Ibid.

[40]Kevin Sack, "Unintended Consequence for Dialysis Patients as Drug Rule Changes," *New York Times*, May 11, 2012, http://www.nytimes.com/2012/05/11/health/policy/dialysis-rule-changes-followed-by-transfusion-increases.html.

[41]Pollak, "Drugs Were Wasted to Buoy Profit."

[42]Hirth, et al., "The Initial Impact of Medicare's New Prospective Payment System."

[43]Ibid.

[44]Ibid.

[45]Pollak, "Drugs Were Wasted to Buoy Profit."

[46]Sack, "Unintended Consequence for Dialysis Patients."

[47]Ibid.

[48]Ibid.

[49]Scott Bronstein and Drew Griffin, "Dialysis Company Accused of Giant Medicare Fraud," *CNN.com*, November 30, 2012, http://www.cnn.com/2012/11/30/health/medicare-fraud-case/index.html.

[50]Jennifer Brown, "Denver-Based DaVita Sets Aside $300 Million to Settle Kickback Probes," *Denver Post*, May 9, 2013, http://www.denverpost.com/ci_23210434/denver-based-davita-sets-aside-300m-settle-kickback#ixzz2lauSuELW.

[51]U.S. Department of Justice, "DaVita to Pay $450 Million to Resolve Allegations That It Sought Reimbursement for Unnecessary Drug Wastage," news release, June 24, 2015, https://www.justice.gov/opa/pr/davita-pay-450-million-resolve-allegations-it-sought-reimbursement-unnecessary-drug-wastage.

## Chapter 6

[1]"See the Billboard Featuring a Mechanic with Integrity and Pass It On," *Values.com*, http://www.values.com/inspirational-sayings-billboards/26-Integrity.

[2]Cheryl Clark, "1 in 5 ICU Patients Get 'Futile' Care," *HealthLeaders Media,* September 10, 2013, http://healthleadersmedia.com/content.cfm?content_id=296097&page=1&topic=PHY##.

[3]Sarah Jane Reed and Steven Pearson, "Antibiotic Use for Acute Bronchitis, Choosing Wisely—Recommendation Analysis: Prioritizing Opportunities for Reducing Inappropriate Care," Institute for Clinical and Economic Review, 2016, https://icer-review.org/wp-content/uploads/2016/01/FINAL-Antibiotics-November-28.pdf; "High Rates of Unnecessary Prescribing of Antibiotics for Sore Throat and Bronchitis Observed across the United States," Brigham and Women's Hospital, October 3, 2013, http://www.brighamandwomens.org/about_bwh/publicaffairs/news/pressreleases/PressRelease.aspx?PageID=1566.

[4]Sarah Wickline Wallan, "CDC: Many Flu Patients Still Getting Antibiotics at Outpatient Clinics," *MedPage Today*, October 13, 2015, http://www.medpagetoday.com/MeetingCoverage/IDWeek/54070?xid=nl_mpt_DHE_20151014&eun=g452253d0r.

[5]Ibid. (quoting Michael Barnett and Jeffrey Linder, "Antibiotic Prescribing to Adults with Sore Throat in the United States, 1997–2010," *JAMA Internal Medicine* 174, no. 1 (January 1, 2014): 138–40.)

[6]Jessica Glenza, "Doctors in US Incorrectly Prescribe Antibiotics in Nearly a Third of Cases," *Guardian*, May 3, 2016, https://www.theguardian.com/society/2016/may/03/us-doctors-antibiotic-prescriptions study; American College of Physicians website, "Antibiotic Resistance," https://web.archive.org/web/20090305101402/http://www.acponline.org/patients_families/diseases_conditions/antibiotic_resistance/.

[7]Shannon Brownlee, "Why Doctors Uselessly Prescribe Antibiotics for a Common Cold," *Time*, April 16, 2012, http://ideas.time.com/2012/04/16/why-doctors-uselessly-prescribe-antibiotics-for-a-common-cold/#ixzz2iTWarHY2.

[8]Michael L. Barnett and Jeffrey A Linder, "Antibiotic Prescribing to Adults with Sore Throat in the United States, 1997–2010," *JAMA Internal Medicine* 174, no. 1 (2014): 138–40, https://jamanetwork.com/journals/jamainternalmedicine/fullarticle/1745694.

[9]Ibid.

[10]Joel J. Heidelbaugh, Margaret Riley, and Judith M. Habetler, "10 Billing & Coding Tips to Boost Your Reimbursement," *Journal of Family Practice*, November 2008, http://www.mdedge.com/jfponline/article/63368/practice-management/10-billing-coding-tips-boost-your-reimbursement.

[11]Laurence Baker, M. Kate Bundorf, and Anne Royalty, "Private Insurers' Payments for Routine Physician Office Visits Vary Substantially across the United States," *Health Affairs* 32, no. 9 (September 1, 2013): 1583–90, https://www.healthaffairs.org/doi/abs/10.1377/hlthaff.2013.0309.

[12]Heidelbaugh, Riley, and Habetler, "10 Billing & Coding Tips to Boost Your Reimbursement."

[13]Rita F. Redberg, "Squandering Medicare's Money," *New York Times*, May 25, 2011, http://www.nytimes.com/2011/05/26/opinion/26redberg.html.

[14]David H. Newman, "Believing in Treatments That Don't Work," *New York Times*, April 12, 2009, http://well.blogs.nytimes.com/2009/04/02/the-ideology-of-health-care/.

[15]See J. B. Thorlund, C. B. Juhl, E. M. Roos, and L. S. Lohmander, "Arthroscopic Surgery for Degenerative Knee: Systematic Review and Meta-Analysis of Benefits and Harms," *BMJ* 350 (2015): h2747, http://www.bmj.com/content/350/bmj.h2747. CMS and private insurers reduced coverage for knee surgeries shown to be ineffective. Thereafter, the rate of arthroscopic knee surgery for osteoarthritis declined. But an offsetting increase occurred in the frequency of the same surgery for other conditions, such as meniscal damage. The authors speculated that "physicians may have begun to perform more meniscectomies in patients with osteoarthritis to circumvent insurers' coverage restrictions." David Howard, Robert Brophy, and Stephen Howell, "Evidence of No Benefit from Knee Surgery for Osteoarthritis Led to Coverage Changes and Is Linked to Decline in Procedures," *Health Affairs* 31, no. 10 (2012): 2242–49, https://www.healthaffairs.org/doi/abs/10.1377/hlthaff.2012.0644.

[16]Newman, "Believing in Treatments That Don't Work."

[17]Ibid.

[18]Justin W. Timbie, D. Steven Fox, Kristin V. Busum, and Eric C. Schneider, "Five Reasons That Many Comparative Effectiveness Studies Fail to Change Patient Care and Clinical Practice," *Health Affairs* 31, no. 10 (October 2012): 2168–75, https://www.healthaffairs.org/doi/abs/10.1377/hlthaff.2012.0150.

[19]Gina Kolata, "Good or Useless, Medical Scans Cost the Same," *New York Times*, March 1, 2009, http://www.nytimes.com/2009/03/02/health/02scans.html.

[20]Ibid.

[21]Ibid.

[22]Richard J. Ablin and Ronald Piana, *The Great Prostate Hoax: How Big Medicine Hijacked the PSA Test and Caused a Public Health Disaster* (New York: St. Martin's Press, 2014).

[23]Ibid.

[24]Ibid.

[25]Kolata, "Good or Useless."

[26]Rob Stein, "Healthy Men Don't Need PSA Testing for Prostate Cancer, Panel Says," *Washington Post*, October 6, 2011, https://www.washingtonpost.com/national/health-science/healthy-men-dont-need-psa-testing-for-prostate-cancer-panel-says/2011/10/06/gIQAAxFMRL_story.html?utm_term=.78b94ef45849. See also Gerald L. Andriole, David Crawford, Robert L. Grubb III, et al.,

"Mortality Results from a Randomized Prostate-Cancer Screening Trial," *New England Journal of Medicine* 360, no. 13 (March 26, 2009): 1310–19, http://www.nejm.org/doi/full/10.1056/NEJMoa0810696.

[27]Tara Parker-Pope, "Mammogram's Role as Savior Is Tested," *New York Times*, October 24, 2011, http://well.blogs.nytimes.com/2011/10/24/mammograms-role-as-savior-is-tested/.

[28]Ibid.

[29]Nikola Biller-Andorno and Peter Jüni, "Abolishing Mammography Screening Programs? A View from the Swiss Medical Board," *New England Journal of Medicine* 370, no. 21 (May 22, 2014): 1965–67, http://www.nejm.org/doi/full/10.1056/NEJMp1401875.

[30]David J. Beard, Jonathan L. Rees, Jonathan A. Cook, et al., "Arthroscopic Subacromial Decompression for Subacromial Shoulder Pain (CSAW): A Multi-centre, Pragmatic, Parallel Group, Placebo-Controlled, Three-Group, Randomized Surgical Trial," *Lancet*, November 20, 2017, http://dx.doi.org/10.1016/S0140-6736(17)32457-1. See also Patti Neighmond, "Popular Surgery to Ease Chronic Shoulder Pain Called into Question," *NPR*, November 20, 2017, https://www.npr.org/sections/health-shots/2017/11/20/565406503/popular-surgery-to-ease-chronic-shoulder-pain-called-into-question?utm_campaign%E2%80%A6.

[31]Ablin and Piana, *The Great Prostate Hoax*.

[32]Vinay Prasad, Victor Gall, and Adam Cifu, "The Frequency of Medical Reversal," *JAMA Internal Medicine* 171, no. 18 (October 10, 2011): 1675–76, https://jamanetwork.com/journals/jamainternalmedicine/fullarticle/1105961.

[33]Vinay Prasad, Andrae Vandross, Caitlin Toomey, et al., "A Decade of Reversal: An Analysis of 146 Contradicted Medical Practices," *Mayo Clinic Proceedings* 88, no. 8 (August 2013): 790–98, http://www.mayoclinicproceedings.org/article/S0025-6196(13)00405-9/abstract.

[34]Cheryl Clark, "'Perverse Incentives' Perpetuate Use of Disproven Medical Treatments," *HealthLeaders Media*, August 6, 2013, http://healthleadersmedia.com/content.cfm?content_id=294909&page=1&topic=HEP.

[35]E. Haavi Morreim, "The Futility of Medical Necessity," *Regulation* 24, no. 2 (Summer 2001): 22–26.

[36]"One of the many anomalies of medical economics is that 'demand,' normally set by consumers, is in medicine largely determined by the producer, the physician, who decides whether hospitalization, prescriptions, tests, surgery, referrals, and further visits are needed." Paul Starr, "Medicine and the Waning of Professional Sovereignty," *Daedalus* 107, no. 1 (1978): 175–93.

[37]Mark A. Hall and Gerald F. Anderson, "Health Insurers' Assessment of Medical Necessity," *Pennsylvania Law Review* 140, no. 5 (May 1992): 1637–712, 1638.

[38]U.S. Bipartisan Commission on Comprehensive Health Care (The Pepper Commission), *A Call for Action: Final Report* (Washington: Government Printing Office, 1990), p. 41, https://catalog.hathitrust.org/Record/003025536.

[39]Sanjaya Kumar and David B. Nash, *Demand Better! Revive Our Broken Healthcare System*, 1st edition (Bozeman, MT: Second River Healthcare Press, 2011), reprinted in Sanjaya Kumar and David B. Nash, "Health Care Myth Busters: Is There a High Degree of Scientific Certainty in Modern Medicine?," *Scientific American*, March 25, 2011, http://www.scientificamerican.com/article/demand-better-health-care-book/.

[40]"What Conclusions Has Clinical Evidence Drawn about What Works, What Doesn't Based on Randomized Controlled Trial Evidence?," *BMJ Clinical Evidence*, http://clinicalevidence.bmj.com/x/set/static/cms/efficacy-categorisations.html.

[41]Michele G. Sullivan, "Urologists Back PSA Screening; Rail Against USPSTF's Position," *Family Practice News*, May 25, 2012, http://www.family-practicenews.com/index.php?id=2934&type=98&tx_ttnews[tt_news]=134177&cHash=da03e20e36; Steven Salzburg, "PSA Tests Might Hurt a Lot More Than You Think," *Forbes*, January 24, 2012, http://www.forbes.com/sites/stevensalzberg/2012/06/24/psa-tests-might-hurt-a-lot-more-than-you-think/. See also Sarah Kliff, "Many Doctors Think PSA Tests Don't Work. But They'll Keep Doing Them Anyway," *Washington Post*, May 29, 2012, http://www.washingtonpost.com/blogs/ezra-klein/post/many-doctors-think-psa-tests-dont-work-but-theyll-keep-doing-them-anyway/2012/05/29/gJQAOl0qyU_blog.html.

[42]Maggie Mahar, "The Doctor Who Invented PSA Test Calls It 'A Profit-Driven Public Health Disaster'…Why This Is Good News," *Health Beat,* March 11, 2010, http://www.healthbeatblog.com/2010/03/the-doctor-who-invented-psa-test-calls-it-a-profitdriven-public-health-disaster-why-this-is-good-new/.

[43]W. Douglas Weaver, Timothy J. Gardner, and Joseph D. Babb, "The Role of Appropriate Use Criteria for Coronary Revascularization," *Journal of the American College of Cardiology* 53, no. 6 (2009): 554–55, http://dx.doi.org/10.1016/j.jacc.2009.01.001.

[44]Manesh R. Patel, Gregory J. Dehmer, John W. Hirshfeld, Peter K. Smith, and John A. Spertus, "ACCF/SCAI/STS/AATS/AHA/ASNC 2009 Appropriateness Criteria for Coronary Revascularization," *Journal of the American College of Cardiology* 53, no. 6 (2009): 530–53, https://ac.els-cdn.com/S0735109708033457/1-s2.0-S0735109708033457-main.pdf?_tid3D2ccfa0f4-fc65-11e7-93cf-00000aab0f27&acdnat3D1516289893_27eca5fdfc-44273283dedaa933b6f6ac; Weaver, Gardner, and Babb, "The Role of Appropriate Use Criteria."

[45]Pranav Puri, Bobette Patterson, and Jennifer Carroll, "The Economic Impact of Implementation of Appropriate Use Criteria on Volume of PCI Cases and Medical Cost Savings at a Large Community Hospital: 2 Year Trends," *Journal of the American College of Cardiology* 65, no. 10, Supplement, 17 (2015): A1582, http://dx.doi.org/10.1016/S0735-1097(15)61582-0.

[46]Paul S. Chan, Manesh R. Patel, Lloyd W. Klein, et al., "Appropriateness of Percutaneous Coronary Intervention," *JAMA* 306, no. 1 (2011): 53–61, http://jamanetwork.com/journals/jama/fullarticle/1104058.

[47]Robert C. Hendel, Manesh R. Patel, Joseph M. Allen, et al., "Appropriate Use of Cardiovascular Technology: 2013 ACCF Appropriate Use Criteria Methodology Update: A Report of the American College of Cardiology Foundation Appropriate Use Criteria Task Force," *Journal of the American College of Cardiology* 61, no. 12, (2013):1305–17, http://dx.doi.org/10.1016/j.jacc.2013.01.025.

[48]Peter Waldman, "Doctors Use Euphemism for $2.4 Billion in Needless Stents," *Bloomberg*, October 29, 2013, http://www.bloomberg.com/news/articles/2013-10-30/doctors-use-euphemism-for-2-4-billion-in-needless-stents.

[49]Chan et al., "Appropriateness of Percutaneous Coronary Intervention."

[50]Opinion and Order, Amarin Pharma et al. v. U.S. FDA et al., 15 Civ. 3588 (PAE) (SDNY August 7, 2015).

[51]Marc A. Rodwin, "Rooting Out Institutional Corruption to Manage Inappropriate Off-Label Drug Use," *Journal of Law, Medicine & Ethics* 41, no. 3 (2012): 654, 656 (citing David C. Radley, Stan N. Finkelstein, and Randall S. Stafford, "Off-Label Prescribing among Office-Based Physicians," *Archives of Internal Medicine* 166, no. 9 (2006): 1021–26). See also Tewodros Eguale, David L. Buckeridge, Nancy E. Winslade, et al., "Drug, Patient, and Physician Characteristics Associated with Off-Label Prescribing in Primary Care," *Archives of Internal Medicine* 172, no. 10 (2012): 781–88.

[52]Marc A. Rodwin, "Rooting Out Institutional Corruption to Manage Inappropriate Off-Label Drug Use," *Journal of Law, Medicine & Ethics* 41, no. 3 (2012): 654–64.

[53]Larry Husten, "No Benefit for a Commonly Used Cardiac Device," *Forbes*, April 29, 2015, http://www.forbes.com/sites/larryhusten/2015/04/29/no-benefit-for-a-commonly-used-cardiac-device/. The study referred to is Patrick Mismetti, Silvy Laporte, Olivier Pellerin, et al., "Effect of a Retrievable Inferior Vena Cava Filter Plus Anticoagulation vs. Anticoagulation Alone on Risk of Recurrent Pulmonary Embolism: A Randomized Clinical Trial," *JAMA* 313, no. 16 (2015): 1627–35, https://jamanetwork.com/journals/jama/fullarticle/2279714.

[54]R. H. White, E. Geraghty, A. Brunson, et al., "High Variation between Hospitals in Vena Cava Filter Use for Venous Thromboembolism," *JAMA Internal Medicine* 173, no. 7 (2013): 506–12, https://jamanetwork.com/journals/jamainternalmedicine/fullarticle/1669098.

[55]Vinay Prasad, Jason Rho, and Adam Cifu, "The Inferior Vena Cava Filter: How Could a Medical Device Be So Well Accepted without Any Evidence of Efficacy?," *JAMA Internal Medicine* 173, no. 7 (2013): 493–95, https://jamanetwork.com/journals/jamainternalmedicine/article-abstract/1669099. See also V. Prasad, J. Rho, and A. Cifu, "Further Thoughts on Why There Are Good Data Supporting the Inferior Vena Cava Filter," *JAMA Internal Medicine* 174, no. 1 (2014): 164–65, doi:10.1001/jamainternmed.2013.13176.

[56]Mitchell H. Katz, "Inferior Vena Cava Filters: The Harms Are Clear, the Benefits Less So: Comment on 'The Inferior Vena Cava Filter,'" *JAMA Internal Medicine* 173, no. 7 (2013): 495, https://jamanetwork.com/journals/jamainternalmedicine/fullarticle/1669106.

[57]American Medical Association, "2013 Reimbursement for IVC Filter Placement, Repositioning and Retrieval," 2012, Bio2Medical, http://www.bio2medical.com/wp-content/uploads/2013/07/Codes-for-Website-Chart1.pdf.

[58]Peter Waldman, "Doctors Use Euphemism for $2.4 Billion in Needless Stents," *Bloomberg*, October 30, 2013, https://www.bloomberg.com/news/articles/2013-10-30/doctors-use-euphemism-for-2-4-billion-in-needless-stents.

[59]Robert Preidt, "Older Men Gain Little from PSA Test: Study," *Consumer Health-Day*, October 4, 2013, http://consumer.healthday.com/cancer-information-5/mis-cancer-news-102/older-men-gain-little-from-psa-test-study-680775.html; Charles Bankhead, "Prostate Biopsy Triggers Tx in Older Men," *MedPage Today*, April 15, 2013, http://www.medpagetoday.com/HematologyOncology/ProstateCancer/38464.

[60]Shannon Brownlee, "Newtered: Gingrich's Congress Emasculated the One Agency Capable of Controlling Health Care Costs and Improving Quality," *Washington Monthly*, October 2007, http://www.washingtonmonthly.com/features/2007/0710.brownlee.html.

[61]Sanjaya Kumar and David B. Nash, *Demand Better! Revive Our Broken Healthcare System*, 1st ed. (Bozeman, MT: Second River Healthcare Press, 2011), reprinted in Sanjaya Kumar and David B. Nash, "Health Care Myth Busters: Is There a High Degree of Scientific Certainty in Modern Medicine?," *Scientific American,* March 25, 2011, http://www.scientificamerican.com/article/demand-better-health-care-book/.

[62]Ibid.

[63]Ibid.

[64]See Gina Kolata, "Mammogram Debate Took Group by Surprise," *New York Times,* November 20, 2009, http://www.nytimes.com/2009/11/20/health/20prevent.html?_r=0.

[65]Lisa Szabo, "Mammogram Coverage Won't Change, Companies Say," *USAToday,* November 19, 2009, http://usatoday30.usatoday.com/news/health/2009-11-19-1Amammogram19_ST_N.htm.

[66]Tiffany O'Callaghan, "Mammogram Recommendations Spark Controversy, Confusion," *TIME.com,* November 17, 2009, http://healthland.time.com/2009/11/17/new-mammogram-recommendations-spark-controversy-and-confusion/#ixzz2ijlVZFwX.

[67]Ibid.

[68]Stephanie Condon, "GOP Rep. on Mammograms: 'This Is How Rationing Begins,'" *CBSNews.com,* November 18, 2009, http://www.cbsnews.com/8301-503544_162-5699555-503544.html.

[69]Ibid.

[70]Ibid.

[71]Ibid. Democratic Congresswoman Rosa DeLauro defended the Task Force. "If we can cut through the Republicans' political gamesmanship on this issue, the new breast cancer recommendations, as always, were an attempt to put the best possible evidence in the hands of women and their doctors, so they can assess their own risk and benefit."

[72]Randolph E. Schmid, "Mammograms Still Vital in Saving Lives, Health and Human Services Secretary Kathleen Sebelius Says," *Nola.com,* November 18, 2009, http://www.nola.com/health/index.ssf/2009/11/mammograms_still_vital_in_savi.html.

[73]U.S. Department of Health and Human Services, "Statement from Secretary Kathleen Sebelius Regarding Breast Cancer Awareness Month," October 5, 2010, http://www.hhs.gov/news/press/2010pres/10/20101005a.html.

[74]Merrill Goozner, "So Much for Comparative Effectiveness," *The Health Care Blog,* November 20, 2009, http://thehealthcareblog.com/blog/2009/11/20/so-much-for-comparative-effectiveness/.

[75]U.S. Preventive Services Task Force, "Grade Definitions After May 2007," http://www.uspreventiveservicestaskforce.org/Page/Name/grade-definitions#grade-definitions-after-may-2007.

[76]The official assessment can be found at U.S. Preventive Services Task Force, "Grade Definitions after May 2007."

[77]Maggie Mertens, "Senate Passes Mikulski's Overhaul Amendment on Women's Health," *NPR News,* December 3, 2009, http://www.npr.org/sections/health-shots/2009/12/senate_passes_womens_health_am.html.

[78]Nicholas Bagley, "Who Says PCORI Can't Do Cost Effectiveness?," *The Incidental Economist* (blog), October 14, 2013, http://theincidentaleconomist .com/wordpress/who-says-pcori-cant-do-cost-effectiveness/.

[79]Katharine Cooper Wulff, Franklin G. Miller, and Steven D. Pearson, "Can Coverage Be Rescinded When Negative Trial Results Threaten a Popular Procedure? The Ongoing Saga of Vertebroplasty," *Health Affairs* 30, no. 12 (2011): 2269–76.


CHAPTER 7

[1]Frances Robles and Eric Lipton, "Political Ties of Top Billers for Medicare," *New York Times*, April 9, 2014, http://www.nytimes.com/2014/04/10/business/ doctor-with-big-medicare-billings-is-no-stranger-to-scrutiny.html.

[2]Ibid.

[3]Phil Kerpen, "Menendez Has Set a New Low for Blatant Corruption in the U.S.," *N.Y. Post*, September 30, 2017, http://nypost.com/2017/09/30/menendez-has-set-a-new-low-for-blatant-corruption-in-the-us/.

[4]Carol D. Leonnig and Jerry Markon, "Sen. Menendez Contacted Top Officials in Friend's Medicare Dispute," *Washington Post*, February 6, 2013, http://www.wash-ingtonpost.com/politics/sen-menendez-contacted-top-officials-in-friends-medi-care-dispute/2013/02/06/e01bf928-6fd4-11e2-aa58-243de81040ba_story.html.

[5]Ibid.

[6]Ibid; Jonathan Tamari, "Justice Filing Confirms Justice Dept. Investigation," *Philly.com*, January 31, 2014, http://www.philly.com/philly/news/politics/ Menendez-filing-confirms-Justice-Dept-investigation.html.

[7]Julia Edwards, "Senator Menendez of New Jersey Indicted on Corruption Charges," *Washington Post*, April 1, 2015; Herb Jackson, "Menendez Says He's 'Angry and Ready to Fight' after Being Indicted on Corruption Charges," *Record*, April 1, 2015; Herb Jackson, "Salomon Melgen, Sen. Menendez's Friend, Indicted in Medicare Fraud Scheme," *Record*, April 14, 2015.

[8]Carl Hiaasen, "It Wasn't Corruption—It Was a Bro-Mance," *Miami Herald*, April 18, 2015, http://www.miamiherald.com/opinion/opn-columns-blogs/ carl-hiaasen/article18797418.html#storylink=cpy.

[9]Curt Anderson, "Florida Eye Doctor Salomon Melgen Found Guilty of Medicare Fraud," *Time.com*, April 28, 2017, http://time.com/4760046/ salomonmelgeneyedoctormedicarefraudguilty/.

[10]Adam Berger, "Retina Surgeon's AMD Regimen at Center of Medicare Fraud Case," *Ophthalmology Times*, May 27, 2017, http://modernretina.modernmedicine .com/modern-retina/news/retina-surgeon-s-amd-regimen-center-medicare-fraud-case.

[11]Nicholas Pugliese, "Mistrial Declared in Bob Menendez Trial after Jury Deadlocks," *USA Today*, November 16, 2017, https://www.usatoday.com/story/news/politics/2017/11/16/jury-bob-menendez-trial-says-its-deadlocked/870635001/.

[12]Brian Klepper, "Congress Has a Little Drug Problem," *Health Care Blog*, March 16, 2016, http://thehealthcareblog.com/blog/2016/03/16/congress-has-a-drug-problem/.

[13]Peter Schweizer, "Politicians' Extortion Racket," *New York Times*, October 21, 2013, http://nyti.ms/15YFkwi; Thomas J. DiLorenzo, "Regulatory Extortion," *Independent Institute*, March 1, 2000, http://www.independent.org/publications/article.asp?id=184.

[14]Laura Meckler, "Obama's Health Expert Gets Political," *Wall Street Journal*, July 24, 2009, http://www.wsj.com/articles/SB124839406488477649.

[15]Peter Baker, "Obama Was Pushed by Drug Industry, E-mails Suggest," *New York Times*, June 8, 2012, http://www.nytimes.com/2012/06/09/us/politics/e-mails-reveal-extent-of-obamas-deal-with-industry-on-health-care.html?pagewanted=all&_r=1. See also David D. Kirkpatrick, "White House Affirms Deal on Drug Costs," *New York Times*, August 5, 2009, at http://www.nytimes.com/2009/08/06/health/policy/06insure.html; Tom Hamburger, "Obama Gives Powerful Drug Lobby a Seat at the Table," *Los Angeles Times*, August 4, 2009, http://www.latimes.com/health/la na healthcare-pharma4-2009aug04-story.html; Paul Blumenthal, "The Legacy of Billy Tauzin: The White House-PhRMA Deal," *Sunlight Foundation*, February 12, 2010, https://sunlightfoundation.com/blog/2010/02/12/the-legacy-of-billy-tauzin-the-white-house-phrma-deal/.

[16]Michael F. Cannon, "A Closer Look at Those Industry Deals," *Kaiser Health News*, July 16, 2009, https://khn.org/news/071609cannon/.

[17]Chris Frates, "Payoffs for States Get Reid to 60," *Politico*, December 19, 2009, http://www.politico.com/story/2009/12/payoffs-for-states-get-reid-to-60-030815.

[18]Shelley Wood, "Stents, ICDs, Inappropriate? Then, under New Audit Program, CMS Won't Pay," *Medscape*, December 3, 2011, http://www.medscape.com/viewarticle/791095. See also Sana M. Al-Khatib, Anne Hellkamp, Jeptha Curtis, et al., "Non–Evidence-Based ICD Implantations in the United States," *JAMA* 305, no. 1 (2011): 43–49, https://jamanetwork.com/journals/jama/fullarticle/644551; Brenda Goodman, "Study: Implanted Cardiac Defibrillators Overused," *WebMD Health News*, January 4, 2011, http://www.webmd.com/heart-disease/news/20110104/study-overuse-of-implanted-cardiac-defibrillators.

[19]Denise Grady, "Many Defibrillators Implanted Unnecessarily, Study Says," *New York Times*, January 4, 2011, http://www.nytimes.com/2011/01/05/health/05device.html?_r=0.

[20]Larry Husten, "CMS Tightening the Screws on Unnecessary Procedures in Florida and 10 Other States," *Forbes,* December 4, 2011, http://www.forbes.com/sites/larryhusten/2011/12/04/cms-tightening-the-screws-on-unnecessary-procedures-in-florida-and-10-other-states/.

[21]Ibid.; Walter Eisner, "Wall Street's 'Friday Mediscare,'" *Orthopedics This Week,* December 12, 2011, http://ryortho.com/2011/12/wall-streetrsquos-ldquofriday-mediscarerdquo/.

[22]Joe Carlson, "Scaling Back Scrutiny: Fla. Hospitals Welcome Prepayment Review Shift," *Modern Healthcare,* January 21, 2012, http://www.modernhealthcare.com/article/20120121/MAGAZINE/301219960.

[23]Rosemary Gibson and Janardan Prasad Singh, *Medicare Meltdown: How Wall Street and Washington Are Ruining Medicare and How to Fix It* (Lanham, MD: Rowman & Littlefield, 2013), p. 57.

[24]For more information about the SGR, see Medicare Payment Advisory Commission "Medicare Sustainable Growth Rate System Fact Sheet," March 2012, http://www.medpac.gov/documents/fact-sheets/mar12_sgrfactsheet.pdf?sfvrsn=0. For information on a proposed alternative to the SGR, see Letter from Douglas W. Elmendorf, Director of Congressional Budget Office, to Michael B. Enzi, Ranking Member, Committee on Health, Education, Labor, and Pensions, U.S. Senate, June 21, 2010, https://www.cbo.gov/sites/default/files/111th-congress-2009-2010/reports/06-21-high-risk_insurance_pools.pdf.

[25]William B. Millard, "SGR Out, MACRA In," *Annals of Emergency Medicine* 67, no. 2 (2016): A15–A22, https://www.emra.org/uploadedFiles/EMRA/Events/LAC17_Journal-Club_Annals-%20MACRA.pdf.

[26]Richard Himmelfarb, *Catastrophic Politics: The Rise and Fall of the Medicare Catastrophic Coverage Act of 1988* (University Park: Pennsylvania State University Press, 1995).

[27]Thomas Waldron, "Trial Shines Light on 'Bell-Ringing' Concept," *Baltimore Sun,* July 2, 2000, http://articles.baltimoresun.com/2000-07-02/news/0007020077_1_lobbyist-fulton-bill.

[28]Paul Keckley, Saul B. Helman, Chuck Peck, and Kevin Cornish, "Medical Necessity and Unnecessary Care—The Full Story," *Pulse Weekly (Navigant Healthcare),* January 26, 2015, http://www.naviganthrp.com/medical-necessity-unnecessary-care-full-story/.

[29]Donald M. Berwick and Andrew D. Hackbarth, "Eliminating Waste in US Health Care," *JAMA* 307, no. 14, (2012): 1513–16, doi:10.1001/jama.2012.362. See also Debra Sherman, "Stemming the Tide of Overtreatment in U.S. Healthcare," *Reuters,* February 16, 2012, http://www.reuters.com/article/2012/02/16/us-overtreatment-idUSTRE81F0UF20120216.

[30]Institute of Medicine, Mark Smith, Robert Saunders, Leigh Stuckhardt, and J. Michael McGinnis, eds., *Best Care at Lower Cost: The Path to Continuously Learning Health Care in America* (Washington: The National Academies Press, 2012), p. 14, https://www.ncbi.nlm.nih.gov/books/NBK207212/.

[31]Robin Hanson, "Cut Medicine in Half," *Cato Unbound*, September 10, 2007, https://www.cato-unbound.org/2007/09/10/robin-hanson/cut-medicine-half.

[32]Ibid.

[33]"Doctors Speak Out about Unnecessary Care as Cost Put at $800 Billion a Year," *Science Daily*, October 3, 2012, http://www.sciencedaily.com/releases/2012/10/121003083033.htm.

[34]"Early Trends among Seven Recommendations from the Choosing Wisely Campaign," *JAMA Internal Medicine* 175, no. 12 (2015): 1913–20, https://jamanetwork.com/journals/jamainternalmedicine/fullarticle/2457401; Scott Harris, "Disappointing Results Seen Thus Far for Choosing Wisely," *MedPage Today*, October 14, 2015, http://www.medpagetoday.com/PublicHealthPolicy/GeneralProfessionalIssues/54096?xid=nl_mpt_DHE_20151015&.

[35]Shannon Brownlee, "Taking Action to Reduce Overuse," *IHI Improvement Blog*, September 17, 2015, http://www.ihi.org/communities/blogs/_layouts/15/ihi/community/blog/itemview.aspx?List=7d1126ec-8f63-4a3b-9926-c44ea3036813&ID=163.

## CHAPTER 8

[1]Lance Williams, Stephen K. Doig, and Christina Jewett, "Heart Failure Cases Surge among Prime Hospital's Medicare Patients," *California Watch*, November 27, 2011, http://californiawatch.org/health-and-welfare/heart-failure-cases-surge-among-prime-hospital-s-medicare-patients-13703.

[2]Lance Williams, "IE Hospital Investigated for Medicare Fraud," *ABCNews*, November 28, 2011, http://abclocal.go.com/kabc/story?section=news/local/inland_empire&id=8446927.

[3]Williams, Doig, and Jewett, "Heart Failure Cases Surge."

[4]Ibid.

[5]William Heisel, "Kwashiorkor Research Shows Prime Healthcare's Cases Must Be Off Base," *USC Annenberg Center for Health Journalism*, January 23, 2012, http://www.reportingonhealth.org/blogs/2012/01/23/kwashiorkor-research-shows-prime-healthcares-cases-must-be-base.

[6]William Heisel, "Kwashiorkor in Surf City: 5 Tips from California Watch's Medicare Billing Investigation," *USC Annenberg Center for Health Journalism*, March 9, 2011, http://www.reportingonhealth.org/blogs/kwashiorkor-surf-city-5-tips-california-watchs-medicare-billing-investigation.

[7]Lance Williams and Stephen K. Doig, "Prime Hospital Abruptly Stops Billing Medicare for Rare Ailment," *The Center for Investigative Reporting, California Watch*, December 20, 2012, http://californiawatch.org/dailyreport/prime-hospital-abruptly-stops-billing-medicare-rare-ailment-18751.

[8]Lance Williams, Stephen K. Doig, and Christina Jewett, "Hospital's Heart Diagnoses Surge after Pay Changed," *California Watch, SFGate*, November 28, 2011, http://www.sfgate.com/news/article/Hospital-s-heart-diagnoses-surge-after-pay-changed-2296567.php.

[9]Joe Carlson, "$700M in Kwashiorkor Charges Trigger OIG Audit: HHS Finds 217 Cases of Kwashiorkor at Two Hospitals Weren't Legitimate," *Modern Healthcare*, February 12, 2014, http://www.modernhealthcare.com/article/20140212/NEWS/302129957.

[10]The reports are available at The Center for Public Integrity, "Cracking the Codes," https://www.publicintegrity.org/health/medicare/cracking-codes.

[11]Joe Eaton and David Donald, "Hospitals Grab at Least $1 Billion in Extra Fees for Emergency Room Visits," *Center for Public Integrity*, September 20, 2012, https://www.publicintegrity.org/2012/09/20/10811/hospitals-grab-least-1-billion-extra-fees-emergency-room-visits.

[12]Ibid.

[13]Ibid.

[14]Ibid.

[15]Ibid.

[16]Peter K. Lindenauer, Tara Lagu, Meng-Shiou Shieh, Penelope S. Pekow, and Michael B. Rothberg, "Association of Diagnostic Coding with Trends in Hospitalizations and Mortality of Patients with Pneumonia, 2003–2009," *JAMA* 307, no. 12, (2012): 1405–13.

[17]Mary Brophy Marcus, "Reported Decline in U.S. Pneumonia Deaths May Be False: Study," *HealthDay*, April 3, 2012, http://consumer.healthday.com/senior-citizen-information-31/misc-death-and-dying-news-172/reported-decline-in-u-s-pneumonia-deaths-may-be-false-study-663421.html.

[18]John Goodman, "What Health Policy Analysts Can Learn from Development Economics," *Health Affairs Blog*, October 13, 2015, http://healthaffairs.org/blog/2015/10/13/what-health-policy-analysts-can-learn-from-development-economics/; David Himmelstein and Steffie Woolhandler, "Quality Improvement: 'Become Good at Cheating and You Never Need to Become Good at Anything Else,'" *Health Affairs Blog*, August 27, 2015, http://healthaffairs.org/blog/2015/08/27/quality-improvement-become-good-at-cheating-and-you-never-need-to-become-good-at-anything-else/; Joe Carlson, "Faulty Gauge? Readmissions Are Down, but Observational-Status Patients Are Up—and That Could Skew Medicare Numbers," *Modern Healthcare*, June 8, 2013, http://www.modernhealthcare.com/article/20130608/MAGAZINE/306089991.

[19]Ankur Gupta, Larry A. Allen, Deepak L. Bhatt, et al., "Association of the Hospital Readmissions Reduction Program Implementation with Readmission and Mortality Outcomes in Heart Failure," *JAMA Cardiology,* November 12, 2017, https://jamanetwork.com/journals/jamacardiology/article-abstract/2663213. For criticisms of the study, see Casey Ross, "The Data Are In, But Debate Rages: Are Hospital Readmission Penalties a Good Idea?," *STAT*, December 11, 2017, https://www.statnews.com/2017/12/11/hospital-readmissions-debate/.

[20]John Commins, "Lower Readmissions Linked to Higher Risk of Death," *HealthLeaders Media*, November 13, 2017, http://www.healthleadersmedia.com/quality/lower-readmissions-linked-higher-risk-death?spMailingID=12384704&spUserID=MTY3ODg4NjI3Mjk1S0&s%E2%80%A6#.

[21]Ge Bai and Gerard F. Anderson, "Extreme Markup: The Fifty US Hospitals with the Highest Charge-to-Cost Ratios," *Health Affairs* 34, no. 6 (2015): 922–28, https://www.healthaffairs.org/doi/abs/10.1377/hlthaff.2014.1414. See also Lena H. Sun, "50 Hospitals Charge Uninsured More than 10 Times Cost of Care, Study Finds," *Washington Post,* June 8, 2015.

[22]Michael Batty and Benedic Ippolito, "Mystery of the Chargemaster: Examining the Role of Hospital List Prices in What Patients Actually Pay," *Health Affairs* 36, no. 4 (April 2017): 689–96, https://www.healthaffairs.org/doi/abs/10.1377/hlthaff.2016.0986. See also John Gregory, "Hospital Chargemaster Rates Linked to Higher Payments, but Not Higher Quality Care," *Health Exec*, April 4, 2017, http://healthexec.com/topics/finance/hospital-chargemaster-rates-linked-higher-payments-not-higher-quality-care; Glenn A. Melnick and Katya Fonkych, "Hospital Pricing and the Uninsured: Do the Uninsured Pay Higher Prices?," *Health Affairs*, March 2008, http://content.healthaffairs.org/content/27/2/w116.full.pdf. Physicians also use chargemaster pricing. There, the uninsured pay such inflated prices, they appear to be more profitable than insured patients, even after accounting for the uninsured who do not pay. See Jonathan Gruber and David Rodriguez, "How Much Uncompensated Care Do Doctors Provide?," *Journal of Health Economics,* September 2007, https://economics.mit.edu/files/6423. ("Our best estimate is that physicians provide *negative* uncompensated care to the uninsured, earning more on uninsured patients than on insured patients with comparable treatments.")

[23]Rhonda L. Rundle and Anna Wilde Matthews, "Tenet Reaped Outsize Gains from Flaw in Medicare System," *Wall Street Journal*, November 11, 2002, http://www.wsj.com/articles/SB1036780906876999788.

[24]U.S. Department of Justice, "Tenet Healthcare Corporation to Pay U.S. More than $900 Million to Resolve False Claims Act Allegations," June 29, 2006, http://www.justice.gov/archive/opa/pr/2006/June/06_civ_406.html; U.S. Securities and Exchange Commission, "SEC Charges Tenet Healthcare Corporation and Four Former Senior Executives with Concealing Scheme to Meet

Earnings Targets by Exploiting Medicare System," April 2, 2007, https://www .sec.gov/news/press/2007/2007-60.htm.

[25]Fred Mogul, "Feds Dock Beth Israel Medical Center $13M for 'Turbocharging' Medicare," *WNYC*, March 1, 2012, http://www.wnyc.org/story/ 190040-feds-dock-beth-israel-13m-turbocharging-medicare/.

[26]Keith Goldberg, "NYC Hospital Pays $13M for Medicare Turbocharging," *Law360*, March 1, 2012, https://www.law360.com/articles/314845/nyc-hospital-pays-13m-for-medicare-turbocharging.

[27]Nina Bernstein, "Beth Israel to Pay $13 Million for Inflating Medicare Fees," *New York Times*, March 1, 2012, http://www.nytimes.com/2012/03/02/ nyregion/beth-israel-admits-inflating-fees-for-medicare-patients.html.

[28]Office of the U.S. Attorney General, Southern District of New York, "Manhattan U.S. Attorney Recovers $11.75 Million in Medicare False Claims Act Lawsuit Against Lenox Hill Hospital," May 4, 2012, http://www.justice.gov/ archive/usao/nys/pressreleases/May12/lenoxhillsettlement.html.

[29]Christopher Weaver, Anna Wilde Mathews, and Tom McGinty, "Medicare Overpays as Hospital Prices Rise: Soaring Bills for Sickest Patients Can Throw Payment Formula out of Whack," *Wall Street Journal*, April 15, 2015, http://www .wsj.com/articles/medicare-overpays-as-hospital-prices-rise-1429151451.

[30]Ibid.

[31]See Chapter 8 for a longer discussion of federal support for EHRs. See also Brian Schilling, "The Federal Government Has Put Billions into Promoting Electronic Health Record Use: How Is It Going?," The Commonwealth Fund, *Quality Matters*, June/July 2011.

[32]Christopher Cheney, "MU Fraud on the Rise, OIG Warns," *HealthLeaders Media*, February 14, 2014; Brooks Egerton and Miles Moffeit, "Texas Hospitals Got $18 Million from Federal Agency Despite Safety Issues," *Dallas Morning News*, August 2013, http://www.dallasnews.com/investigations/patient-safety/ headlines/20130824-texas-hospitals-got-18-million-from-federal-agency-de-spite-safety-issues.ece?nclick_check=1; Miles Moffeit, "Former Texas Hospital Chain Owner Found Guilty of Medicare Fraud," *Dallas Morning News*, July 24, 2014, http://www.dallasnews.com/news/metro/20140724-former-texas-hospi-tal-chain-owner-found-guilty-of-medicare-fraud.ece.

[33]Reed Abelson, Julie Creswell, and Griff Palmer, "Medicare Bills Rise as Records Turn Electronic," *New York Times*, September 21, 2012, http:// www.nytimes.com/2012/09/22/business/medicare-billing-rises-at-hospitals-with-electronic-records.html?_r=0.

[34]Ibid.

[35]Ibid.

[36]Ibid.

[37]Cristopher S. Brunt, "CPT Fee Differentials and Visit Upcoding under Medicare Part B," *Health Economics* 20, no. 7 (2011): 831–41, http://onlinelibrary .wiley.com/doi/10.1002/hec.1649/abstract.

[38]Abelson, Creswell, and Palmer, "Medicare Bills Rise as Records Turn Electronic."

[39]"Letter from Obama Administration on Healthcare Billing," *New York Times*, September 24, 2012, http://www.nytimes.com/interactive/2012/09/ 25/business/25medicare-doc.html.

[40]AllAboutFrogs.org, "The Scorpion and the Frog," http://allaboutfrogs.org/ stories/scorpion.html.

[41]Matthew Wynia, D. S. Cummins, J. B. VanGeest, and I. B. Wilson, "Physician Manipulation of Reimbursement Rules for Patients—Between a Rock and a Hard Place," *JAMA* 2000, 283(14):1858–65. https://jamanetwork.com/journals/ jama/fullarticle/192577.

[42]Robert Lowes, "Managed Care: Can Lying Be Good Medicine?," *Medical Economics*, October 11, 2002, http://medicaleconomics.modernmedicine. com/medical-economics/news/clinical/obstetrics-gynecology-womens-health/ managed-care-can-lying-be-good-m?page=full.

[43]Cristopher S. Brunt, "CPT Fee Differentials and Visit Upcoding under Medicare Part B," *Health Economics* 20, no. 7 (2011): 831–41, http://onlinelibrary .wiley.com/doi/10.1002/hec.1649/abstract.

[44]Ibid.

[45]Anemona Hartocollis, "Out of Prison, Doctor Hopes to Regenerate His Lost Fame," *New York Times*, May 14, 2006, http://www.nytimes.com/2006/05/14/ nyregion/14doctor.html?pagewanted=all&_r=0.

[46]Ibid.

[47]Eric Konigsberg, "The OB-GYN Who Loves Women," *New York Magazine*, http://nymag.com/nymetro/health/features/3422/.

[48]Ibid.

[49]Jennifer Steinhauer and Sherri Day, "Doctor Convicted of Insurance Fraud in Fertility Procedures," *New York Times*, January 10, 2001, at http://www.nytimes .com/2001/01/10/nyregion/doctor-convicted-of-insurance-fraud-in-fertility- procedures.html.

[50]Christina Bramlet, "IRC Study: Public Less Accepting of Insurance Fraud," April 1, 2013, *PROPERTYCASUALTY360.com*, http://www .propertycasualty360.com/2013/04/01/irc-study-public-less-accepting- of-insurance-fraud.

[51]U.S. Department of Health and Human Services, Office of the Inspector General, "Coding Trends of Medicare Evaluation and Management Serivces," May 2012, OEI-04-10-00180, https://oig.hhs.gov/oei/reports/oei-04-10-00180.pdf.

[52]Laurence Baker, M. Kate Bundorf, and Anne Royalty, "Private Insurers' Payments for Routine Physician Office Visits Vary Substantially across the United States," *Health Affairs* 32, no. 9 (2013): 1583–90, https://www.healthaffairs.org/doi/abs/10.1377/hlthaff.2013.0309.

[53]Todd Spangler, "U.S. Senate Hearing on Medicare Fraud Focuses on Michigan Cancer Doctor," *Detroit Free Press*, March 26, 2014, http://archive.freep.com/article/20140326/NEWS06/303260119/medicare-fraud-senate-michigan-oakland-county-cancer-doctor. See also Charlie Langton, "New Charge Filed Against Disgraced Cancer Doctor Farid Fata," *CBSDetroit*, November 22, 2013, http://detroit.cbslocal.com/2013/11/22/new-charge-filed-against-disgraced-cancer-doctor-farid-fata/.

[54]Robert Allen, "Cancer Doc Patients Say 45 Years in Prison Not Enough," *Detroit Free Press*, July 10, 2015, http://www.freep.com/story/news/local/michigan/oakland/2015/07/10/fata-sentence-handed-down/29952245/.

[55]Trudi Bird, "Michigan Doctor Held on $9 Million Bond for Misdiagnosing Cancer Patients in Medicare Scam," *NY Daily News*, August 16, 2013, http://www.nydailynews.com/news/national/doctor-held-9-million-bond-misdiagnosing-cancer-medicare-scam-article-1.1428639.

[56]Rene Stutzman, "Leesburg Eye Doctor Gets 10 Years in Prison for Fake Eye Operations," *Orlando Sentinel*, March 13, 2017, http://www.orlandosentinel.com/news/breaking-news/os-leesburg-eye-doctor-sentenced-for-fraud-20170310-story.html.

[57]Zachary R. Dowdy, "LI Physician Faces Medicare Fraud Charges," *Newsday*, March 25, 2014, http://www.newsday.com/long-island/nassau/li-physician-faces-medicare-fraud-charges-1.7502319.

[58]John Marzulli, "Brooklyn Surgeon in Medicare Billing Scheme Preyed on 'Elderly,'" *New York Daily News*, July 12, 2016, http://www.nydailynews.com/new-york/nyc-crime/brooklyn-surgeon-extracted-1m-medicare-billing-scheme-article-1.2708302.

[59]U.S. Department of Justice, Office of Public Affairs, "New York Doctor Convicted of Multimillion-Dollar Health Care Fraud," July 29, 2016, https://www.justice.gov/opa/pr/new-york-doctor-convicted-multimillion-dollar-health-care-fraud.

[60]Trudi Bird, "Michigan Doctor Held on $9 Million Bond for Misdiagnosing Cancer Patients in Medicare Scam," *NY Daily News*, August 16, 2013, http://www.nydailynews.com/news/national/doctor-held-9-million-bond-misdiagnosing-cancer-medicare-scam-article-1.1428639.

[61]Robert Pear, "Report Links Dead Doctors to Payments by Medicare," *New York Times*, July 9, 2008, http://www.nytimes.com/2008/07/09/washington/09fraud.html?_r=0.

[62]Ibid.

[63]Associated Press, "Report: Medicare Claims Were Paid in Names of Dead Providers: Related Issues Cost $1B in 2009," *PTManager Blog*, December 16, 2011, http://www.ptmanager.com/ptmanagerblog/2011/12/16/report-medicare-claims-were-paid-in-names-of-dead-providers.html.

[64]Jorgen Wouters, "Doctor Billed the Feds Millions for Treating Dead Patients," *Daily Finance*, June 8, 2011, http://www.dailyfinance.com/2011/06/08/doctor-billed-the-feds-millions-for-treating-dead-patients.

[65]U.S. Department of Justice, Office of Public Affairs, "Administrator and Biller of Illinois Physician Group Convicted in $4.5 Million Medicare Fraud Scheme," May 18, 2015, http://www.justice.gov/opa/pr/administrator-and-biller-illinois-physician-group-convicted-45-million-medicare-fraud-scheme.

[66]U.S. Department of Health and Human Services, Office of Inspector General, "Medicare Recovery Audit Contractors and CMS's Actions to Address Improper Payments, Referrals of Potential Fraud, and Performance," August 2013, OEI-04-11-00680, https://oig.hhs.gov/oei/reports/oei-04-11-00680.pdf.

[67]U.S. Department of Health and Human Services, Office of Inspector General, "Improper Payments for Evaluation and Management Services Cost Medicare Billions in 2010," OEI-04-10-00181, 2014, http://oig.hhs.gov/oei/reports/oei-04-10-00181.pdf.

[68]Charles Ornstein, "Medicare Overpays Billions for Office Visits, Patient Evaluations," *ProPublica*, May 29, 2014, http://www.propublica.org/article/medicare-overpays-billions-for-office-visits-patient-evaluations; Charles Ornstein and Ryann Grochowski Jones, "Top Billing: Meet the Docs Who Charge Medicare Top Dollar for Office Visits," *ProPublica*, May 15, 2014, http://www.propublica.org/article/billing-to-the-max-docs-charge-medicare-top-rate-for-office-visits.

[69]Ibid.

## Chapter 9

[1]Atul Gawande, "The Cost Conundrum," *New Yorker*, June 1, 2009, http://www.newyorker.com/reporting/2009/06/01/090601fa_fact_gawande.

[2]Brooke Murphy, "20 Things to Know about Balance Billing," *Becker's Hospital Review*, February 17, 2016.

[3]Morgan Haefner, "Texas Governor Signs Legislation on Surprise Billing, Mediation Efforts," *Becker's Hospital Review*, May 31, 2017, http://www.beckershospitalreview.com/finance/texas-governor-signs-legislation-on-surprise-billing-mediation-efforts.html.

[4]Consumer Reports National Research Center, "Surprise Medical Bills Survey: 2015 Nationally-Representative Online Survey," May 5, 2015, http://consumersunion.org/wp-content/uploads/2015/05/CY-2015-SURPRISE-MEDICAL-BILLS-SURVEY-REPORT-PUBLIC.pdf.

[5]Karen Politz, "Surprise Medical Bills," Kaiser Family Foundation, March 17, 2016, http://kff.org/private-insurance/issue-brief/surprise-medical-bills/.

[6]Zack Cooper and Fiona Scott Morton, "Out-of-Network Emergency-Physician Bills—An Unwelcome Surprise," *New England Journal of Medicine* 375 (November 17, 2016): 1915–18, http://www.nejm.org/doi/full/10.1056/NEJMp1608571.

[7]Christopher Garmon and Benjamin Chartock, "One in Five Inpatient Emergency Department Cases May Lead to Surprise Bills," *Health Affairs* 36, no. 1 (2017): 77–181.

[8]Zack Cooper, Fiona Scott Morton, and Nathan Shekita, "Surprise! Out-of-Network Billing for Emergency Care in the United States," NBER Working Paper no. 23623, July 2017, National Bureau of Economic Research, http://www.nber.org/papers/w23623.

[9]Haley Sweetland Edwards, "The Hidden Cost of 'Surprise' Medical Bills," *Time*, March 3, 2016.

[10]Ge Bai and Gerard F. Anderson, "Extreme Markup: The Fifty US Hospitals with the Highest Charge-to-Cost Ratios," *Health Affairs* 34, no. 6 (2015): 922–28, https://www.healthaffairs.org/doi/abs/10.1377/hlthaff.2014.1414. See also Lena H. Sun "50 Hospitals Charge Uninsured More than 10 Times Cost of Care, Study Finds," *Washington Post*, June 8, 2015.

[11]Brooke Murphy, "20 Things to Know about Balance Billing," *Becker's Hospital Review*, February 17, 2016.

[12]Ge Bai and Gerard F. Anderson, "Variation in the Ratio of Physician Charges to Medicare Payments by Specialty and Region," *JAMA* 317, no. 3 (2017): 315–18, https://jamanetwork.com/journals/jama/fullarticle/2598253. See also Andrew M. Seaman, "Doctors May Accept Low Fee from Medicare, but Not from All Patients," *Reuters*, January 17, 2017, http://www.reuters.com/article/us-health-cost-medical-idUSKBN15136T.

[13]Margot Sanger-Katz and Reed Abelson, "First Comes the Emergency. Then Comes the Surprise Out-of-Network Bill," *New York Times*, November 16, 2016, http://nyti.ms/2f1P1la.

[14]Elisabeth Rosenthal, "After Surgery, Surprise $117,000 Medical Bill from Doctor He Didn't Know," *New York Times*, September 20, 2014, https://www.nytimes.com/2014/09/21/us/drive-by-doctoring-surprise-medical-bills.html.

[15]Ibid.

[16]Haley Sweetland Edwards, "How You Could Get Hit with a Surprise Medical Bill," *Time*, March 7, 2016.

[17]Betsy Imholz, "Letter to the Editor," *New York Times*, July 4, 2016, http://www.nytimes.com/2016/07/04/opinion/when-the-cost-of-a-medical-emergency-adds-up.html.

[18]Brooke Murphy, "20 Things to Know about Balance Billing," *Becker's Hospital Review*, February 17, 2016.

[19]Sanger-Katz and Abelson, "First Comes the Emergency."

[20]Bob Herman, "Billing Squeeze: Hospitals in Middle as Insurers and Doctors Battle over Out-of-Network Charges," *Modern Healthcare*, August 29, 2015, http://www.modernhealthcare.com/article/20150829/MAGAZINE/308299987.

[21]Sweetland Edwards, "Surprise Medical Bills."

[22]Ayla Ellison, "Patients Hit with Surprise Bills for 22% of In-Network ER Visits," *Becker's Hospital Review E-weekly*, November 17, 2016.

[23]Murphy, "20 Things to Know."

[24]Mark Hall, Paul Ginsburg, and Steven M Lieberman, "How to Get Rid of Surprise Medical Bills," *Brookings*, October 13, 2016, https://www.brookings.edu/opinions/how-to-get-rid-of-surprise-medical-bills/.

[25]Herman, "Billing Squeeze."

[26]Sweetland Edwards, "Surprise Medical Bills."

[27]Michael F. Cannon, "Ascertaining Costs and Benefits of Colonoscopy More Difficult Than the Procedure Itself," *JAMA Internal Medicine*, June 21, 2016, https://object.cato.org/sites/cato.org/files/articles/cannon-jama-internal-medicine.pdf.

[28]Ilene MacDonald, "1 in 4 Physician Practices Now Hospital-Owned," *FierceHealthcare*, September 7, 2016, http://www.fiercehealthcare.com/practices/1-4-physician-practices-now-hospital-owned.

[29]Avalere Health, "Medicare Payment Differentials across Outpatient Settings of Care," February 2016, http://www.physiciansadvocacyinstitute.org/Portals/0/assets/docs/Payment-Differentials-Across-Settings.pdf.

[30]Ibid.

[31]Tammy Worth, "Hospital Facility Fees: Why Cost May Give Independent Physicians an Edge," *Medical Economics*, August 6, 2014, http://medicaleconomics.modernmedicine.com/medical-economics/content/tags/facility-fees/hospital-facility-fees-why-cost-may-give-independent-ph?page=full.

[32]Statement of Mark E. Miller, Executive Director, Medicare Payment Advisory Commission, Before the Committee on Ways and Means, U.S. House of Representatives, Hospital Policy Issues, July 22, 2015, http://www.medpac.gov/docs/default-source/congressional-testimony/testimony-hospital-policy-issues-ways-and-means-.pdf?sfvrsn=0.

[33]Margot Sanger-Katz, "When Hospitals Buy Doctors' Offices, and Patient Fee Soar," *New York Times*, February 6, 2015, http://nyti.ms/1zeXsM9.

[34]Worth, "Hospital Facility Fees."

[35]Joseph Burns, "Medicare, Insurers Questioning Payment Differences Based on Where Care is Delivered," *Covering Health* (blog), August 1, 2014, http://healthjournalism.org/blog/2014/08/medicare-insurers-questioning-payment-differences-based-on-where-care-is-delivered/.

[36]Gina Kolata, "Private Oncologists Being Forced Out, Leaving Patients to Face Higher Bills," *New York Times*, November 23, 2014, https://www.nytimes.com/2014/11/24/health/private-oncologists-being-forced-out-leaving-patients-to-face-higher-bills.html.

[37]Sanger-Katz, "When Hospitals Buy Doctors' Offices."

[38]Ames Alexander, Karen Garloch, and David Raynor, "As Doctors Flock to Hospitals, Bills Spike for Patients," *Charlotte Observer*, April 22, 2015, http://www.charlotteobserver.com/news/special-reports/prognosis-profits/article9085619.html#.VNKv3mR4pSU.

[39]Robert A. Berenson, Suzanne F. Delbanco, Stuart Guterman, et al., "Refining the Framework for Payment Reform," Robert Wood Johnson Foundation, Urban Institute, September 2016, https://www.brookings.edu/wp-content/uploads/2016/09/rwjf_moni_payment-reform_berenson.pdf.

[40]Merritt Hawkins, "2016 Physician Inpatient/Outpatient Revenue Survey," 2016, https://www.merritthawkins.com/uploadedFiles/MerrittHawkins/Surveys/Merritt_Hawkins-2016_RevSurvey.pdf.

[41]Cooper, Morton, and Shekita, "Surprise! Out-of-Network Billing."

[42]Julie Creswell, Reed Abelson, and Margot Sanger-Katz, "The Company Behind Many Surprise Emergency Room Bills," *New York Times*, July 24, 2017, https://www.nytimes.com/2017/07/24/upshot/the-company-behind-many-surprise-emergency-room-bills.html.

[43]Cooper, Morton, and Shekita, "Surprise! Out-of-Network Billing."

[44]Creswell, Abelson, and Sanger-Katz, "Surprise Emergency Room Bills."

[45]Ibid.

[46]Jeff Falk, "Study: Freestanding Emergency Departments in Texas Deliver Costly Care, 'Sticker Shock,'" *Rice University News & Media*, March 23, 2017, http://news.rice.edu/2017/03/23/study-freestanding-emergency-departments-in-texas-deliver-costly-care-sticker-shock/.

[47]Ibid.

[48]Ibid.

[49]Jenny Deam, "Academic Study Questioning ER Pricing Sparks Fight: Industry Challenges Data in Report Led by Houston Health Economist," *Houston Chronicle*, May 10, 2017, http://www.houstonchronicle.com/business/medical/article/Academic-study-questioning-ER-pricing-sparks-fight-11137336.php.

[50]Joe Cantlupe, "More to the Story: Annals of Emergency Medicine Halts Urgent Care Study Publication over Data in Controversial Decision," *Health Data Buzz*, May 8, 2017, https://healthdatabuzz.com/2017/05/08/more-to-the-story-annals-of-emergency-medicine-journal-halts-urgent-care-study-publication-over-data-in-controversial-decision/.

[51]Ibid.

[52]Ibid.

[53]Vivian Ho, Leanne Metcalfe, Cedric Dark, et al., "Comparing the Utilization and Costs of Care in Freestanding Emergency Departments, Hospital Emergency Departments, and Urgent Care Centers," *Annals of Emergency Medicine* 70, no. 6 (2017), http:// dx.doi.org/10.1016/j.annemergmed.2016 .12.006.

[54]Critics of the study include Paul D. Kivela, "Original Allegations about Data Integrity by Emergency Physicians," *Annals of Emergency Medicine* 70, no. 6 (2017), http://dx.doi.org/10.1016/j.annemergmed.2017.08.044; Paul D. Kivela, "Additional Information Regarding Request for Retraction of Ho Article," *Annals of Emergency Medicine* 70, no. 6 (2017), http://dx.doi .org/10.1016/j.annemergmed.2017.08.010; William P. Jaquis, Dean Wilkerson, Michael A. Granovsky, et al., "Emergency Physicians' Rebuttal of Author's Response," *Annals of Emergency Medicine* 70, no. 6 (2017), http://dx.doi .org/10.1016/j.annemergmed.2017.08.011; and Jeremiah D. Schuur, Donald M. Yealy, and Michael L. Callaham, "Comparing Freestanding Emergency Departments, Hospital-Based Emergency Departments, and Urgent Care in Texas: Apples, Oranges, or Lemons?" *Annals of Emergency Medicine* 70, no. 6 (2017), http://dx.doi.org/10.1016/j.annemergmed.2017.04.019; and Renee Y. Hsia, Jaime King, and Brendan G. Carr, "Don't Hate the Player; Hate the Game," *Annals of Emergency Medicine* 70, no. 6 (2017), http://dx.doi.org/10.1016/j .annemergmed.2017.08.062.

For the researchers' response to some of these criticisms, see Vivian Ho, Leanne Metcalfe, Cedric Dark, et al., "Author's Response to Critic's Allegations," *Annals of Emergency Medicine* 70, no. 6 (2017), http://dx.doi.org/10.1016/j .annemergmed.2017.08.017.

## CHAPTER 10

[1]Donald G. McNeil Jr., "Palliative Care Extends Life of Lung Cancer Patients, Study Finds," *New York Times*, August 18, 2010, http://www .nytimes.com/2010/08/19/health/19care.html. See also Stephen R. Connor, Bruce Pyenson, Kathryn Fitch, et al., "Comparing Hospice and Non-hospice Patient Survival among Patients Who Die Within a Three-Year Window," *Journal of Pain and Symptom Management* 33, no. 3 (March 2007): 238–246, http://www.jpsmjournal.com/article/S0885-3924(06)00724-X/ fulltext.

[2]Peter Waldman, "Hospice Providers Took Liberties to Grow Burgeoning Business," *Pittsburgh Post Gazette*, December 11, 2011, http://www.post-gazette.com/news/nation/2011/12/11/Hospice-providers-took-liberties-to-grow-burgeoning-business/stories/201112110227.

[3]Ibid.

[4]Ibid.

[5]Ibid.

[6]John K. Iglehart, "A New Era of For-Profit Hospice Care—The Medicare Benefit," *New England Journal of Medicine* 360 (June 25, 2009): 2701–03, http://www.nejm.org/doi/full/10.1056/NEJMp0902437, http://www.nejm.org/toc/nejm/360/26/.

[7]National Hospice and Palliative Care Organization, "Facts and Figures: Hospice Care in America," 2016, https://www.nhpco.org/sites/default/files/public/Statistics_Research/2016_Facts_Figures.pdf.

[8]John Hargraves and Niall Brennan, "Medicare Hospice Spending Hit $15.8 Billion in 2015, Varied by Locale, Diagnosis," *Health Affairs* 35, no. 10 (October 2016): 1902–07, doi:10.1377/hlthaff.2016.0650.

[9]U.S. Department of Health and Human Services, Office of Inspector General, *HHS OIG Work Plan, FY 2013*, (Washington, 2013), https://oig.hhs.gov/reports-and-publications/archives/workplan/2013/work-plan-2013.pdf.

[10]Ben Hallman and Nicky Forster, "The Business of Dying Has Never Been More Lucrative," *Huffington Post*, July 24, 2015, https://www.huffingtonpost.com/entry/hospice-report_us_55b1307ee4b0a9b94853fc7a.

[11]Iglehart, "A New Era of For-Profit Hospice Care."

[12]See also *Hospice Services: Assessing Payment Adequacy and Updating Payments*, MedPAC Report to the Congress, p. 282, March 2012.

[13]Peter Waldman, "Aunt Midge Not Dying in Hospice Reveals $14 Billion U.S. Market," *Bloomberg.com*, December 5, 2011, http://www.bloomberg.com/news/articles/2011-12-06/hospice-care-revealed-as-14-billion-u-s-market.

[14]Kathleen Tschantz Unroe, Greg A. Sachs, Susan E. Hickman, et al., "Hospice Use among Nursing Home Patients," *Journal of the American Medical Directors Association* 14, no. 4 (April 2013): 254–59, https://www.ncbi.nlm.nih.gov/pmc/articles/PMC3820369/.

[15]Medicare Learning Network, "Hospice Payment System," September 2016, https://www.cms.gov/Outreach-and-Education/Medicare-Learning-Network-MLN/MLNProducts/downloads/hospice_pay_sys_fs.pdf.

[16]Peter Waldman and Gary Putka, "Hospice Turns Months-to-Live Patient into Years of Abusing Drugs," *Bloomberg.com*, December 29, 2011, http://www.bloomberg.com/news/articles/2011-12-30/hospice-turns-months-to-live-patient-into-years-of-abusing-drugs.

[17]Waldman, "Aunt Midge Not Dying in Hospice."

[18]Ibid. See also Peter Waldman, "Preparing Americans for Death Lets Hospices Neglect End of Life," *Bloomberg.com*, July 21, 2011, http://www.bloomberg.com/ news/articles/2011-07-22/preparing-americans-for-death-lets-for-profit-hospices-neglect-end-of-life.

[19]Waldman and Putka, "Months-to-Live Patient."

[20]Waldman, "Preparing Americans for Death."

[21]Randy Dotinga, "Slowly Dying Patients, an Audit and a Hospice's Undoing," *Kaiser Health News*, January 16, 2013, http://khn.org/news/san-diego-hospice/.

[22]Joanne Faryon, "Medicare Audit Forces San Diego Hospice to Close," *KPBS Public Media*, February 13, 2013, http://www.kpbs.org/news/2013/ feb/13/meidcare-audit-forces-sd-hospice-close/.

[23]Paul Sisson, "$112 Million Claim Filed Against SD Hospice," *San Diego Union-Tribune*, June 18, 2013, http://www.sandiegouniontribune.com/news/ health/sdut-hospice-bankruptcy-san-diego-millions-2013jun18-story.html.

[24]Wikipedia, "Diagnosis-Related Group," https://en.wikipedia.org/wiki/ Diagnosis-related_group.

[25]U.S. Department of Health and Human Services, Office of the Inspector General, *Medicare Could Save Millions by Implementing a Hospital Transfer Payment Policy for Early Discharges to Hospice Care*, May 2013, http://oig.hhs.gov/oas/ reports/region1/11200507.pdf.

[26]Tresa Baldas, "Hospice Center Denies Paying Kickbacks for Corrupt Doctor's Referrals," *Detroit Free Press*, November 30, 2016, http://www.freep.com/ story/news/local/michigan/detroit/2016/11/30/hospice-center-denies-paying-kickbacks-cancer-patient-referrals/94677294/.

[27]U.S. Department of Health and Human Services, Centers for Medicare and Medicaid Services, "MLN Matters: Update to Hospice Payment Rates, Hospice Cap, Hospice Wage Index, Quality Reporting Program and the Hospice Price for Fiscal Year (FY) 2015," August 11, 2014, http://www.cms.gov/Outreach-and-Education/ Medicare-Learning-Network-MLN/MLNMattersArticles/Downloads/ MM8876.pdf.

[28]U.S. Department of Justice, Office of Public Affairs, "United States Files False Claims Act Lawsuit Against the Largest For-Profit Hospice Chain in the United States," news release, May 2, 2013, http://www.justice.gov/opa/pr/united-states-files-false-claims-act-lawsuit-against-largest-profit-hospice-chain-united.

[29]U.S. Department of Justice "Chemed Corp. and Vitas Hospice Services Agree to Pay $75 Million to Resolve False Claims Act Allegations Relating to Billing for Ineligible Patients and Inflated Levels of Care," October 30, 2017, https:// www.justice.gov/opa/pr/chemed-corp-and-vitas-hospice-services-agree-pay-75-million-resolve-false-claims-act.

[30]United States' Complaint at ¶ 47, United States v.VITAS Hospice Services, L.L.C., No. 4:13–cv–00449 (W.D. Mo., May 2, 2013).

[31]Tom McLaughlin,"Largest US Hospice Company Sued for Medicare Fraud," *Panama City News Herald*, May 9, 2013, http://www.newsherald.com/news/ crime-public-safety/largest-us-hospice-company-sued-for-medicare-fraud-1 .140101.

[32]Aaron Sharockman, "Rick Scott and the Fraud Case of Columbia/HCA," *PolitiFact Florida*, June 11, 2010, http://www.politifact.com/florida/article/2010/ jun/11/rick-scott-and-fraud-case-columbiahca/.

[33]J. D. Wolverton, "Rick Scott & Health Care Fraud," *Dailykos.com*, October 17, 2010, http://www.dailykos.com/story/2010/10/17/911096/-Rick-Scott-Health-Care-Fraud.

[34]U.S. Department of Health and Human Services, Office of the Inspector General, *Medicare Hospice: Use of General Impatient Care*, OEI-02-10-00490, 2013, http://oig.hhs.gov/oei/reports/oei-02-10-00490.pdf.

[35]U.S. Attorney's Office, Northern District of Illinois, "Illinois Hospice Executive Charged with Federal Health Care Fraud for Allegedly Falsely Elevating Level of Patients' Care," news release, January 27, 2014, https://www.fbi.gov/ chicago/press-releases/2014/illinois-hospice-executive-charged-with-federal-health-care-fraud-for-allegedly-falsely-elevating-level-of-patients-care.

[36]Ibid.

[37]U.S. Department of Justice, U.S. Attorney's Office, Northern District of Illinois, "Director of Lisle-Based Hospice Company Convicted in Scheme to Fraudulently Bill Medicare for Medically Unnecessary Services," news release, March 9, 2016, https://www.justice.gov/usao-ndil/pr/director-lisle-based-hospice-company-convicted-scheme-fraudulently-bill-medicare-0.

[38]Joe Carlson, "Unusual Billing Patterns Spur Probe of Inpatient Hospice Care," *Modern Health Care*, May 6, 2013, http://www.modernhealthcare.com/ article/20130506/NEWS/305069968. See also Office of the Inspector General, "Medicare Hospice: Use of General Inpatient Care," OEI-02-1 0-00490, May 3, 2013, http://oig.hhs.gov/oei/reports/oei-02-10-00490.pdf.

[39]Indictment, United States v. Kolodesh, No. 11-464 (E.D. Pa. August 17, 2011), http://www.justice.gov/archive/usao/pae/News/2011/Oct/kolodesh_ indictment.pdf.

[40]Waldman, "Aunt Midge Not Dying in Hospice."

[41]Ibid.

[42]Kay Lazar and Matt Carroll, "A Rampant Prescription, a Hidden Peril," *Boston Globe*, April 29, 2012, http://www.boston.com/news/local/massachusetts/ articles/2012/04/29/nursing_home_residents_with_dementia_often_given_anti-psychotics_despite_health_warnings/.

[43]Ina Jaffe and Robert Benincasa, "Old and Overmedicated: The Real Drug Problem in Nursing Homes," *NPR*, December 8, 2014, http://www.npr.org/sections/health-shots/2014/12/08/368524824/old-and-overmedicated-the-real-drug-problem-in-nursing-homes.

[44]Jaffe and Benincasa, "Old and Overmedicated."

[45]Jan Goodwin, "Antipsychotics in Nursing Homes," *AARP Bulletin*, July/August 2014, https://www.aarp.org/health/drugs-supplements/info-2014/antipsychotics-overprescribed.html.

[46]U.S. Department of Justice, Office of Public Affairs "U.S. Files Suit Against Johnson & Johnson for Paying Kickbacks to Nation's Largest Nursing Home Pharmacy," news release, January 15, 2015, http://www.justice.gov/opa/pr/us-files-suit-against-johnson-johnson-paying-kickbacks-nation-s-largest-nursing-home-pharmacy.

[47]U.S. Department of Justice, Office of Public Affairs, "Two Atlanta-Based Nursing Home Chains and Their Principals Pay $14 Million to Settle False Claims Act Case," news release, February 26, 2010, http://www.justice.gov/opa/pr/2010/February/10-civ-204.html.

[48]Sava may be a repeat offender. In 2015, the U.S. government joined three whistleblower lawsuits that accuse Sava, which collected more than a billion dollars in payments from Medicare, of charging for rehabilitation services that were not needed and delaying residents' discharges to maximize revenues. See Dani Kass, "DOJ Steps in on FCA Suit Against National Nursing Co.," *Law360*, October 29, 2015, https://www.law360.com/articles/720696.

[49]U.S. Department of Justice, Office of Public Affairs, "Nation's Largest Nursing Home Pharmacy and Drug Manufacturer to Pay $112 Million to Settle False Claims Act Cases," news release, November 3, 2009, http://www.justice.gov/opa/pr/nation-s-largest-nursing-home-pharmacy-and-drug-manufacturer-pay-112-million-settle-false.

[50]U.S. Department of Justice, Office of Public Affairs, "Johnson & Johnson to Pay More than $2.2 Billion to Resolve Criminal and Civil Investigations," news release, November 4, 2013, https://www.justice.gov/opa/pr/johnson-johnson-pay-more-22-billion-resolve-criminal-and-civil-investigations.

[51]U.S. Department of Justice, "Nation's Largest Nursing Home Pharmacy." See also Complaint of the United States, U.S. ex rel. Bernard Lisitza and David Kammerer v. Johnson & Johnson, et al., No. 07-10288-RGS, (D. MA, January 15, 2010), https://www.justice.gov/sites/default/files/opa/legacy/2013/11/04/jj-complaint-ma.pdf.

[52]Ibid.

[53]David S. Hilzenrath, "Justice Suit Accuses Johnson & Johnson of Paying Kickbacks," *Washington Post*, January 16, 2010, http://www.washingtonpost.com/wp-dyn/content/article/2010/01/15/AR2010011503903.html.

[54]Testimony from Daniel R. Levinson, Inspector General, Department of Health and Human Services, before the United States Senate Special Committee on Aging, "Overprescribed: The Human and Taxpayers' Costs of Antipsychotics in Nursing Homes," November 30, 2011, https://oig.hhs.gov/testimony/docs/2011/levinson_testimony_11302011.pdf.

[55]Ibid.

[56]Ibid.

[57]Institute of Medicine, *Improving the Quality of Care in Nursing Homes* (Washington: The National Academies Press, 1986), https://doi.org/10.17226/646.

[58]Harris Meyer, "Drugmakers' Payments Draw Heat," *BusinessWeek*, November 4, 2009, http://www.businessweek.com/bwdaily/dnflash/content/nov2009/db2009114_700374.htm.

[59]U.S. Department of Justice, Office of Public Affairs, "Two Atlanta-Based Nursing Home Chains and Their Principals Pay $14 Million to Settle False Claims Act Case," news release, February 26, 2010, http://www.justice.gov/opa/pr/two-atlanta-based-nursing-home-chains-and-their-principals-pay-14-million-settle-false-claims.

[60]U.S. Department of Justice, "Johnson & Johnson to Pay More than $2.2 Billion."

[61]Kaiser Family Foundation, "Overview of Nursing Facility Capacity, Financing, and Ownership in the United States in 2011," June 28, 2013, http://kff.org/medicaid/fact-sheet/overview-of-nursing-facility-capacity-financing-and-ownership-in-the-united-states-in-2011/.

[62]Kim Sloan, "Former Nursing Home Owner, George Houser, Sentenced to 20 Years in Prison," *Northwest Georgia News*, August 14, 2012, http://www.northwestgeorgianews.com/rome/former-nursing-home-owner-george-houser-sentenced-to-years-in/article_e5323661-e335-5bcd-8df4-67148d50a2fa.html.

[63]U.S. Attorney's Office, Northern District of Georgia, "Former Nursing Home Operator Sentenced to Prison for 20 Years for Health Care Fraud and Tax Fraud," Federal Bureau of Investigation, news release, August 13, 2012, https://www.justice.gov/archive/usao/gan/press/2012/08-14-12.html.

[64]Ibid.

[65]Sloan, "Former Nursing Home Owner Sentenced."

[66]Ibid.

[67]U.S. Attorney's Office, Northern District of Georgia, "Atlanta Man Convicted of Billing for Worthless Services While Operating 'Horrendous' Nursing Homes," news release, April 3, 2012, https://www.justice.gov/archive/usao/gan/press/2012/04-03-12.html.

[68]Caitlin Ostroff, "Rehabilitation Center at Holly Hills Cited for Building Violations," *Miami Herald*, September 27, 2017, http://www.miamiherald.com/news/local/community/broward/article175766806.html. See also Bob Norman, "Hollywood

Nursing Home Should Never Have Been Licensed, State Senator Says," *Local-10News*, October 26, 2017, https://www.local10.com/news/local-10-investigates/hollywood-nursing-home-should-never-have-been-licensed-senator-says.

[69]Ibid.

[70]Bob Norman, "Owner of Nursing Home Where Eight Died Has History of Fraud Allegations: Hospital Involved in Alleged Billion Dollar Scheme," *Local-10News*, September 13, 2017, https://www.local10.com/weather/hurricane-irma/owner-of-nursing-home-where-8-died-has-history-of-fraud-allegations.

[71]Complaint of the United States, U.S.A. v. Jack Jacobo Michel, M.D. et al., 1:04-cv-21579-AJ (S.D. FL—June 30, 2004).

[72]Ibid.

[73]Ibid.

[74]U.S. Department of Justice, "Miami Hospital Pays $15.4 Million to Resolve Fraud Case for Kickbacks and Medically Unnecessary Treatments," news release, November 30, 2006, https://www.justice.gov/archive/opa/pr/2006/November/06_civ_803.html.

[75]Ibid.

[76]Norman, "Owner of Nursing Home Where Eight Died."

[77]Dan Christensen, "Gov Scott, His Lobbyist Pal, a Nursing Home Deal and a Curious Change of Heart at AHCA," FloridaBulldog.org, November 6, 2011, http://www.floridabulldog.org/2017/11/gov-scott-his-lobbyist-pal/.

[78]Ibid.

[79]Amy Sherman, "Rick Scott 'Oversaw the Largest Medicare Fraud' in U.S. History, Florida Democratic Party Says," *PolitiFact Florida*, March 3, 2014, http://www.politifact.com/florida/statements/2014/mar/03/florida-democratic-party/rick-scott-rick-scott-oversaw-largest-medicare-fra/.

[80]Christensen, "Gov Scott, His Lobbyist Pal, a Nursing Home Deal."

[81]Arek Sarkissian, "Nursing Home Deaths: Owner's Hospital Was Paid $48 Million for State Prisoner Health," *News-Press*, September 26, 2107, http://www.news-press.com/story/news/politics/2017/09/26/nursing-home-deaths-owners-hospital-paid-48-million-state-prisoner-health/706489001/.

[82]Norman, "Hollywood Nursing Home Should Never Have Been Licensed."

## Chapter 11

[1]Sean Dooley and Lynn Redmond, "Doctor Jailed for Prescribing Drugs at Starbucks Defends Himself," *ABC News*, November 13, 2013, http://abcnews.go.com/Health/doctor-jailed-illegally-prescribing-drugs-starbucks-defends-actions/story?id=20803865; Hailey Branson-Potts, "O.C. Doctor to Get Sentence for Illegal Pain Prescriptions," *Los Angeles Times*, April 4, 2013, http://articles.latimes.com/2013/apr/04/local/la-me-0405-starbucks-doctor-20130405.

[2]Dooley and Redmond, "Doctor Jailed for Prescribing Drugs at Starbucks."

[3]Branson-Potts, "O.C. Doctor to Get Sentence."

[4]Dooley and Redmond, "Doctor Jailed for Prescribing Drugs at Starbucks."

[5]Ibid.

[6]Paul Jesilow, G. Geis, and H. Pontell, "Fraud by Physicians Against Medicaid." *JAMA* 266, no. 23 (1991): 3318–22.

[7]Parija Kavilanz, "Prescription Drugs Worth Millions to Dealers," *CNNMoney*, June 1, 2011, http://money.cnn.com/2011/06/01/news/economy/prescription_drug_abuse/index.htm.

[8]Lizette Alvarez, "Florida Laws Shutting 'Pill Mills,'" *New York Times*, August 31, 2011, http://www.nytimes.com/2011/09/01/us/01drugs.html.

[9]Partnership for Drug-Free Kids, "Generic OxyContin Hits Black Market," May 24, 2014, http://www.drug-rehabs.com/addiction/oxycontin/black-market/.

[10]Max Blau, "As New and Lethal Opioids Flood U.S. Streets, Crime Labs Race to Identify Them," *STAT*, July 5, 2017, https://www.statnews.com/2017/07/05/opioid-identification-analogs/.

[11]Fred Schulte and Elizabeth Lucas, "Liquid Gold: Pain Doctors Soak Up Profits by Screening Urine for Drugs," *Kaiser Health News*, November 6, 2017, https://khn.org/news/liquid-gold-pain-doctors-soak-up-profits-by-screening-urine-for-drugs/.

[12]Justin Zaremba, "Pharmacist Pleads Guilty to $1.5 Million Health Care Fraud Scheme, Illegally Selling Oxycodone," *NJ.com*, January 25, 2014, http://www.nj.com/morris/index.ssf/2014/01/pharmacist_pleads_guilty_in_15_million_health_care_fraud.html.

[13]"Feds Seize Records from Several Miami Pharmacies," *CBS4 Miami*, October 12, 2011, http://miami.cbslocal.com/2011/10/12/feds-seize-records-from-several-miami-pharmacies/.

[14]Rebecca R. Ruiz, "U.S. Charges 412, Including Doctors, in $1.3 Billion Health Fraud," *New York Times*, July 13, 2017, https://www.nytimes.com/2017/07/13/us/politics/health-care-fraud.html.

[15]Lizette Alvarez, "Florida Laws Shutting 'Pill Mills,'" *New York Times*, August 31, 2011, http://www.nytimes.com/2011/09/01/us/01drugs.html.

[16]Centers for Disease Control and Prevention, "Opioid Painkiller Prescribing Infographic," *CDC Vital Signs*, July 1, 2014, https://www.cdc.gov/vitalsigns/opioid-prescribing/infographic.html.

[17]"The $272 Billion Swindle: Why Thieves Love America's Health-Care System," *The Economist*, May 31, 2014, https://www.economist.com/news/united-states/21603078-why-thieves-love-americas-health-care-system-272-billion-swindle.

[18]Associated Press, "Drug Wholesalers Shipped 780M Pain Pills to West Virginia," *NBCWashington,* December 18, 2016, http://www.nbcwashington .com/news/local/Drug-Wholesalers-Shipped-780M-Pain-Pills-to-West-Virginia-407331135.html.

[19]Eric Eyre, "Drug Firms Poured 780M Painkillers into WV Amid Rise of Overdoses," *Charleston Gazette-Mail,* December 17, 2016, http://www.wvgazettemail .com/news-health/20161217/drug-firms-poured-780m-painkillers-into-wv-amid-rise-of-overdoses.

[20]Centers for Disease Control and Prevention, National Center for Health Statistics, "Drug Overdose Mortality by State," February 22, 2017, https://www .cdc.gov/nchs/pressroom/sosmap/drug_poisoning_mortality/drug_poisoning .htm. See also Michael B. Sauter, "10 States with the Most Drug Overdoses," *24/7 Wall St.com,* June 24, 2016, http://247wallst.com/special-report/2016/06/24/10-states-with-the-most-drug-overdoses/3/.

[21]Associated Press, "28 ODs in 4 Hours: How the Heroin Epidemic Choked a W.Va. City," *CBSNews.com,* September 4. 2016, http://www.cbsnews.com/ news/4-hours-in-huntington-va-how-the-heroin-epidemic-choked-a-city/.

[22]Christopher Ingraham, "Drugs Are Killing So Many People in West Virginia That the State Can't Keep Up with the Funerals," *Washington Post,* March 7, 2017, https://www.washingtonpost.com/news/wonk/wp/2017/03/07/drugs-are-killing-so-many-people-in-west-virginia-the-state-cant-keep-up-with-the-funerals/?utm_term=.b839358e5cfb.

[23]Gina Kolata and Sarah Cohen, "Drug Overdoses Propel Rise in Mortality Rates of Young Whites," *New York Times,* January 16, 2016, http://www.nytimes. com/2016/01/17/science/drug-overdoses-propel-rise-in-mortality-rates-of-young-whites.html?action=click&contentCollection=Health&module= RelatedCoverage&region=EndOfArticle&pgtype=article.

[24]Memorandum Opinion and Order, United States v. Charles York Walker Jr., No. 2:17-cr-00010, (S.D. W.Va. June 26, 2017), http://www.wvsd.uscourts .gov/sites/default/files/opinions/ORD%20-%20Walker%20-%20Plea%20 Rejection%20FINAL%20COPY.pdf.

[25]Jake Zuckerman, "WV Governor Signs Medical Marijuana into Law," *Charleston Gazette-Mail,* April 19, 2017, http://www.wvgazettemail.com/ news-politics/20170419/wv-governor-signs-medical-marijuana-into-law.

[26]Ronnie Cohen, "Would Legalizing Medical Marijuana Help Curb the Opioid Epidemic?," *Reuters.com,* March 27, 2017, http://www.reuters.com/article/ us-health-addiction-medical-marijuana-idUSKBN16Y2HV.

[27]"Convictions of 'Dr. Feelgood' Stand," *Patriot Ledger,* April 15, 2009, http://www.patriotledger.com/apps/pbcs.dll/article?AID=/20090415/ News/304159546.

[28]Tracy Weber and Charles Ornstein, "Fraud Rx: Medicare Makes Moves to Tighten Oversight of Dirty Doctors," *Pacific Standard*, February 7, 2014, http://www.psmag.com/health-and-behavior/fraud-rx-medicare-makes-moves-tighten-oversight-dirty-doctors-73910.

[29]Charles Ornstein, "Florida Doctor Pleads Guilty to Fraud—Years after Complaints about His Prescribing," *ProPublica*, June 23, 2016, https://www.propublica.org/article/florida-doctor-pleads-guilty-fraud-years-after-complaints-prescribing.

[30]U.S. Government Accountability Office, GAO-09-1004T, "Medicaid: Fraud and Abuse Related to Controlled Substances Identified in Selected States," 2009, http://www.gao.gov/products/GAO-09-1004T.

[31]U.S. Government Accountability Office, GAO-12-104T, "Medicare Part D: Instances of Questionable Access to Prescription Drugs," 2011, http://www.gao.gov/products/GAO-12-104T.

[32]Ibid.

[33]Ibid.

[34]U.S. Government Accountability Office, "Medicare Part D."

[35]Anupam B. Jena, Dana Goldman, Lesley Weaver, and Pinar Karaca-Mandic, "Opioid Prescribing by Multiple Providers in Medicare: Retrospective Observational Study of Insurance Claims," *BMJ* 348 (2014): g1393.

[36]Lenny Bernstein, "Half a Million Medicare Recipients Were Prescribed Too Many Opioid Drugs Last Year," *Washington Post,* July 13, 2017, https://www.washingtonpost.com/news/to-your-health/wp/2017/07/13/half-a-million-medicare-recipients-were-prescribed-too-many-opioid-drugs-last-year/?utm_term=.d0e0cc25aca6&wpisrc=nl_sb_smartbrief.

[37]Tracy Weber, Charles Ornstein, and Jennifer LaFleur, "Medicare Drug Program Fails to Monitor Prescribers, Putting Seniors and Disabled at Risk," *ProPublica*, May 11, 2013, http://www.propublica.org/article/part-d-prescriber-checkup-mainbar.

[38]Tracy Weber and Charles Ornstein, "'Let the Crime Spree Begin': How Fraud Flourishes in Medicare's Drug Plan," *ProPublica*, December 19, 2013, http://www.propublica.org/article/how-fraud-flourishes-in-medicares-drug-plan.

[39]Shantanu Agrawal and Peter Budetti, "Physician Medical Identity Theft," *JAMA* 307, no. 5 (2012): 459–60.

[40]Weber and Ornstein, "Let the Crime Spree Begin."

[41]Deepak Chitnis, "Indian American Pharmacist in Michigan Mukesh Khunt Convicted for Healthcare Fraud," *American Bazaar*, March 13, 2014, http://www.americanbazaaronline.com/2014/03/13/indian-american-pharmacist-michigan-mukesh-khunt-convicted-healthcare-fraud/; U.S. Attorney's Office,

Eastern District of Michigan, "Jury Convicts 38th Defendant in Health Care Fraud Scheme," July 21, 2014, https://www.fbi.gov/detroit/press-releases/2014/jury-convicts-38th-defendant-in-health-care-fraud-scheme.

[42]Charles Ornstein, "Even after Doctors Are Sanctioned or Arrested, Medicare Keeps Paying," *ProPublica*, April 16, 2014, http://www.propublica.org/article/even-after-doctors-are-sanctioned-or-arrested-medicare-keeps-paying.

[43]Tracy Weber and Charles Ornstein, "Caught Up in a Medicare Drug Fraud," *ProPublica*, December 31, 2013, http://www.propublica.org/article/caught-up-in-a-medicare-drug-fraud.

[44]Charles Ornstein, "Following Abuses, Medicare Tightens Reins on Its Drug Program," *NPR.org*, May 20, 2014, http://www.npr.org/sections/health-shots/2014/05/20/314227055/following-abuses-medicare-tightens-reins-on-its-drug-program.

[45]Charles Ornstein, "Fraud Still Plagues Medicare Drug Program, Watchdog Finds," *ProPublica*, June 23, 2015, http://www.propublica.org/article/fraud-still-plagues-medicare-drug-program-watchdog-finds.

## CHAPTER 12

[1]See Centers for Medicare and Medicaid Services, "CFO Audit: Improvement in Medicare," news release, March 26, 1999, http://cms.hhs.gov/media/press/release.asp?Counter=358. See also David A. Hyman, "HIPAA and Health Care Fraud: An Empirical Perspective," *Cato Journal* 22 (2002).

[2]Interview with Dr. Malcolm K. Sparrow, *AARP Bulletin*, October 1997, http://www.aarp.org/bulletin/oct97/sparrow1.htm. See also Malcolm K. Sparrow, *License to Steal: How Fraud Bleeds America's Health Care System,* 2nd edition (Boulder, CO: Westview Press, 2000).

[3]U.S. Department of Health and Human Services, Centers for Medicare and Medicaid Services Office of Enterprise Data and Analytics, *2016 CMS Statistics*, March 2017, https://www.cms.gov/Research-Statistics-Data-and-Systems/Statistics-Trends-and-Reports/CMS-Statistics-Reference-Booklet/Downloads/2016_CMS_Stats.pdf.

[4]Centers for Medicare and Medicaid Services, *CMS Releases Prescriber-Level Medicare Data for First Time*, April 30, 2015, https://www.cms.gov/Newsroom/MediaReleaseDatabase/Fact-sheets/2015-Fact-sheets-items/2015-04-30.html.

[5]"The $272 Billion Swindle: Why Thieves Love America's Health-Care System," *The Economist*, May 31, 2014, https://www.economist.com/news/united-states/21603078-why-thieves-love-americas-health-care-system-272-billion-swindle.

[6]U.S. Department of Justice, "Annual Report of the Departments of Health and Human Services and Justice, Health Care Fraud and Abuse Program FY 2014," March 19, 2015, (Appendix at 90), http://oig.hhs.gov/publications/docs/hcfac/FY2014-hcfac.pdf.

[7]U.S. Department of Health and Human Services, "Departments of Justice and Health and Human Services Announce over $27.8 Billion in Returns from Joint Efforts to Combat Health Care Fraud," news release, March 19, 2015, http://www.hhs.gov/news/press/2015pres/03/20150319a.html. Similar figures appear in earlier reports. See U.S. Department of Health and Human Services, Office of Inspector General, "Reports and Publications (Health Care Fraud and Abuse Control Program Report section)," http://oig.hhs.gov/reports-and-publications/hcfac/index.asp.

[8]Weber and Ornstein, "Let the Crime Spree Begin."

[9]Tristram Korten, "How to Commit Medicare Fraud in Six Easy Steps," Fast Company, December 2011, http://www.fastcompany.com/1795066/how-commit-medicare-fraud-six-easy-steps.

[10]U.S. Department of Justice, Office of Public Affairs, "Justice Department Recovers over $4.7 Billion From False Claims Act Cases in Fiscal Year 2016," December 14, 2016, https://www.justice.gov/opa/pr/justice-department-recovers-over-47-billion-false-claims-act-cases-fiscal-year-2016.

[11]Jack Cloherty and Pierre Thomas, "Biggest Medicare Fraud in History Busted, Say Feds," ABC News, February 28, 2012, http://abcnews.go.com/Blotter/biggest-medicare-fraud-history-busted-feds/story?id=15809129; U.S. Department of Justice, Office of Public Affairs, "Dallas Doctor Arrested for Alleged Role in Nearly $375 Million Health Care Fraud Scheme," February 28, 2012, http://www.justice.gov/opa/pr/dallas-doctor-arrested-alleged-role-nearly-375-million-health-care-fraud-scheme.

[12]Kevin Krause, "Former Rockwall Doctor Guilty of Nation's Biggest Home Health Care Fraud," Dallas Morning News, April 13, 2016, http://crimeblog.dallasnews.com/2016/04/formerrockwalldoctorguiltyofnationsbiggesthomehealthcarefraud.html/; Kevin Krause, "Doctor with History of Maiming Patients Sentenced to 35 Years in $373 Million Home Health Scheme," Dallas Morning News, August 10, 2017, https://www.dallasnews.com/news/crime/2017/08/09/doctor-maimed-patients-bilked-taxpayers-record-370-million-gets-35-years-prison.

[13]Ibid.

[14]Bradford Pearson, "North Texas Men Convicted of Healthcare Fraud," D CEO Healthcare, October 22, 2013, http://healthcare.dmagazine.com/2013/10/22/north-texas-men-convicted-of-healthcare-fraud/.

[15]U.S. Department of Justice, Office of Public Affairs, "Two Owners of Miami Home Health Company Each Sentenced to More Than Six Years in Prison for $20 Million Health Care Fraud Scheme," news release, June 21, 2012, http://www .justice.gov/opa/pr/two-owners-miami-home-health-company-each-sentenced-more-six-years-prison-20-million-health; U.S. Department of Justice, Office of Public Affairs, "Owner and Employee of Miami Home Health Company Plead Guilty in $22 Million Health Care Fraud Scheme," news release, January 26, 2012, http://www.justice.gov/opa/pr/owner-and-employee-miami-home-health-company-plead-guilty-22-million-health-care-fraud-scheme.

[16]U.S. Department of Justice, Office of Public Affairs, "Doctor and Home Health Agency Owner Plead Guilty in Connection with Detroit Fraud Scheme," news release, May 8, 2012, http://www.justice.gov/opa/pr/doctor-and-home-health-agency-owner-plead-guilty-connection-detroit-fraud-scheme.

[17]U.S. Attorney's Office, District of Columbia, "More Than 20 People Arrested Following Investigations into Widespread Health Care Fraud in D.C. Medicaid Program," news release, February 20, 2014, https://www.fbi.gov/washingtondc/ press-releases/2014/more-than-20-people-arrested-following-investigations-into-widespread-health-care-fraud-in-d.c.-medicaid-program.

[18]Barbara Martinez, "Home Care Yields Medicare Bounty," *Wall Street Journal*, April 26, 2010, http://www.wsj.com/news/articles/SB10001424052748703625304575116040870004462. See also Michael Lipkin, "Amedisys to Pay $150M to Settle DOJ Medicare Billing Suits," *Law360*, April 23, 2014, http://www.law360 .com/articles/531089/amedisys-to-pay-150m-to-settle-doj-medicare-billing-suits.

[19]Martinez, "Home Care Yields Medicare Bounty."

[20]U.S. Attorney's Office, Southern District of Florida, "Three Individuals Charged in $1 Billion Medicare Fraud and Money Laundering Scheme," July 22, 2016, https://www.justice.gov/usao-sdfl/pr/three-individuals-charged-1-billion-medicare-fraud-and-money-laundering-scheme.

[21]Yedidya Borenstein, "Philip Esformes Charged in Unprecedented $1B Medicare Fraud Case in Miami," *Jewish Voice*, July 27, 2015, http.//jewishvoiceny.com/index .php?option=com_content&view=article&id=15247:philip-esformes-charged-in-unprecedented-1b-medicare-fraud-case-in-miami&catid=110&Itemid=774; Dan Mangan, "$1 Billion Alleged Medicare Fraud, Money Laundering Scheme Leads to Florida Arrests," *CNBC.com*, July 22, 2016, http://www.cnbc.com/2016/07/22/1-billion-alleged-medicare-fraud-money-laundering-scheme-leads-to-florida-arrests. html; Alex Zielinski, "Elder Care Company Placed Thousands of Seniors into Nursing Homes to Defraud Medicare and Medicaid," *ThinkProgress*, July 25, 2016, https:// thinkprogress.org/elder-care-company-placed-thousands-of-seniors-into-nursing-homes-to-defraud-medicare-and-medicaid-3b074ef2de2b.

[22]U.S. Attorney's Office, Southern District of Florida, "Three Individuals Charged."

[23]Bill Singer, "UPDATE: The Epidemic of Florida Medicare Fraud," *Forbes*, September 19, 2011, http://www.forbes.com/sites/billsinger/2011/09/19/update-the-epidemic-of-florida-medicare-fraud/.

[24]Ibid.

[25]U.S. Department of Justice, Office of Public Affairs, "Miami–Area Psychiatrist Pleads Guilty for Role in $200 Million Medicare Fraud Scheme," news release, June 30, 2011, http://www.justice.gov/opa/pr/miami-area-psychiatrist-pleads-guilty-role-200-million-medicare-fraud-scheme.

[26]Jay Weaver, "Miami Man Gets 15 Years in Nation's Biggest Medicare Therapy Scam," *Miami Herald*, October 21, 2014, http://www.miamiherald.com/news/local/community/miami-dade/article3208683.html.

[27]Dan Eggen, "Health–Care Exec's Medicare Fraud Scheme Included Lobbying Washington," *Washington Post*, October 5, 2011, https://www.washingtonpost.com/politics/health-executive-lobbied-in-washington-to-advance-medicare-fraud-scheme/2011/09/28/gIQA7dRXNL_story.html.

[28]U.S. Attorney's Office, Southern District of Florida, "South Florida Doctor and Other Professionals Charged with Health Care Fraud at Biscayne Milieu Health Center Inc.," news release, October 2, 2014, https://www.fbi.gov/miami/press-releases/2014/south-florida-doctor-and-other-professionals-charged-wth-health-care-fraud-at-biscayne-milieu-health-center-inc.

[29]U.S. Department of Justice, Office of Public Affairs, "Eight Individuals and a Corporation Convicted at Trial in Florida in $50 Million Medicare Fraud," news release, August 24, 2012, https://www.justice.gov/opa/pr/eight-individuals-and-corporation-convicted-trial-florida-50-million-medicare-fraud.

[30]U.S. Department of Justice, Office of Public Affairs, "Jury Convicts All Seven Defendants in $97 Million Medicare Fraud Scheme," news release, March 12, 2014, http://www.justice.gov/opa/pr/jury-convicts-all-seven-defendants-97-million-medicare-fraud-scheme.

[31]U.S. Department of Justice, Office of Public Affairs, "Former President of Riverside General Hospital Sentenced to 45 Years in Prison in $158 Million Medicare Fraud Scheme," news release, June 9, 2015, http://www.justice.gov/opa/pr/former-president-riverside-general-hospital-sentenced-45-years-prison-158-million-medicare.

[32]Terri Langford, "FBI Arrests Historic Houston Hospital's CEO, Son, 5 Others," *Houston Chronicle*, October 4, 2012, http://www.chron.com/news/houston-texas/article/FBI-arrests-historic-Houston-hospital-s-CEO-son-3918870.php.

[33]Kent Moore, "Changes Coming to Medicare Payments for Durable Medical Equipment," *Family Practice Management*, May 14, 2013, http://blogs.aafp.org/fpm/gettingpaid/entry/changes_coming_to_medicare_payment.

[34]U.S. Government Accountability Office, GAO-12-820, *Health Care Fraud: Types of Providers Involved in Medicare, Medicaid, and the Children's Health Insurance Program Cases*, 2012, http://www.gao.gov/assets/650/647849.pdf (table 5).

[35]Lindsay Wise, "Medicare Fraud Targets Seniors, Scooters: 'I Don't Need It. I Don't Want It,'" *McClatchyDC*, May 7, 2013, http://www.mcclatchydc.com/news/politics-government/congress/article24748903.html.

[36]Jay Weaver, "Prosecutors Called Their Business 'All-Fraud,'" *Miami Herald*, August 4, 2008, http://www.miamiherald.com/news/special-reports/watchdog-report/article1929737.html.

[37]"Former Pastor Sentenced for Role in $11 Million Medicare Fraud Scheme," *Arizona Daily Independent*, October 20, 2013, https://arizonadailyindependent.com/2013/10/20/former-pastor-sentenced-for-role-in-11-million-medicare-fraud-scheme/.

[38]U.S. Department of Justice, Office of Public Affairs, "Los Angeles Church Pastor Sentenced to Serve 36 Months in Prison for $14.2 Million Medicare Fraud Scheme," February 27, 2012, http://www.justice.gov/opa/pr/los-angeles-church-pastor-sentenced-serve-36-months-prison-142-million-medicare-fraud-scheme.

[39]U.S. Attorney's Office, District of Kansas, "Texas Man Convicted of Medicare Fraud in Kansas," February 16, 2012, https://www.fbi.gov/kansascity/press-releases/2012/texas-man-convicted-of-medicare-fraud-in-kansas.

[40]Wise, "Medicare Fraud Targets Seniors."

[41]"Woman Arrested for Health Care Fraud," *12 News KBMT & K-JAC*, October 18, 2011, http://www.12newsnow.com/story/15724681/woman-arrested-for-health-care-fraud.

[42]Statement by Daniel R. Levinson, Office of the Inspector General, U.S. Department of Health and Human Services (HHS) on Preventing Health Care Fraud: New Tools and Approaches to Combat Old Challenges before U.S. Senate Committee on Finance, March 2, 2011, http://www.hhs.gov/asl/testify/2011/03/t20110302i.html.

[43]Statement by Lewis Morris, Chief Counsel, Office of Inspector General, U.S. Department of Health and Human Services, on Reducing Fraud, Waste, and Abuse in Medicare before Committee on Ways and Means, Subcommittee on Health and Subcommittee on Oversight, United States House of Representatives, June 15, 2010, http://www.hhs.gov/asl/testify/2010/06/t20100615c.html.

[44]Terri Langford, "Private Ambulances Take Medicare, Taxpayers for a Ride," *Houston Chronicle*, July 26, 2013, http://www.chron.com/news/houston-texas/article/Some-Ems-companies-taking-Medicare-for-a-ride-2220817.php.

[45]"Editorial: Medicare Fraud Must End," *Houston Chronicle*, October 20, 2011, http://www.chron.com/opinion/editorials/article/Medicare-fraud-must-end-2228816.php.

[46]Langford, "Private Ambulances."

[47]Ibid.

[48]Matthew Spina, "Rural/Metro Faces Accusations of Overbilling in NY," *Buffalo News*, January 16, 2012, http://www.boundtreeuniversity.com/news/1220552-Rural-Metro-faces-accusations-of-overbilling-in-NY/. See also U.S. Attorney's Office, District of Arizona, "Rural/Metro to Pay $2.8 Million to Resolve False Claims Allegations," December 26, 2013, http://www.justice.gov/usao-az/pr/attachment2013-099ruralmetrosettlement-agreement-pdf.

[49]Rebecca LeFever, "Harrisburg Company, Owner and York Employee Face Medicare Fraud Charges," *Ydr.com*, January 13, 2012, http://www.ydr.com/ci_19735405. See also U.S. Attorney's Office, Middle District of Pennsylvania, "Health Care Fraud," June 2, 2015, http://www.justice.gov/usao-mdpa/health-care-fraud.

[50]Susan Trautsch, "Ambulance Transport Company Settles on Alleged Medicare Fraud," *South Carolina Radio Network*, December 2, 2010, http://www.southcarolinaradionetwork.com/2010/12/02/ambulance-transport-provider-settles-on-alleged-medicare-fraud/.

[51]Tony Gonzalez, "Health Fraud Prosecutions Net $100 Million in Tennessee This Year," *Kingsport Times-News*, December 4, 2011, http://www.timesnews.net/article/9039090/health-fraud-prosecutions-net-100-million-in-tennessee-this-year. See also U.S. Attorney's Office, Middle District of Tennessee, "Former Owners of Murfreesboro Ambulance Service Sentenced to Federal Prison for Defrauding Medicare," January 17, 2014, https://www.fbi.gov/memphis/press-releases/2014/former-owners-of-murfreesboro-ambulance-service-sentenced-to-federal-prison-for-defrauding-medicare.

[52]Michael Owens, "Saltville Rescue Squad Accused of Fraud," *HeraldCourier.com*, February 3, 2012, http://www.heraldcourier.com/news/saltville-rescue-squad-accused-of-fraud/article_1772200b-757a-5aae-ac07-86fc207f85ab.html; Laurence Hammack, "Saltville Rescue Squad President Convicted of Health Care Fraud," *Roanoke Times*, September 19, 2012, http://www.roanoke.com/webmin/news/saltville-rescue-squad-president-convicted-of-health-care-fraud/article_742d438b-ff0a-5a92-b1e3-7d3e3a998ab7.html.

[53]U.S. Department of Justice, Office of Public Affairs, "New York City Ambulance Companies Pay U.S. $2.85 Million to Resolve Claims for Fraudulent Medicare Appeals," June 4, 2010, http://www.justice.gov/opa/pr/new-york-city-ambulance-companies-pay-us-285-million-resolve-claims-fraudulent-medicare.

[54]Linnet Myers, "FBI: Medical Fraud Luring Crime Rings," *Chicago Tribune*, March 22, 1995, http://articles.chicagotribune.com/1995-03-22/news/9503220190_1_health-care-fraud-fbi-director-louis-freeh-medical-fraud.

[55]Lewis Morris, "Combating Fraud in Health Care: An Essential Component of Any Cost Containment Strategy," *Health Affairs* 28, no. 5 (2009): 1351–56, https://www.healthaffairs.org/doi/abs/10.1377/hlthaff.28.5.1351.

[56]U.S. Department of Justice, Office of Public Affairs, "Members and Associates of Organized Crime Enterprise, Others Indicted for Health Care Fraud Crimes Involving More Than $163 Million," October 13, 2010, http://www.justice.gov/opa/pr/73-members-and-associates-organized-crime-enterprise-others-indicted-health-care-fraud-crimes.

[57]Daniel Beekman, "10 Yrs. for Armenian Mobster," *NY Daily News*, August 15, 2013, http://www.nydailynews.com/new-york/10-yrs-armenian-mobster-article-1.1428461.

[58]Chris Adams, "Even as Prosecutions Rise, Medicare Fraud Often Runs Rampant," *Kansas City Star*, March 26, 2014, http://www.kansascity.com/news/local/article343418/Even-as-prosecutions-rise-Medicare-fraud-often-runs-rampant.html.

[59]Ibid.

[60]Statement of Aghaegbuna 'Ike' Odello, Hearing on Improved Efforts to Combat Health Care Fraud, before the Subcommittee on Health of the Committee on Ways and Means, March 2, 2011, http://waysandmeans.house.gov/hearing-on-improving-efforts-to-combat-health-care-fraud/.

[61]Jay Weaver, "A Former Scam Artist Tells How It Works," *Miami Herald*, August 5, 2008, http://www.miamiherald.com/news/special-reports/watchdog-report/article1929762.html.

[62]Jay Weaver, "Feds Fear Medicare Fraud Suspect May Flee Abroad," *Miami Herald*, May 6, 2012, http://www.miamiherald.com/2012/05/05/2784943/feds-fear-medicare-fraud-suspect.html.

[63]Christie Smythe and Henry Meyer, "Russian Diplomats Accused of Bilking Medicaid," *Bloomberg.com*, December 6, 2013, http://www.bloomberg.com/news/articles/2013-12-06/russian-diplomats-accused-of-bilking-medicaid.

[64]Paul Rubin, "Rent a Patient," *Phoenix New Times*, April 24, 2003, http://www.phoenixnewtimes.com/news/rent-a-patient-6408607.

[65]Paul Rubin, "Out of Patients," *Phoenix New Times*, May 29, 2003, http://www.phoenixnewtimes.com/content/printView/6408437.

[66]Kristen Hallam, "Health Insurers Allege 'Rent-A-Patient' Fraud," *Washington Post*, March 12, 2005, http://www.washingtonpost.com/wp-dyn/articles/A28484-2005Mar11.html.

[67]U.S. Department of Justice, Office of Public Affairs, "Detroit-Area Clinic Owner Pleads Guilty in Connection with Medicare Fraud Scheme," news release, December 6, 2011, http://www.justice.gov/opa/pr/detroit-area-clinic-owner-pleads-guilty-connection-medicare-fraud-scheme.

[68]Alex Robinson, "Second Doc Pleads Guilty in Flushing Clinic Fraud," *TimesLedger*, March 4, 2014, http://www.timesledger.com/stories/2014/9/medicarefraud2_tl_2014_02_28_q.html.

[69]Kelli Kennedy, "Professional Patients Aid Massive Medicare Fraud in Fla.," *Boston Globe*, December 25, 2008, http://www.boston.com/news/nation/articles/2008/12/25/professional_patients_aid_massive_medicare_fraud_in_fla/?page=full.

[70]Ibid.

[71]Jay Weaver, "Medicare Fraud Rampant in South Florida," *Miami Herald*, August 3, 2008, http://www.miamiherald.com/news/special-reports/watchdog-report/article1929719.html.

[72]Ibid.

[73]U.S. Department of Health and Human Services, "Medicare Fraud Strike Force Charges 90 Individuals for Approximately $260 Million in False Billing," news release, May 13, 2014, http://www.hhs.gov/news/press/2014pres/05/20140513b.html.

[74]Marilyn May, "Medicare Fraud Takedown: A Closer Look," *Healio.com*, June 30, 2015, http://www.healio.com/ophthalmology/regulatory-legislative/news/online/%7B449aca05-0903-4b0b-af9e-458c9a83ea04%7D/medicare-fraud-takedown-a-closer-look.

[75]Ibid.

[76]Rebecca R. Ruiz, "U.S. Charges 412, Including Doctors, in $1.3 Billion Health Fraud," *New York Times*, July 13, 2017, https://mobile.nytimes.com/2017/07/13/us/politics/health-care-fraud.html; Jesse Pound, "Austin, Houston Doctors among 35 Texans Charged in $1.3 Billion Medicare Fraud Sting," *San Antonio Express-News*, July 13, 2017, http://www.expressnews.com/business/article/Austin-Houston-doctors-among-35-Texans-charged-11287987.php.

CHAPTER 13

[1]The website for the Heart Attack Grill Restaurant, http://www.heartattackgrill.com.

[2]Marshall Allen and *ProPublica*, "How Many Die from Medical Mistakes in U.S. Hospitals?" *Scientific American*, September 20, 2013, http://www.scientificamerican.com/article/how-many-die-from-medical-mistakes-in-us-hospitals/.

[3]Committee on Quality of Health Care in America and Institute of Medicine, *To Err Is Human: Building a Safer Health System*, ed. Linda T. Kohn, 1st edition (Washington: National Academies Press, 2000).

[4]HealthGrades, "Patient Safety in American Hospitals," 2004, www.ihf-fih.org/sp/content/download/530/4009/file/Patient%20Safety%20in%20American%20Hospitals.pdf.

[5]John T. James, "A New, Evidence-Based Estimate of Patient Harms Associated with Hospital Care," *Journal of Patient Safety* 9, no. 3 (September 2013): 122–28, doi:10.1097/PTS.0b013e3182948a69.

[6]Martin A. Makary and Michael Daniel, "Medical Error—The Third Leading Cause of Death in the US," *BMJ* 353 (2016): i2139, doi:https://doi.org/10.1136/bmj.i2139.

[7]Ibid. See also Hannah Nichols, "The Top 10 Leading Causes of Death in the United States," *Medical News Today*, February 23, 2017, https://www.medicalnewstoday.com/articles/282929.php.

[8]John T. James, "A New, Evidence-Based Estimate of Patient Harms Associated with Hospital Care," *Journal of Patient Safety* 9, no. 3 (September 2013): 122–28, doi:10.1097/PTS.0b013e3182948a69.

[9]John C. Goodman, Pamela Villarreal, and Biff Jones, "The Social Cost of Adverse Medical Events, and What We Can Do about It," *Health Affairs* 30, no. 4 (2011): 590–95, doi:10.1377/hlthaff.2010.1256.

[10]David C. Classen, Roger Resar, Frances Griffin, et al., "'Global Trigger Tool' Shows That Adverse Events in Hospitals May Be Ten Times Greater than Previously Measured." *Health Affairs* 30, no. 4 (2011): 581–89, doi:10.1377/hlthaff.2011.0190. See also Cheryl Clark, "1 in 3 Hospitalized Patients Suffers an Adverse Event," *HealthLeaders Media,* April 7, 2011, http://www.healthleadersmedia.com/print/QUA 264653/1-in-3-Hospitalized-Patients-Suffers-an-Adverse-Event (quoting David Classen, MD).

[11]Jill Van Den Bos, Karan Rustagi, Travis Gray, et al., "The $17.1 Billion Problem: The Annual Cost of Measurable Medical Errors," *Health Affairs* 30, no. 4 (2011): 596–603, doi:10.1377/hlthaff.2011.0084.

[12]Goodman, Villareal, and Jones, "The Social Cost of Adverse Medical Events."

[13]Barbara Starfield, "Is US Health Really the Best in the World?," *JAMA* 284, no. 4 (2000): 483–85, doi:10.1001/jama.284.4.483 (citing studies).

[14]Catharine Paddock, "Medicare Will Not Pay for Hospital Mistakes and Infections, New Rule," *Medical News Today,* August 20, 2007, http://www.medicalnewstoday.com/articles/80074.php. A study published in 2014 suggests that hospitals are doing better at preventing HAIs. See Shelley S. Magill, Jonathan R. Edwards, Wendy Bamberg, et al., "Multistate Point-Prevalence Survey of Health Care–Associated Infections," *New England Journal of Medicine* 370, no. 13 (2014): 1198–208, doi:10.1056/NEJMoa1306801.

[15]Peter Pronovost, Dale Needham, Sean Berenholtz, et al., "An Intervention to Decrease Catheter-Related Bloodstream Infections in the ICU," *New England Journal of Medicine* 355, no. 26 (2006): 2725–32, doi:10.1056/NEJMoa061115. The protocol also encouraged physicians to avoid the femoral artery and to remove catheters that were no longer needed.

[16]Ibid., 2729. The contents of the checklist are described in slightly different ways in different places. See, for example, Nancy Kass, Peter J. Pronovost, Jeremy Sugarman, et al., "Controversy and Quality Improvement: Lingering Questions

about Ethics, Oversight, and Patient Safety Research," *Joint Commission Journal on Quality and Patient Safety/Joint Commission Resources* 34, no. 6 (June 2008): 349–53. The actual Johns Hopkins checklist, and many others, can be found at http://gawande.com/the-checklist-manifesto.

[17]Atul Gawande, "The Checklist," *New Yorker*, December 10, 2007, http://www.newyorker.com/magazine/2007/12/10/the-checklist.

[18]Ibid.

[19]Atul Gawande, "A Lifesaving Checklist," *New York Times*, December 30, 2007, http://www.nytimes.com/2007/12/30/opinion/30gawande.html.

[20]Ibid.

[21]David Maxfield, Joseph Grenny, Ramon Lavandero, and Linda Groah, "The Silent Treatment: Why Safety Tools and Checklists Aren't Enough," 2011, http://silenttreatmentstudy.com/silent/The%20Silent%20Treatment.pdf.

[22]Gawande, "The Checklist."

[23]Gawande, "A Lifesaving Checklist."

[24]Gawande, "The Checklist."

[25]Peter Pronovost and Eric Vohr, *Safe Patients, Smart Hospitals: How One Doctor's Checklist Can Help Us Change Health Care from the Inside Out*, 1st ed. (New York: Plume, 2011).

[26]Ibid.

[27]Cheryl Clark, "How One Hospital Zapped Infection Rates," *HealthLeaders Media*, March 8, 2013, http://healthleadersmedia.com/content.cfm?topic=QUA&content_id=289932##.

[28]Reed Abelson, "Go to the Wrong Hospital and You're 3 Times More Likely to Die," *New York Times*, December 14, 2016, https://www.nytimes.com/2016/12/14/business/hospitals-death-rates-quality-vary-widely.html.

[29]Ibid.

[30]J. K. Wall, "The Low Hanging Fruit Is Lying on the Ground," *The Health Care Blog*, July 29, 2015, http://thehealthcareblog.com/blog/2015/07/29/the-low-hanging-fruit-is-lying-on-the-ground/.

[31]Molly Joel Coye, "No Toyotas in Health Care: Why Medical Care Has Not Evolved to Meet Patients' Needs," *Health Affairs* 20, no. 6 (2001): 44–56.

[32]Charles Ornstein, "Accreditors Can Keep Their Hospital Inspection Reports Secret, Feds Decide," *ProPublica*, August 3, 2017, https://www.propublica.org/article/accreditors-can-keep-their-hospital-inspection-reports-secret-feds-decide.

[33]David A. Hyman and Charles Silver, "The Poor State of Health Care Quality in the U.S.: Is Malpractice Liability Part of the Problem or Part of the Solution?," *Cornell Law Review* 90, no. 4 (2005): 893.

[34]Ornstein, "Accreditors."

[35]The figures and quotations in this paragraph are taken from Cheryl Clark, "Hospitals Profit on Bloodstream Infections," *HealthLeaders Media,* May 23, 2013, http://healthleadersmedia.com/content.cfm?topic=QUA&content_id=292493. The citation for the study is Eugene Hsu, Della Lin, Samuel J. Evans, et al., "Doing Well by Doing Good: Assessing the Cost Savings of an Intervention to Reduce Central Line-Associated Bloodstream Infections in a Hawaii Hospital," *American Journal of Medical Quality: The Official Journal of the American College of Medical Quality* 29, no. 1 (2014): 13–19, doi:10.1177/1062860613486173.

[36]Hsu et al., "Doing Well by Doing Good."

[37]Ibid.

[38]Sunil Eappen, Bennett H. Lane, Barry Rosenberg, et al., "Relationship between Occurrence of Surgical Complications and Hospital Finances," *JAMA* 309, no. 15 (2013): 1599–606, doi:10.1001/jama.2013.2773. The surgeries included in the study were craniotomy, colorectal resection, total or partial hip replacement, knee arthroplasty, coronary artery bypass graft, spinal surgery (laminectomy, excision of intervertebral disk, or spinal fusion), hysterectomy (abdominal or vaginal), appendectomy, and cholecystectomy or common bile duct exploration.

[39]Dan C. Krupka, Warren S. Sandberg, and William B. Weeks, "The Impact on Hospitals of Reducing Surgical Complications Suggests Many Will Need Shared Savings Programs with Payers," *Health Affairs* 31, no. 11 (November 2012): 2571–578, doi:10.1377/hlthaff.2011.0605.

[40]Thomas C. Tsai, Felix Greaves, Jie Zheng, et al., "Better Patient Care at High-Quality Hospitals May Save Medicare Money and Bolster Episode-Based Payment Models," *Health Affairs* 35, no. 9 (2016): 1681–89, doi:10.1377/hlthaff.2016.0361.

[41]Sheila Leatherman, Donald Berwick, Debra Iles, et al., "The Business Case for Quality: Case Studies and an Analysis," *Health Affairs* 22, no. 2 (2003): 17–30, doi:10.1377/hlthaff.22.2.17. In the mid-2000s, the Commonwealth Fund published a series of studies emphasizing the lack of a business case for quality in the health care sector. They can be found at http://www.commonwealthfund.org/Search.aspx?searchtype=Publications&search=Business+Case+&filefilter=1.

[42]David A. Asch, Mark V. Pauly, and Ralph W. Muller, "Asymmetric Thinking about Return on Investment," *New England Journal of Medicine* 374, no. 7 (2016): 606–08.

[43]L. Silvia Munoz-Price, Kristopher Arheart, Patrice Nordmann, et al., "Eighteen Years of Experience with Acinetobacter Baumannii in a Tertiary Care Hospital," *Critical Care Medicine* 41, no. 12 (2013): 2733–42.

[44]L. Silvia Munoz-Price, Philip Carling, Timothy Cleary, et al., "Control of a Two-Decade Endemic Situation with Carbapenem-Resistant Acinetobacter Baumannii: Electronic Dissemination of a Bundle of Interventions," *American Journal of Infection Control* 42, no. 5 (2014): 466–71, doi:10.1016/j.ajic.2013.12.024.

[45]Alexandra Wilson Pecci, "Nurses' Unlikely Infection Control Tool Quashes HAI," *HealthLeaders Media*, May 13, 2014, http://www.healthleadersmedia.com/nurse-leaders/nurses-unlikely-infection-control-tool-quashes-hai?page=0%2C1#.

[46]Ibid.

[47]Ibid.

[48]See Rene Letourneau, "9 in 10 Health Plans Still Tied to FFS Model," *HealthLeaders Media,* March 27, 2013, http://www.healthleadersmedia.com/content/HEP-290546/9-in-10-Health-Plans-Still-Tied-to-FFS-Model.

[49]David A. Hyman and Charles Silver, "Healthcare Quality, Patient Safety, and the Culture of Medicine: 'Denial Ain't Just a River in Egypt," *New England Law Review* 46, no. 3 (2012).

[50]J. K. Wall, "The Low Hanging Fruit Is Lying on the Ground," *Health Advice and More* (blog), July 29, 2015, https://healthadviceandmore.wordpress.com/2015/07/29/the-low-hanging-fruit-is-lying-on-the-ground/ (quoting Indiana University management professor Mohan Tatikonda).

[51]Steve Cohen, "Can Obamacare Improve Patient Safety? Tort Reform Hasn't," *Forbes*, October 26, 2013, http://www.forbes.com/sites/stevecohen/2013/10/26/can-obamacare-improve-patient-safety-tort-reform-hasnt/. We chronicled the history of the improvement of anesthesia safety in Hyman and Silver, "Poor State of Health Care Quality."

[52]David A. Hyman and Charles Silver, "Healthcare Quality, Patient Safety, and the Culture of Medicine: 'Denial Ain't Just a River in Egypt,'" *New England Law Review* 46, no. 3 (2012).

[53]Jeffrey B. Cooper, "Getting into Patient Safety: A Personal Story," Agency for Healthcare Research and Quality, August 2006, http://www.webmm.ahrq.gov/perspective.aspx?perspective ID=29.

[54]Bob Wachter, "Bureaucracy Run Amok: Can Checklists Kill?," *The Hospital Leader*, January 11, 2008, http://thehospitalleader.org/bureaucracy-run-amok-can-checklists-kill/.

[55]Gawande, "A Lifesaving Checklist."

[56]Gawande, "The Checklist."

[57]Ibid.

[58]Ibid.

[59]Grace M. Lee, Christine W. Hartmann, Denise Graham, et al., "Perceived Impact of the Medicare Policy to Adjust Payment for Health-Care Associated Infections," *American Journal of Infection Control* 40, no. 4 (2012). See also Catharine Paddock, "Medicare Will Not Pay for Hospital Mistakes and Infections, New Rule," *Medical News Today*, August 20, 2007, http://www.medicalnewstoday.com/articles/80074.php; and Vanessa Fuhrmans, "Insurers Stop Paying for Care Linked to Errors," *Wall Street Journal*, January 15, 2008, http://online.wsj.com/news/articles/SB120035439914089727.

Whether the new Medicare policy has reduced the rate at which infections occur is being debated. Compare Grace M. Lee, Ken Kleinman, Stephen B. Soumerai, et al., "Effect of Nonpayment for Preventable Infections in U.S. Hospitals," *New England Journal of Medicine* 367, no. 15 (2012): 1428–37, doi:10.1056/NEJMsa1202419, with Caroline P. Thirukumaran, Laurent G. Glance, Helena Temkin-Greener, et al., "Impact of Medicare's Nonpayment Program on Hospital-Acquired Conditions," *Medical Care* 55, no. 5 (2017): 447–55, doi:10.1097/MLR.0000000000000680.

## Chapter 14

[1]Johnny Fontane, "The Godfather Wiki," http://godfather.wikia.com/wiki/Johnny_Fontane.

[2]Akanksha Jayanthi, "More than $31B Distributed in MU Payments to Date," *Becker's Health IT & CIO Review*, August 28, 2015, http://www.beckershospitalreview.com/healthcare-information-technology/more-than-31b-distributed-in-mu-payments-to-date.html; Chun-Ju Saiao, Ashish K. Jha, Jennifer King, et al., "Office-Based Physicians Are Responding to Incentives and Assistance by Adopting and Using Electronic Health Records," *Health Affairs* 32, no. 8 (2013): 1470–77, https://www.healthaffairs.org/doi/full/10.1377/hlthaff.2013.0323; Marsha R. Gold, Catherine G. McLaughlin, Kelly J. Devers, et al., "Obtaining Providers' 'Buy-In' and Establishing Effective Means of Information Exchange Will Be Critical to HITECH's Success," *Health Affairs* 31, no. 3 (2012): 3514–26, https://www.healthaffairs.org/doi/abs/10.1377/hlthaff.2011.0753; Mitch Wagner, "U.S. Allocates $1.2 Billion for Electronic Medical Records," *InformationWeek HealthCare*, August 21, 2009, http://www.informationweek.com/healthcare/electronic-health-records/us-allocates-$12-billion-for-electronic-medical-records/d/d-id/1082464?; Jeff Overly, "E-Records to Draw Health Fraud Scrutiny after OIG Report," *Law360.com,* January 8, 2014, http://0-www.law360.com.tallons.law.utexas.edu/articles/499522/e-records-to-draw-health-fraud-scrutiny-after-oig-report.

[3]Stephen T. Mennemeyer, Nir Menachemi, Saurabh Rahurkar, and Eric W. Ford, "Impact of the HITECH Act on Physicians' Adoption of Electronic Health Records," *Journal of the American Medical Informatics Association* 23, no. 2 (2015): 375–79, https://doi.org/10.1093/jamia/ocv103.

[4]Cheryl Clark, "It's Impossible to Know What $1B in Federal Quality Spending Buys," *HealthLeaders Media*, February 20, 2014, http://www.healthleadersmedia.com/quality/its-impossible-know-what-1b-federal-quality-spending-buys.

[5]Ibid.

[6]Institute of Medicine, "Report Brief, Crossing the Quality Chasm: A New Health System for the 21st Century," *National Academy of Sciences*, March 2001, https://iom.nationalacademies.org/~/media/Files/Report%20Files/2001/Crossing-the-Quality-Chasm/Quality%20Chasm%202001%20%20report%20brief.pdf.

[7]Dylan Tweney, "Infoporn: How Flatscreen TVs Get Cheaper," *Wired*, April 26, 2011, http://www.wired.com/magazine/2011/04/st_infoporn_lcds/.

[8]Jeffrey A. Hart, "Flat Panel Displays," in *Innovation in Global Industries: U.S. Firms Competing in a New World (Collected Studies)*, ed. Jeffrey T. Macher and David C. Mowery (Washington: The National Academies Press, 2008), http://pubs.acs.org/cen/coverstory/83/8326electronics.html.

[9]"Adopting Technological Innovation in Hospitals: Who Pays and Who Benefits?," *American Hospital Association,* October 2006, http://www.aha.org/content/00-10/061031-adoptinghit.pdf.

[10]David Goldhill, *Catastrophic Care: How American Health Care Killed My Father—and How We Can Fix It* (New York: Alfred A. Knopf, 2013), p. 85.

[11]David Dranove, "Unleashing Innovation in Healthcare Markets," *Code Red* (blog), January 14, 2013, http://dranove.wordpress.com/2013/01/14/unleashing-innovation-in-healthcare-markets/.

[12]Barak D. Richman, Krishna Udayakumar, Will Mitchell, and Kevin A. Schulman, "Lessons from India in Organizational Innovation: A Tale of Two Heart Hospitals," *Health Affairs* 27, no. 5 (2008): 1260–70, https://www.healthaffairs.org/doi/full/10.1377/hlthaff.27.5.1260.

[13]Goldhill, *Catastrophic Care*, p. 85.

[14]Judith H. Hibbard, Jessica Greene, Shoshanna Sofaer, et al., "An Experiment Shows That a Well-Designed Report on Costs and Quality Can Help Consumers Choose High-Value Health Care," *Health Affairs* 31, no. 3, (2012): 560–68, https://www.healthaffairs.org/doi/pdf/10.1377/hlthaff.2011.1168.

[15]Ha T. Tu and Johanna Lauer, "Word of Mouth and Physician Referrals Still Drive Health Care Provider Choice," HSC Research Brief no. 9, *Center for Studying Health System Change,* December 2008, http://www.hschange.com/CONTENT/1028/.

[16]New York State Department of Health, "Adult Cardiac Surgery in New York State," https://www.health.ny.gov/statistics/diseases/cardiovascular.

[17]Dana B. Mukamel, David L. Weimer, Jack Zwanziger, et al., "Quality Report Cards, Selection of Cardiac Surgeons, and Racial Disparities: A Study of the Publication of the New York State Cardiac Surgery Reports," *Inquiry* 41, no. 4, (2004/2005): 435–46.

[18]Eric C. Schneider and Arnold M. Epstein, "Influence of Cardiac-Surgery Performance Reports on Referral Practices and Access to Care. A Survey of Cardiovascular Specialists," *New England Journal of Medicine* 335, no. 4, (1996): 251–56; E. L. Hannan, Cathy C. Stone, Theodore L. Biddle, and Barbara A. DeBuono, "Public Release of Cardiac Surgery Outcomes Data in New York: What Do New York State Cardiologists Think of It?," *American Heart Journal* 134, no. 6 (1997): 1120–28, http://www.sciencedirect.com/science/article/pii/S0002870397700346.

[19]Ashish K. Jha and Arnold M. Epstein, "The Predictive Accuracy of the New York State Coronary Artery Bypass Surgery Report-Card System," *Health Affairs* 25, no. 3 (2006): 844–55, doi:10.1377/hlthaff.25.3.844.

[20]David L. Brown, Arnold M. Epstein, and Eric C. Schneider, "Influence of Cardiac Surgeon Report Cards on Patient Referral by Cardiologists in New York State after 20 Years of Public Reporting," *Circulation: Cardiovascular Quality and Outcomes* 6, no. 6 (2013): 643–48.

[21]Laurence F. McMahon, "What to Do When It's You: Bill Clinton and Hospital Report Cards," *American Journal of Managed Care* 10, no. 10 (2004): 664, http://www.ajmc.com/journals/issue/2004/2004-10-vol10-n10/oct04-1900p664#sthash.na3O5bRD.dpuf.

[22]Xerox, *Variation in Payment for Hospital Care in Rhode Island*, prepared for the Rhode Island Office of the Health Insurance Commissioner and the Rhode Island Executive Office of Health and Human Services, December 19, 2012, http://www.ohic.ri.gov/documents/Hospital-Payment-Study-Final-General-Dec-2012.pdf.

[23]Massachusetts Office of Attorney General, "Examination of Health Care Cost Trends and Cost Drivers," June 22, 2011, http://www.mass.gov/ago/docs/healthcare/2011-hcctd.pdf; Massachusetts Division of Health Care Finance and Policy, "Massachusetts Health Care Cost Trends: Price Variation in Health Care Services," June 3, 2011, http://archives.lib.state.ma.us/bitstream/handle/2452/113870/ocn753988593-main_report.pdf?sequence=1&isAllowed=y. See also Freedman Health Care, "Re-examining the Health Care Cost Drivers and Trends in the Commonwealth: A Review of State Reports (2008–2015)," February 2016, http://www.mahp.com/assets/pdfs/MAHP-freedman-report.pdf.

[24]Massachusetts Health Policy Commission, "Provider Price Variation: Stakeholder Discussion Series Summary Report," July 2016, http://www.mass .gov/anf/budget-taxes-and-procurement/oversight-agencies/health-policy-commission/publications/2016-ppv-summary-report.pdf.

[25]Massachusetts Division of Health Care Finance and Policy, "Massachusetts Health Care Cost Trends: Price Variation in Health Care Services," June 3, 2011, http://archives.lib.state.ma.us/bitstream/handle/2452/113870/ocn753988593-main_report.pdf?sequence=1&isAllowed=y.

[26]Chapin White, James D. Reschovsky, and Amelia M. Bond, "Understanding Differences between High- and Low-Price Hospitals: Implications for Efforts to Rein in Costs," *Health Affairs* 33, no. 2 (2014): 324–31.

[27]Massachusetts Health Policy Commission, "Provider Price Variation," p. 1; David Seltz, David Auerbach, Kate Mills, Marian Wrobel, and Aaron Pervin, "Addressing Price Variation in Massachusetts," *Health Affairs Blog,* May 12, 2016, http://healthaffairs.org/blog/2016/05/12/addressing-price-variation-in-massachusetts/.

[28]Dave Barkholz, "Data Suggest New York Hospital Prices Depend on Leverage, not Quality," *Modern Healthcare*, December 19, 2016, http://www.modernhealthcare .com/article/20161219/NEWS/161219910?template=print.

[29]Ibid. See also Gorman Actuarial, "Why Are Hospital Prices Different? An Examination of New York Hospital Reimbursement," *New York State Health Foundation*, December 2016, http://nyshealthfoundation.org/resources-and-reports/resource/an-examination-of-new-york-hospital-reimbursement.

[30]Maggie Mahar, "'The Third Rail of Payment Reform'—Tackling Wide Variations in How Much Providers Charge," *HealthBeat* (blog), September 29, 2012, http://www.healthbeatblog.com/2012/09/the-third-rail-of-payment-reform-tackling-wide-variations-in-how-much-providers-charge/#sthash.kr6aMA5R.pdf.

[31]Joseph Neff, Ames Alexander, and Karen Garloch, "Prognosis Profits: North Carolina's Urban Hospitals Pile Up the Cash," *News Observer,* April 22, 2012, http://www.newsobserver.com/news/special-reports/prognosis-profits/article16924640.html.

[32]Mahar, "The Third Rail of Payment Reform" (quoting Anna Mathews, "Same Doctor Visit, Double the Cost," *Wall Street Journal*, August 26, 2012).

## PART 2

[1]Sean P. Keehan, Devin A. Stone, John A. Poisal, et al., "National Health Expenditure Projections, 2016–25: Price Increases, Aging Push Sector to 20 Percent of Economy," *Health Affairs* 36, no.3 (2017): 553–63.

## CHAPTER 15

[1]The Pew Charitable Trusts, "Household Expenditures and Income," March 30, 2016, http://www.pewtrusts.org/en/research-and-analysis/issue-briefs/2016/03/household-expenditures-and-income. See also U.S. Department of Labor, Bureau of Labor Statistics, *Consumer Expenditures—2012,* September 10, 2013, http://www.bls.gov/news.release/cesan.nr0.htm.

[2]Dan Munro, "Top Ten Healthcare Quotes for 2012," *Forbes.com,* December 23, 2012, http://www.forbes.com/sites/danmunro/2012/12/23/top-ten-healthcare-quotes-for-2012-2/.

[3]Ibid.

[4]The Henry J. Kaiser Family Foundation, *2014 Employer Health Benefits Survey,* September 10, 2014, http://kff.org/report-section/ehbs-2014-summary-of-findings/.

[5]Kevin F. Hallock, "The Relationship between Company Size and CEO Pay," *WorkSpan,* February 2011, https://author.ilr.cornell.edu/ICS/InsightsAndConvenings/upload/02-11-Research-for-the-real-world.pdf; Kevin F. Hallock and Linda Barrington, "A Look at CEO Pay," The GailFosler Group, December 9, 2010, http://www.gailfosler.com/a-look-at-ceo-pay.

[6]Nicholas D. Kristof, "The Wrong Side of History," *New York Times,* November 18, 2009, http://www.nytimes.com/2009/11/19/opinion/19kristof.html?_r=0.

[7]David A. Hyman, *Medicare Meets Mephistopheles* (Washington: Cato Institute, 2006).

[8]Martin S. Feldstein, "The Rising Price of Physicians' Services," *Review of Economics and Statistics* 52, no. 2, (1970): 121–33, http://www.jstor.org/stable/1926113?seq=1#page_scan_tab_contents.

[9]Michael A. Morrisey, *Health Insurance* (Chicago: Health Administration Press, 2008).

[10]Feldstein, "The Rising Price of Physicians' Services."

[11]Martin S. Feldstein, *The Rising Cost of Hospital Care,* National Center for Health Services Research and Development (Washington: Information Resources Press, 1971). See also Martin Feldstein and Bernard Friedman, "Tax Subsidies, the Rational Demand for Insurance, and the Health Care Crisis," *Journal of Public Economics* 7, no. 2 (1977): 155–78.

[12]Ibid.

[13]Amy N. Finkelstein, "The Aggregate Effects of Health Insurance: Evidence from the Introduction of Medicare," *Quarterly Journal of Economics* 122, no. 1 (2007): 1–37.

[14]Blue Cross Blue Shield, "Report Finds Significant Cost Variations in Knee and Hip Replacement Procedures across the U.S.," https://www.bcbs.com/learn/bcbs-blog/report-finds-significant-cost-variations-knee-and-hip-replacement-procedures-across.

[15]"Australian Medical Association Criticises Proposal for Up-Front General Practitioner Fee," *ABCNews* Australia, December 29, 2013, http://www.abc.net .au/news/2013-12-29/ama-criticises-proposals-for-new-gp-fee/5177522.

[16]For a survey of the studies that presents a decidedly more optimistic assessment of the connection between insurance and health than we do, see Benjamin D. Sommers, Atul A. Gawande, and Katherine Baicker, "Health Insurance Coverage and Health—What the Recent Evidence Tells Us," *New England Journal of Medicine* 377 (August 10, 2017): 586–93, http://www.nejm.org/doi/full/10.1056/ NEJMsb1706645#t=article.

[17]Katherine Baicker, Sarah L. Taubman, Heidi L. Allen, et al., "The Oregon Experiment—Effects of Medicaid on Clinical Outcomes," *New England Journal of Medicine* 368, no. 18 (2013): 1713–22, http://www.nejm.org/doi/full/10.1056/ NEJMsa1212321#t=article. An article appeared the year before in an economics journal: Amy N. Finkelstein, Sarah Taubman, Bill Wright, et al., "The Oregon Health Insurance Experiment: Evidence from the First Year," *Quarterly Journal of Economics* 127, no. 3 (2012): 1057–106, https://academic.oup.com/qje/article-abstract/127/3/1057/1923446?redirectedFrom=PDF.

[18]Sarah L. Taubman, Heidi L. Allen, Bill J. Wright, et al., "Medicaid Increases Emergency-Department Use: Evidence from Oregon's Health Insurance Experiment Science," *Science* 343, no. 6168 (2014): 263–68, http://science.sciencemag .org/content/343/6168/263.

[19]Amy N. Finkelstein, Sarah L. Taubman, Heidi L. Allen, et al., "Effect of Medicaid Coverage on ED Use—Further Evidence from Oregon's Experiment," *New England Journal of Medicine* 375, no. 16 (2016): 1505–07, doi:10.1056/ NEJMp1609533.

[20]Frank R. Lichtenberg, "The Effects of Medicare on Health Care Utilization and Outcomes," in *Frontiers in Health Policy Research,* vol. 5, ed. Alan M. Garber (Cambridge: MIT Press, 2002), pp. 27–52, http://www.nber.org/chapters/c9857 .pdf.

[21]Martin S. Feldstein, "The Welfare Loss of Excess Health Insurance," *Journal of Political Economy* 81, no. 2 (1973): 251–80.

[22]U.S. Department of Commerce, U.S. Census Bureau, "Table HIB-1. Health Insurance Coverage Status and Type of Coverage by Sex, Race and Hispanic Origin: 1999 to 2012," http://www.census.gov/data/tables/time-series/demo/ health-insurance/historical-series/hib.html.

[23]U.S. Department of Commerce, U.S. Census Bureau, "Current Population Survey, 1988 to 2013 Annual Social and Economic Supplements," https://www .census.gov/prod/techdoc/cps/cpsmar13.pdf.

[24]Ibid.

[25]Centers for Medicare and Medicaid Services, Office of the Actuary, National Health Statistics Group; U.S. Department of Commerce, Bureau of

Economic Analysis; and U.S. Bureau of the Census, "National Health Expenditures; Aggregate and Per Capita Amounts, Annual Percent Change and Percent Distribution: Selected Calendar Years 1960-2011," 2011.

[26]Alexander J. Ryu, Teresa B. Gibson, M. Richard McKellar, and Michael E. Chernew, "The Slowdown in Health Care Spending in 2009–11 Reflected Factors Other than the Weak Economy and Thus May Persist," *Health Affairs* 32, no.5 (2013): 835–40.

[27]Jeff Overley, "ACA Sign-Ups Hit 8M in Win for Health Care Industry," *Law360.com*, April 22, 2014, http://www.law360.com/articles/528830/aca-sign -ups-hit-8m-in-win-for-health-care-industry.

[28]Robert Pear, "Health Insurance Companies Seek Big Rate Increases for 2016," *New York Times,* July 3, 2015, http://www.nytimes.com/2015/07/04/us/ health-insurance-companies-seek-big-rate-increases-for-2016.html?emc=edit_ th_20150704&nl=todaysheadlines&nlid=15782921.

[29]Brian Blase, "Medicaid Not Big Enough? Obama Administration Proposes $100 Billion More Spending," *Forbes.com*, April 4, 2016, http://www.forbes.com/ sites/theapothecary/2016/04/04/medicaid-not-big-enough-obama-administration- proposes-100-billion-more-spending/#3046fc741e0f.

[30]Caroline Humer and Rodrigo Campos, "Trump Says Pharma 'Getting Away with Murder,' Stocks Slide," *Reuters,* January 22, 2017, https://www.reuters .com/article/us-usa-trump-drugpricing/trump-says-pharma-getting away- with-murder-stocks-slide-idUSKBN14V24J.

[31]David Besanko, David Dranove, and Craig Garthwaite, "Insurance and the High Prices of Pharmaceuticals," NBER Working Paper no. 22353, National Bureau of Economic Research, June 2016.

[32]Ibid., p. 31.

[33]Wayne Winegarden, "The Economic Costs of Pharmacy Benefit Managers: A Review of the Literature," Pacific Reasearch Institute, 2017, http://www pacificresearch.org/wp-content/uploads/2017/06/PBM_Lit_Final.pdf.

[34]Julie Appleby, "Filling a Prescription? You Might Be Better off Paying Cash," *CNN*, June 23, 2016, http://www.cnn.com/2016/06/23/health/prescription- drug-prices-pbm/index.html.

## CHAPTER 16

[1]American Medical Association, "AMA Urges Members of Congress to Oppose AHCA," March 22, 2017, https://www.ama-assn.org/ama-urges- members-congress-oppose-ahca; Sy Mukherjee, "These 3 Powerful Groups Are Slamming the GOP's Obamacare Replacement Plan," *Fortune*, March 8, 2017, http://fortune.com/2017/03/08/gop-healthcare-plan-aarp-ama-aha/; American Academy of Pediatrics, "AAP Statement Opposing House Passage of American

Health Care Act," May 4, 2017, https://www.aap.org/en-us/about-the-aap/aap-press-room/Pages/AHCAHousePassage.aspx; Mary Norine Walsh, "Cardiology Societies React to AHCA Bill," *Cardiology Today*, May 4, 2017, https://www.healio.com/cardiology/practice-management/news/online/%7Ba1296b1a-ba49-4b6e-9f00-5eb33f06691a%7D/cardiology-societies-react-to-ahca-bill; American Nurses Association, "American Nurses Association Strongly Opposes New Health Care Reform Bill," March 8, 2017, http://www.nursingworld.org/FunctionalMenuCategories/MediaResources/PressReleases/ANA-Strongly-Opposes-New-Health-Care-Reform-Bill.html.

[2]A typical mainstream critique appears in Matthew Fiedler, Henry J. Aaron, Loren Adler, and Paul B. Ginsburg, "Moving in the Wrong Direction—Health Care under the AHCA," *New England Journal of Medicine* 376 (2017): 2405–07, doi:10.1056/NEJMp1706848.

[3]Michael F. Cannon, "The House GOP Leadership's Health Care Bill Is ObamaCare-Lite—Or Worse," *Cato At Liberty* (blog), March 7, 2017, https://www.cato.org/blog/house-gop-leaderships-health-care-bill-obamacare-lite-or-worse.

[4]Ashley Kirzinger, Bryan Wu, and Mollyann Brodie, "Kaiser Health Tracking Poll: Health Care Priorities for 2017," Kaiser Family Foundation, January 6, 2017, http://www.kff.org/health-costs/poll-finding/kaiser-health-tracking-poll-health-care-priorities-for-2017/.

[5]"Tax Expenditures," in "Some Background," chap. 2 in *Tax Policy Center's Briefing Book*, http://www.taxpolicycenter.org/briefing-book/what-are-largest-tax-expenditures. See also U.S. Department of Treasury, *Tax Expenditures* (FY2016), https://www.treasury.gov/resource-center/tax-policy/Documents/Tax-Expenditures-FY2016.pdf; Committee for a Responsible Federal Budget, "The Tax Break-Down: Cafeteria Plans and Flexible Spending Accounts," September 12, 2013, http://crfb.org/blogs/tax-break-down-cafeteria-plans-and-flexible-spending-accounts.

[6]Bruce Bartlett, "Taxing Medicare Benefits," *New York Times*, September 17, 2013, http://economix.blogs.nytimes.com/2013/09/17/taxing-medicare-benefits/?_r=0.

[7]Ibid. See also *Bad Breaks All Around: The Report of The Century Foundation Working Group on Tax Expenditures* (New York: The Century Foundation Press, 2002), https://s3-us-west-2.amazonaws.com/production.tcf.org/app/uploads/2002/09/01153641/20020901-bad-breaks-all-around-8.pdf.

[8]Martin Feldstein and Bernard Friedman, "Tax Subsidies, the Rational Demand for Insurance, and the Health Care Crisis," *Journal of Public Economics* 7, no. 2 (1977): 155–78.

[9]Cannon, "ObamaCare-Lite—Or Worse."

[10]Eric Bradner, "Democrats' Medicare-for-All Litmus Test," *CNN.com*, April 3, 2017, http://www.cnn.com/2017/04/03/politics/medicare-for-all-democrats-bernie-sanders/index.html; Alexander Burns and Jennifer Medina, "The Single-Payer Party? Democrats Shift Left on Health Care," *New York Times*, June 3, 2017, https://www.nytimes.com/2017/06/03/us/democrats-universal-health-care-single-payer-party.html?emc=edit_th_20170604&nl=todaysheadlines&nlid=15782921&_r=0.

[11]Kristen Bialik, "More Americans Say Government Should Ensure Health Care Coverage," Pew Research Center, January 3, 2017, http://www.pewresearch.org/fact-tank/2017/01/13/more-americans-say-government-should-ensure-health-care-coverage/.

[12]Joseph Wood, "Insurance Is Not the Problem. It's Also Not the Solution," *The Health Care Blog*, March 16, 2017, http://thehealthcareblog.com/blog/2017/03/16/theyllnevercare-insurance-is-not-the-problem-its-also-not-the-solution/.

[13]Bernie Sanders, "Medicare-for-All: Leaving No One Behind," *BernieSanders.com*, https://berniesanders.com/issues/medicare-for-all/.

[14]Elisabeth Rosenthal, "As Hospital Prices Soar, a Stitch Tops $500," *New York Times*, December 2, 2013, sec. Health, http://www.nytimes.com/2013/12/03/health/as-hospital-costs-soar-single-stitch-tops-500.html.

[15]Diane Archer, "Medicare Is More Efficient Than Private Insurance," *Health Affairs Blog*, September 20, 2011, http://healthaffairs.org/blog/2011/09/20/medicare-is-more-efficient-than-private-insurance/.

[16]"Total Number of Medicare Beneficiaries," *Kaiser Family Foundation*, https://www.kff.org/medicare/state-indicator/total-medicare-beneficiaries/?currentTimeframe=0&sortModel=%7B%22colId%22:%22Location%22,%22sort%22:%22asc%22%7D.

[17]Robert A. Book, "Medicare Administrative Costs Are Higher, Not Lower, Than for Private Insurance," *The Heritage Foundation*, June 25, 2009, http://www.heritage.org/health-care-reform/report/medicare-administrative-costs-are-higher-not-lower-private-insurance.

[18]Ibid.

[19]Robert Book, "Medicare-For-All Would Increase, Not Save, Administrative Costs," *Forbes*, September 20, 2017, https://www.forbes.com/sites/theapothecary/2017/09/20/medicare-for-all-would-increase-not-save-administrative-costs/#2f73830f60ba.

[20]Ibid.

[21]Sanders, "Medicare-for-All."

[22]Ibid.

[23]Martin S. Feldstein, "Why Is Growth Better in the United States Than in Other Industrial Countries," NBER Working Paper no. 23221, National Bureau of Economic Research, March 2017, http://www.nber.org/papers/w23221.

[24]David Squires and Chloe Anderson, "U.S. Health Care from a Global Perspective: Spending, Use of Services, Prices, and Health in 13 Countries," *Commonwealth Fund*, October 2015, http://www.commonwealthfund.org/~/media/files/publications/issue-brief/2015/oct/1819_squires_us_hlt_care_global_perspective_oecd_intl_brief_v3.pdf.

[25]Sanders, "Medicare-for-All."

[26]Centers for Medicare and Medicaid Services, *National Health Expenditure Data*, https://www.cms.gov/Research-Statistics-Data-and-Systems/Statistics-Trends-and-Reports/NationalHealthExpendData/NationalHealthAccountsHistorical.html.

[27]Jonathan Chait, "Obama's Agenda and the Deficit," *New Republic*, July 18, 2010, https://newrepublic.com/article/76344/the-future-the-obama-agenda.

[28]Ezra Klein, "Cost Control and the ACA," *Washington Post*, July 19, 2010, http://voices.washingtonpost.com/ezra-klein/2010/07/cost_control_and_the_aca.html.

[29]John Holahan, Lisa Clemans-Cope, Matthew Buettgens, et al., "The Sanders Single-Payer Health Care Plan: The Effect on National Health Expenditures and Federal and Private Spending," *The Urban Institute*, May 2016, http://www.urban.org/sites/default/files/publication/80486/200785-The-Sanders-Single-Payer-Health-Care-Plan.pdf.

[30]Michael Tanner, "Embracing the Hard Realities of Health-Care Reform," *National Review*, June 7, 2017, http://www.nationalreview.com/article/448350/health-care-reform-reality-check-single-payer-model-economically-ruinous.

[31]Holahan et al., "The Sanders Single-Payer Health Care Plan."

[32]Chris Conover, "Why Bernie Sanders' Health Plan Will Cost at Least 40% More Than Advertised," *Forbes.com*, January 20, 2016, https://www.forbes.com/sites/theapothecary/2016/01/20/why-bernie-sanders-health-plan-will-cost-at-least-40-more-than-advertised/#33c90ba14426.

[33]Alan Cole and Scott Greenberg, "Details and Analysis of Senator Bernie Sanders's Tax Plan," *The Tax Foundation*, January 28, 2016, https://taxfoundation.org/details-and-analysis-senator-bernie-sanders-s-tax-plan/.

[34]Danielle Kurtzleben, "Study: Sanders' Proposals Would Add $18 Trillion to Debt over 10 Years," *NPR.org*, May 9, 2016, http://www.npr.org/2016/05/09/477402982/study-sanders-proposals-would-add-18-trillion-to-debt-over-10-years.

## CHAPTER 17

[1]Barbara Hijek, "Meet Dr. Stein, the Big Daddy of Vasectomies," *Sun Sentinel*, June 6, 2009, http://www.sun-sentinel.com/sfl-mtblog-2009-06-meet_the_big_daddy_of_vasectom_1-story.html; *VasWeb*, "Vasectomy & Reversal Centers of Florida," http://www.vasweb.com.

[2]Heather Sullivan, "Vasectomy Madness: Procedures Rise during March Madness," *NBC12*, March 12, 2012, http://www.nbc12.com/story/17138054/vasectomy-madness-procedures-rise-during-march-madness.

[3]Lindley Estates, "Va. Doctor Running Vasectomy Special Ahead of March Madness," *Free Lance-Star*, March 16, 2016, http://www.richmond.com/news/virginia/va-doctor-running-vasectomy-special-ahead-of-march-madness/article_fe711d0b-f39c-5553-8e01-15947bddcbad.html.

[4]*VasWeb*, "Fees," http://www.vasweb.com/vasectomy.html#Fees.

[5]David A. Hyman and Charles Silver, "Just What the Patient Ordered: The Case for Result-Based Compensation Arrangements," *Journal of Law, Medicine & Ethics* 29, no. 2 (2001): 170–73.

[6]*Missbutterbean*, "2017 Cost of Flu Shots: CVS, Walgreens, Rite Aid, Walmart, Costco, Sam's Club, & More," January 13, 2017, http://www.missbutterbean.com/2017-flu-shots/; G.E. Miller, "Where to Get Free or the Cheapest Flu Shots," *20 Something Finance*, January 1, 2015, http://20somethingfinance.com/where-to-get-cheap-or-free-flu-shots/.

[7]*Ariba Medical Spa*, "Services We Offer," http://www.aribamedicalspa.com/#!services/c14e8.

[8]Lou Carlozo, "How Much Does a Vasectomy Cost? Part 1: From $300 to $3,500 Plus," *Clear Health Costs*, December 21, 2012, https://clearhealthcosts.com/blog/2012/12/how-much-does-a-vasectomy-cost-from-300-to-3500-plus/.

[9]*CG Cosmetic Surgery*, "Miami Summer Sale on Breast Implants," February 26, 2011, https://www.cgcosmetic.com/blog/2011/02/26/summer-sale-breast-implants/.

[10]*Westlake Plastic Surgery*, "Breast Augmentation Special," https://westlakeplasticsurgery.com/breast-augmentation-special?lmc_track=5123776186.

[11]Liz Segre, "Lasik Eye Surgery Cost," *AllAboutVision.com*, July 27, 2017, http://www.allaboutvision.com/visionsurgery/cost.htm; *QualSight*, "LASIK Cost—How Much Is LASIK," https://www.qualsight.com/how-much-is-lasik; Anna Helhoski, "How Much Does Lasik Cost?," *NerdWallet.com*, February 18, 2015, http://www.nerdwallet.com/blog/health/healthcare-price-transparency/how-much-does-lasik-cost/.

[12]Ha T. Tu and Jessica H. May, "Self-Pay Markets in Health Care: Consumer Nirvana or Caveat Emptor?," *Health Affairs* 26, no. 2 (2007): w217–w226, doi:10.1377/hlthaff.26.2.w217.

[13]Devon Herrick, "The Market for Medical Care Should Work Like Cosmetic Surgery," National Center for Policy Analysis, May 21, 2013, http://www.ncpa.org/pub/st349.

[14]To his credit, Ezekiel Emanuel makes testable predictions about the impact of the ACA, one of which is that the prices commercial insurers pay for CT scans and MRIs "should decline by 25% to 50% by 2020." Ezekiel Emanuel, *Reinventing American Health Care* (New York: PublicAffairs, 2014), p. 301.

[15]Devon Herrick, "Why Can't the Market for Medical Care Work Like Cosmetic Surgery?" National Center for Policy Analysis, June 17, 2013, http://healthblog.ncpa.org/why-cant-the-market-for-medical-care-work-like-cosmetic-surgery/.

[16]Devon M. Herrick, "The Market for Medical Care Should Work Like Cosmetic Surgery," National Center for Policy Analysis, Policy Report no. 349, May 2013, http://www.ncpa.org/pdfs/st349.pdf.

[17]Iva Roze Skoch, "Why Is IVF So Expensive in the United States?," *Newsweek*, July 21, 2010, http://www.newsweek.com/why-ivf-so-expensive-united-states-74385.

[18]"Missouri, Women Under 35; Best IVF Clinics in Missouri for Women Under 35 Using Fresh Embryos," *FertilitySuccessRates.com*, https://fertilitysuccessrates.com/report/Missouri/women-under-35/data.html.

[19]"Treatment Costs: MCRM Dispels the Myths of IVF Costs," *MCRM Fertility*, http://www.mcrmfertility.com/new-patients/treatment-costs.aspx (visited December 7, 2016).

[20]"Cost Comparison: National Cycle Costs vs. WINFertility's Treatment Bundle," *WINFertility*, http://www.winfertility.com/how-we-are-different/ivf-cost-comparison/.

[21]Marshall Allen, "A Hospital Charged $1,877 to Pierce a 5-Year-Old's Ears. This Is Why Health Care Costs So Much," *ProPublica*, November 28, 2017, https://www.propublica.org/article/a-hospital-charged-to-pierce-ears-why-health-care-costs-so-much?utm_campaign=KHN%3A%20First%20Edition&%E2%80%A6.

[22]Sarah Kliff, "A Woman Had a Baby. Then Her Hospital Charged Her $39.95 to Hold It," *Vox,* October 4, 2016, https://www.vox.com/2016/10/4/13160624/medical-bills-birth-delivery.

[23]Dylan Stableford, "Snakebite Victim Charged $89,000 for 18-Hour Hospital Stay," *Yahoo News*, January 28, 2014, http://news.yahoo.com/snake-bite-89000-162515519.html.

[24]Elisabeth Rosenthal, "As Hospital Prices Soar, a Stitch Tops $500," *New York Times*, December 2, 2013, sec. Health, http://www.nytimes.com/2013/12/03/health/as-hospital-costs-soar-single-stitch-tops-500.html.

[25]Steven Brill and Brady McCombs, "Bitter Pill: Why Medical Bills Are Killing Us," *Time*, April 4, 2013, http://time.com/198/bitter-pill-why-medical-bills-are-killing-us/.

[26]Nina Bernstein, "How to Charge $546 for Six Liters of Saltwater," *New York Times*, August 25, 2013, http://www.nytimes.com/2013/08/27/health/exploring-salines-secret-costs.html.

[27]Jim Landers, "DMN Reporter Got His Knees Replaced—but Was the Stiff Price a Good Deal?," *Dallas Morning News*, July 16, 2015, https://www.dallasnews.com/business/health-care/2015/07/16/dmn-reporter-got-his-knees-replaced—but-was-the-stiff-price-a-good-deal.

[28]Ge Bai and Gerard F. Anderson, "Extreme Markup: The Fifty US Hospitals with the Highest Charge-to-Cost Ratios," *Health Affairs* 34, no. 6 (2015): 922–28, https://www.healthaffairs.org/doi/abs/10.1377/hlthaff.2014.1414.

[29]Brill and McCombs, "Bitter Pill."

[30]*ScriptSave WellRx*, "Compare Pharmacy Prescription Drug Prices," https://www.wellrx.com/prescriptions.

[31]Tricia Romano, "The Hunt for an Affordable Hearing Aid," *New York Times*, October 22, 2013, http://well.blogs.nytimes.com/2012/10/22/the-hunt-for-an-affordable-hearing-aid/.

[32]Andis Robeznieks, "Retailers Making Big Push into Healthcare," *Modern Healthcare*, May 4, 2014, http://www.modernhealthcare.com/article/20130504/MAGAZINE/305049991.

[33]Susan Thurston, "More Adults Getting Flu Shots at Their Local Pharmacy or Retail Outlet," *Tampa Bay Times*, October 13, 2012, http://www.tampabay.com/news/business/retail/more-adults-getting-flu-shots-at-their-local-pharmacy-or-retail-outlet/1256143.

[34]Ibid.

[35]Christopher Cheney, "Behind the CVS Health Rebranding Strategy," *HealthLeaders Media*, September 8, 2014, http://healthleadersmedia.com/page-1/led-308131/Behind-the-CVS-Health-Rebranding-Strategy##; Christopher Cheney, "CVS Ramps Up Retail Clinics with Provider Affiliations," *Health-Leaders Media*, July 22, 2014, http://healthleadersmedia.com/content.cfm?content_id=306633&page=1&topic=QUA; Ayla Ellison, "CVS vs. Walgreens, Who Wins the Healthcare Collaboration Battle?," *Becker Hospital Review*, August 28, 2014, http://www.beckershospitalreview.com/hospital-transactions-and-valuation/cvs-vs-walgreens-who-wins-the-healthcare-collaboration-battle.html; Hiroko Tabuchi, "How CVS Quit Smoking and Grew into a Health Care Giant," *New York Times*, July 11, 2015, http://www.nytimes.com/2015/07/12/business/how-cvs-quit-smoking-and-grew-into-a-health-care-giant.html?_r=0.

[36]John Commins, "CVS Health Posts Strong Retail, Omnicare Outlook," *HealthLeaders Media*, February 10, 2016, http://www.healthleadersmedia.com/health-plans/cvs-health-posts-strong-retail-omnicare-outlook.

[37]"IBM Watson, CVS Deal: IBM and CVS Partner to Predict Patient Health," *HNGN.com*, July 31, 2015, http://www.hngn.com/articles/114717/20150731/ibm-watson-cvs-deal-partners-predict-patient-health.htm.

[38]*CVSHealth*, "CVS Health and IBM Tap Watson to Develop Care Management Solutions for Chronic Disease," July 30, 2015, https://cvshealth.com/newsroom/press-releases/cvs-health-and-ibm-tap-watson-develop-care-management-solutions-chronic-disease.

[39]Charles Duhigg, "How Companies Learn Your Secrets," *New York Times*, February 15, 2012, http://www.nytimes.com/2012/02/19/magazine/shopping-habits.html?pagewanted=1&_r=1&hp.

[40]Ibid.

[41]Sheryl Kraft, "How Health Care Will Look with a Physician Shortage," *Chicago Tribune*, November 4, 2015, http://www.chicagotribune.com/lifestyles/health/scdoctorshortagehealth111120151105story.html.

[42]John Commins, "Doctors in Demand: New Physicians Flooded with Job Offers," *HealthLeaders Media*, September 19, 2017, http://www.healthleadersmedia.com/physician-leaders/doctors-demand-new-physicians-flooded-job-offers?spMailingID=11954869&spUserID=MTY3ODg4NjI3Mjk1S0&spJobID=1241608301&spReportId=MTI0MTYwODMwMQS2#.

[43]Jenny Gold, "In Cities, the Average Doctor Wait-Time Is 18.5 Days," *Washington Post*, January 29, 2014, http://www.washingtonpost.com/news/wonkblog/wp/2014/01/29/in-cities-the-average-doctor-wait-time-is-18-5-days/.

[44]Ibid.

[45]"Retail Health Clinics: State Legislation and Laws," National Conference of State Legislatures, November 2014, http://www.ncsl.org/research/health/retail-health-clinics-state-legislation-and-laws.aspx.

[46]"AMA Calls for Investigation of Retail Health Clinics," *Medical News Today*, June 26, 2007, http://www.medicalnewstoday.com/articles/75308.php.

[47]"AMA Lays Down Guidelines for Retail Clinics," *Managed Care Magazine Online*, July 1, 2006, accessed August 24, 2015, http://www.managedcaremag.com/archives/0607/0607.news_retailclinics.html. For a list of regulations enacted by state, see "Retail Clinics: State Legislation and Laws," National Conference of State Legislatures, January 1, 2016.

[48]For an example, see Hilary Daniel and Shari Erickson for the Medical Practice and Quality Committee of the American College of Physicians, "Retail Health Clinics: Executive Summary of a Policy Position Paper from the American College of Physicians," *Annals of Internal Medicine* 163, no. 11 (2015): 869–70. doi:10.7326/M15-0571.

[49]Lydia DePillis, "In a Fight between Nurses and Doctors, the Nurses Are Slowly Winning," *Washington Post*, March 18, 2016, https://www.washingtonpost.com/news/wonk/wp/2016/03/18/in-a-fight-between-nurses-and-doctors-the-nurses-are-slowly-winning/?utm_term=.cec3fa8815fb.

[50]Ryan Basen, "AMA Does Not Want PA Autonomy," *MedPage Today*, June 15, 2017, https://www.medpagetoday.com/meetingcoverage/ama/66039.

[51]Lara C. Pullen, "AMA Does Not Want Pharmacists to Prescribe Medication," *Medscape*, June 22, 2012, http://www.medscape.com/viewarticle/766252.

[52]"Health Care on Aisle 7: The Growing Phenomenon of Retail Clinics," RAND Health, no. RB-9491-1, 2010.

[53]Benjamin J. McMichael, "Occupational Licensing and Legal Liability: The Effect of Regulation and Litigation on Nurse Practitioners, Physician Assistants, and the Healthcare System," PhD Disseration, Graduate School of Vanderbilt University, May 2015, https://law.vanderbilt.edu/phd/students/files/McMichael.pdf.

[54]Andis Robeznieks, "Retailers Making Big Push into Healthcare," *Modern Healthcare*, May 4, 2014, http://www.modernhealthcare.com/article/20130504/MAGAZINE/305049991.

[55]Sarah Wickline Wallan, "ACP: Retail Clinics Need Scope of Practice Limits," *MedPage Today*, October 15, 2015, https://www.medpagetoday.com/primarycare/generalprimarycare/54114; Catharine Paddock, "AMA Calls for Investigation of Retail Health Clinics," *Medical News Today*, June 26, 2007, http://www.medicalnewstoday.com/articles/75308.php.

[56]James D. Woodburn, Kevin L. Smith, and Glen D. Nelson, "Quality of Care in the Retail Health Care Setting Using National Clinical Guidelines for Acute Pharyngitis," *American Journal of Medical Quality* 22, no. 6 (2007): 457–62, doi:10.1177/1062860607309626.

[57]Richard Jacoby, Albert G. Crawford, Paresh Chaudhari, and Neil I. Goldfarb, "Quality of Care for 2 Common Pediatric Conditions Treated by Convenient Care Providers," *American Journal of Medical Quality* 26, no. 1 (February 2011): 53–58, doi:10.1177/1062860610375106.

[58]Andrew Sussman, Lisette Dunham, Kristen Snower, et al., "Retail Clinic Utilization Associated with Lower Total Cost of Care," *American Journal of Managed Care* 19, no. 4 (April 2013): e148–157, http://www.ajmc.com/journals/issue/2013/2013-1-vol19-n4/retail-clinic-utilization-associated-with-lower-total-cost-of-care.

[59]Gardiner Harris, "When the Nurse Wants to Be Called 'Doctor,'" *New York Times*, October 1, 2011, http://www.nytimes.com/2011/10/02/health/policy/02docs.html.

[60]Ateev Mehrotra, Hangsheng Liu, John L. Adams, et al., "Comparing Costs and Quality of Care at Retail Clinics with That of Other Medical Settings for 3 Common Illnesses," *Annals of Internal Medicine* 151, no. 5 (September 1, 2009): 321–28, http://annals.org/aim/article-abstract/744702/comparing-costs-quality-care-retail-clinics-other-medical-settings-3.

[61]Lisa Girion, "Doctors' List Puts a Price on Care," *Los Angeles Times,* May 28, 2007, http://articles.latimes.com/2007/may/28/business/fi-prices28.

[62]Jim Epstein, "Oklahoma Doctors vs. Obamacare," *Reason.com*, November 15, 2012, http://reason.com/reasontv/2012/11/15/the-obamacare-revolt-oklahoma-doctors-fi.

[63]Ibid.

[64]Ibid.

[65]Chad Terhune, "Many Hospitals, Doctors Offer Cash Discount for Medical Bills," *Los Angeles Times*, May 27, 2012, accessed August 25, 2015, http://articles.latimes.com/2012/may/27/business/la-fi-medical-prices-20120527.

[66]Melinda Beck, "How to Cut Your Health-Care Bill: Pay Cash," *Wall Street Journal*, February 15, 2016, http://www.wsj.com/articles/how-to-cut-your-health-care-bill-pay-cash-1455592277.

[67]David Belk, "Are You Paying Way Too Much for Your Medications?" *Huffington Post*, December 14, 2013, https://www.huffingtonpost.com/david-belk/health-care-costs_b_4066552.html.

[68]David Belk, "Medications: What Your Pharmacist Won't Tell You," *True Cost of Healthcare* (blog), 2016, http://truecostofhealthcare.org/medications/.

[69]Charles Ornstein and Katie Thomas, "Prescription Drugs May Cost More with Insurance than without It," *New York Times*, December 9, 2017, https://www.nytimes.com/2017/12/09/health/drug-prices-generics-insurance.html?emc=edit_th_20171210&nl=todaysheadlines&nlid=15782921&_r=1.

[70]Shannon Brownlee, "CVS Clinics Hurt America's Health Care," *Providence Journal*, September 17, 2014, http://www.providencejournal.com/article/20140917/OPINION/309179890.

[71]Kimberly Lankford, "Pay Cash for Your Health Care," *Kiplinger's Personal Finance*, February 2015, http://www.kiplinger.com/article/insurance/T027-C000-S002-pay-cash-for-your-health-care.html#JZUq2QCPKmq3V9e0.99.

[72]Ibid.

[73]Steve Hargreaves, "Cash-Only Doctors Abandon the Insurance System," *CNN.com*, June 11, 2013, http://money.cnn.com/2013/06/11/news/economy/cash-only-doctors/.

[74]Ibid.

[75]Ibid.

[76]Alex Nixon, "Doctors Flock to Concierge Practices: 'The Downside Is It Costs Extra Money, So It's Not for Everyone...,'" *Concierge Medicine Today*, February 3, 2014, http://conciergemedicinetoday.org/2014/02/03/doctors-flock-to-concierge-practices-the-downside-is-it-costs-extra-money-so-its-not-for-everyone/.

[77]Steve Hargreaves, "Cash-Only Doctors Abandon the Insurance System," *CNNMoney*, June 11, 2013, http://money.cnn.com/2013/06/11/news/economy/cash-only-doctors/index.html.

[78]Nancy Baum, "Physician Ownership in Hospitals and Outpatient Facilities," *Center for Healthcare Research and Transformation,* 2013, http://www.chrt.org/document/physician-ownership-in-hospitals-and-outpatient-facilities/.

[79]Centers for Medicare and Medicaid Services, "Physician-Owned Hospitals," *CMS.gov,*https://www.cms.gov/medicare/fraud-and-abuse/physicianselfreferral/physician_owned_hospitals.html.

[80]Tanya Albert Henry, "Physician-Owned Hospitals Seize Their Moment," *Amednews.com,* April 29, 2013, http://www.amednews.com/article/20130429/government/130429948/4/.

[81]Ryan Marling, "How Amazon Can Position Itself as the Pharmacy of the Future," *The Health Care Blog,* June 7, 2017, http://thehealthcareblog.com/blog/2017/06/07/howamazoncanpositionitselfasthepharmacyofthefuture/.

[82]Art Carden, "What Would Louis XIV Have Paid for a Sonicare?," *Forbes.com,* May 26, 2011, reprinted at http://www.independent.org/newsroom/article.asp?id=3086.

[83]Phil Gramm, 142nd Cong. Rec. S9923 (September 5, 1996).

## CHAPTER 18

[1]Patients Beyond Borders, "Medical Tourism Statistics & Facts," http://www.patientsbeyondborders.com/medical-tourism-statistics-facts. Reliable figures on the size of the medical tourism market are hard to come by. Estimates of the number of travelers and the dollar value of the market vary greatly because data are incomplete or differing definitions of medical services are employed. See David Reisman, *Trade in Health: Economics, Ethics and Public Policy* (Cheltenham: Edward Elgar, 2014).

[2]Beth Howard, "Should You Have Surgery Abroad?," *AARP The Magazine,* November 2014, http://www.aarp.org/health/conditions-treatments/info-2014/medical-tourism-surgery-abroad.html.

[3]David Reisman, *Trade in Health: Economics, Ethics and Public Policy* (Cheltenham: Edward Elgar, 2014).

[4]*Patients Beyond Borders*, "Medical Tourism Statistics & Facts," http://www.patientsbeyondborders.com/medical-tourism-statistics-facts.

[5]Joanna Gaines and Duc B. Nguyen, "Medical Tourism," chap. 2(21) in *Centers for Disease Control and Prevention, Health Information for International Travel 2016* (New York: Oxford University Press, 2015), http://wwwnc.cdc.gov/travel/yellowbook/2016/the-pre-travel-consultation/medical-tourism.

[6]Joint Commission International, "Who Is JCI," http://www.jointcommissioninternational.org/about-jci/who-is-jci/, visited December 3, 2016.

[7]Ketaki Gokhale, "Heart Surgery in India for $1,583 Costs $106,385 in U.S.," *Bloomberg.com,* July 28, 2013, http://www.bloomberg.com/news/2013-07-28/heart-surgery-in-india-for-1-583-costs-106-385-in-u-s-.html.

[8]Ibid.

[9]J. Geeta Anand, "The Henry Ford of Heart Surgery," *Wall Street Journal*, November 25, 2009, http://www.wsj.com/articles/SB125875892887958111.

[10]Chris Morris, "'Production Line' Heart Surgery," *BBC News*, August 2, 2010, http://www.bbc.com/news/health-10837726.

[11]Tarun Khanna, V. Kasturi Rangan, and Merlina Manocaran, "Narayana Hrudayalaya Heart Hospital: Cardiac Care for the Poor (A)," *Harvard Business School Case 505-078*, June 2005 (revised August 2011), http://www.hbs.edu/faculty/Pages/item.aspx?num=32452.

[12]Devon M. Herrick, "Medical Tourism: Global Competition in Health Care, National Center for Policy Analysis," NCPA Policy Report no. 304, August 2007, www.ncpa.org/pub/st/st304.

[13]Ketaki Gokhale, "Heart Surgery in India for $1,583 Costs $106,385 in U.S.," *Bloomberg.com*, July 28, 2013, http://www.bloomberg.com/news/2013-07-28/heart-surgery-in-india-for-1-583-costs-106-385-in-u-s-.html.

[14]"Top 10 Procedures," *Narayana Health*, http://www.narayanahealth.org/top-10-procedures.

[15]Khanna, Rangan, and Manocaran, "Narayana Hrudayalaya Heart Hospital."

[16]Helen Nyambura-Mwaura and Samuel Gebre, "India Health-Care Providers Look to Tap Africa 'Growth Wave,'" *Bloomberg.com*, November 24, 2016, https://www.bloomberg.com/news/articles/2016-11-25/africans-seeking-health-care-in-india-draw-hospitals-to-kenya.

[17]Saritha Rai, "Indian Surgeon Known for Walmart-izing Heart Surgery Brings Affordable Healthcare Closer to Americans," *Forbes*, February 25, 2014, https://www.forbes.com/sites/saritharai/2014/02/25/indian-surgeon-known-for-walmart-izing-heart-surgery-brings-affordable-healthcare-closer-to-americans/#4164c40d4081.

[18]Nyambura-Mwaura and Gebre, "India Health-Care Providers."

[19]Khanna, Rangan, and Manocaran, "Narayana Hrudayalaya Heart Hospital."

[20]Nyambura-Mwaura and Gebre, "India Health-Care Providers."

[21]Khanna, Rangan, and Manocaran, "Narayana Hrudayalaya Heart Hospital."

[22]Adam Plowright, "Inside India's 'No-Frills' Hospitals, Where Heart Surgery Costs Just $800," *Business Insider*, April 21, 2013, http://www.businessinsider.com/inside-indias-no-frills-hospitals-where-heart-surgery-costs-just-800-2013-4; Joe Carter, "What India's $800 Heart Surgery Can Teach Us about Healthcare in the U.S.," *Acton Institute PowerBlog*, June 25, 2013, http://blog.acton.org/archives/56543-what-800-heart-surgery-can-teach-us-about-healthcare.html.

[23]Plowright, "Inside India's 'No-Frills' Hospitals."

[24]G. Ananthakrishnan, "Boom Time for Medicare," *Hindu*, April 30, 2006, http://www.hindu.com/thehindu/mag/2006/04/30/stories/2006043000010100.htm.

[25]Barak Richman, Krishna Udayakumar, Will Mitchell, and Kevin A. Schulman, "Lessons from India in Organizational Innovation: A Tale of Two Heart Hospitals," *Health Affairs* 27, no. 5 (2008): 1260–70, https://www.healthaffairs.org/doi/abs/10.1377/hlthaff.27.5.1260.

[26]Ibid.

[27]Ibid.

[28]Ibid.

[29]Deloitte Center for Health Solutions, "Medical Tourism Consumers in Search of Value Produced," 2008, http://www.academia.edu/9144718/Medical_Tourism_Consumers_in_Search_of_Value_Produced_by_the_Deloitte_Center_for_Health_Solutions.

[30]Reenita Das, "Medical Tourism Gets a Facelift ... and Perhaps a Pacemaker," *Forbes*, August 19, 2014, 2015, http://www.forbes.com/sites/reenitadas/2014/08/19/medical-tourism-gets-a-facelift-and-perhaps-a-pacemaker/; P. Keckley and H. Underwood, "Medical Tourism: Update and Implications," Deloitte Center for Health Solutions, 2009, http://www.coa.org/docs/deloitte-studymedicaltourism_111209_web.pdf.

[31]Astrid Galavan, "Facing Rising Dental Costs, Seniors Head to Mexico," *Associated Press*, August 9, 2015, http://www.businessinsider.com/ap-facing-rising-dental-costs-seniors-head-to-mexico-2015-8; Scott Carney, "Inside India's Rent-a-Womb Business," *Mother Jones*, April 2010, http://www.motherjones.com/politics/2010/02/surrogacy-tourism-india-nayna-patel; David M. Frankford, Linda K. Bennington, and Jane Greene Ryan, "Womb Outsourcing: Commercial Surrogacy in India," *MCN, The American Journal of Maternal/Child Nursing* 40, no. 5 (2015): 284–90; Johanna Hanefeld, Richard Smith, Daniel Horsfall, and Neil Lunt, "What Do We Know about Medical Tourism? A Review of the Literature with Discussion of Its Implications for the UK National Health Service as an Example of a Public Health Care System," *Journal of Travel Medicine* 21, no. 6 (December 2014): 410–17, https://academic.oup.com/jtm/article/21/6/410/1843042.

[32]David Reisman, *Trade in Health: Economics, Ethics and Public Policy* (Cheltenham: Edward Elgar, 2014).

[33]David A. Hyman and Charles Silver, "It Was on Fire When I Lay Down on It: Defensive Medicine, Tort Reform, and Healthcare Spending," in *The Oxford Handbook of U.S. Health Law*, ed. I. Glenn Cohen, Allison K. Hoffman, and William M. Sage (Oxford: Oxford University Press, 2017).

[34]Reisman, *Trade in Health*, p. 73.

[35]Ibid., p. 74.

[36]Elisabeth Rosenthal, "The Growing Popularity of Having Surgery Overseas," *New York Times*, August 6, 2013, http://www.nytimes.com/2013/08/07/us/the-growing-popularity-of-having-surgery-overseas.html.

[37]Bill Brody, "Nighthawks: Global Outsourcing Comes to Radiology," *Johns Hopkins Medicine, Crossroads*, September 9, 2004, http://www.hopkinsmedicine.org/about/Crossroads/09_09_04.html.

[38]Devon M. Herrick, "Medical Tourism: Global Competition in Health Care, National Center for Policy Analysis," NCPA Policy Report no. 304, August 2007, www.ncpa.org/pub/st/st304

[39]See John C. Goodman, "What Medical Tourism Tells Us about Our Healthcare System," *Beacon*, http://blog.independent.org/2013/05/08/what-medical-tourism-tells-us-about-our-healthcare-system/; Devon Herrick, "Medical Tourism: Have Insurance Card, Will Travel," National Center for Policy Analysis, September 22, 2010, http://www.ncpa.org/pub/ba724.

[40]C. Walters, "Get on a Plane, Go to Your Surgery," *Consumerist*, September 11, 2009, http://consumerist.com/2009/09/11/get-on-a-plane-go-to-your-surgery/; Joanne Wojcik, "Employers Consider Short-Haul Medical Tourism," *Business Insurance*, August 23, 2009, http://www.businessinsurance.com/article/20090823/ISSUE01/308239988.

[41]"Medical Tourism Takes a Domestic Twist," *Employee Benefit News*, August 30, 2015, http://ebn.benefitnews.com/news/medical-tourism-domestic-twist-2712341-1.html.

[42]Goodman, "What Medical Tourism Tells Us about Our Health Care System."

[43]"Domestic Medical Tourism Offers More Bang for Buck," *Healthcare Reform Magazine*, January 23, 2014, http://www.healthcarereformmagazine.com/us-domestic-medical-travel/domestic-medical-tourism-more-bang/.

[44]Bruce Einhorn, "Hannaford's Medical-Tourism Experiment," *Bloomberg Business*, November 9, 2008, http://www.bloomberg.com/bw/stories/2008-11-09/hannafords-medical-tourism-experimentbusinessweek-business-news-stock-market-and-financial-advice.

[45]M. P. McQueen, "Paying Workers to Go Abroad for Health Care," *Wall Street Journal*, September 30, 2008, sec. Business, http://www.wsj.com/news/articles/SB122273570173688551.

[46]Scott Hensley, "Medical Tourism Starts at Home," *WSJ Health Blog*, September 10, 2008, http://blogs.wsj.com/health/2008/09/10/medical-tourism-starts-at-home/; "Medical Tourism—Inside and Outside the US Creating Pricing Competition among Hospitals," *The Medical Quack*, November 24, 2009, http://ducknetweb.blogspot.com/2009/11/medical-tourism-inside-and-outside-us.html.

[47]John Goodman, "Employers Opt for Medical Tourism," *NCPA.org Health Policy Blog*, October 17, 2012, http://healthblog.ncpa.org/employers-opt-for-medical-tourism/.

[48]"Wal-Mart Offers No-Cost Heart, Spine, and Transplant Surgeries to Employees," *Massdevice*, October 12, 2012, http://www.massdevice.com/wal-mart-offers-no-cost-heart-spine-transplant-surgeries-employees/.

[49]David Reisman, *Trade in Health: Economics, Ethics and Public Policy* (Cheltenham: Edward Elgar, 2014).

[50]James C. Robinson and Timothy T. Brown, "Increases in Consumer Cost Sharing Redirect Patient Volumes and Reduce Hospital Prices for Orthopedic Surgery," *Health Affairs* 32, no. 8 (August 1, 2013): 1392–97, doi:10.1377/hlthaff.2013.0188.; "Stunning Results from California," *NCPA.org Health Policy Blog*, August 7, 2013, http://healthblog.ncpa.org/stunning-results-from-california/; James C. Robinson and Timothy T. Brown, "Changes in Patient Volumes, Allowed Charges, Consumer Cost Sharing, and CalPERS Payments for Orthopedic Surgery Associated with Reference Pricing," Berkeley Center for Health Technology, https://www.calpers.ca.gov/docs/board-agendas/201306/pension/item-7-attach-1.pdf.

[51]Associated Press, "Employers Offer Cash to Push Shopping around for Health Care," *New York Times*, October 14, 2015.

## CHAPTER 19

[1]Zach Carter, "The Spoilsmen: How Congress Corrupted Patent Reform," *Huffington Post*, August 4, 2011, http://www.huffingtonpost.com/2011/08/04/patent-reform-congress_n_906278.html; Dean Baker, "Issues in Trade and Protectionism," Center for Economic and Policy Research, November 2009, http://cepr.net/documents/publications/trade-and-protectionism-2009-11.pdf.

[2]*Global Intellectual Property Center*, "Prizes and Patent Pools. Viable Alternatives to the Patent System?" (undated), http://www.theglobalipcenter.com/sites/default/files/reports/documents/Prizes__Patent_Pools.pdf. The Global Intellectual Property Center is an arm of the U.S. Chamber of Commerce.

[3]Dean Baker, "Issues in Trade and Protectionism," *Center for Economic and Policy Research*, November 2009, http://cepr.net/documents/publications/trade-and-protectionism-2009-11.pdf.

[4]Daniel F. Spulber, "Public Prizes versus Market Prices: Should Contests Replace Patents?," *Journal of the Patent and Trademark Office Society* 97, no. 4 (2015): 690–735. For a fully developed alternative that retains the use of patents while also breaking the link between incentives to innovate and sales, see Stan Finkelstein and Peter Temin, *Reasonable RX: Solving the Drug Price Crisis* (Upper Saddle River, NJ: FT Press, 2008).

[5]To avoid incentivizing inventors to run up their costs, the prize formula could cap compensable costs at an identified level or step down the multiplier as costs increase.

[6]Pharmaceutical Research and Manufacturers of America, "2015 Biopharmaceutical Research Industry Profile," April 2015, http://phrmacdn.connections media.com/sites/default/files/pdf/2015_phrma_profile.pdf.

[7]Matthew Herper, "The Cost of Creating a New Drug Now $5 Billion, Pushing Big Pharma to Change," *Forbes.com*, August 11, 2013, http://www.forbes .com/sites/matthewherper/2013/08/11/how-the-staggering-cost-of-inventing-new-drugs-is-shaping-the-future-of-medicine/#5d7766486bfc.

[8]David Belk, "The Pharmaceutical Industry," *True Cost of Healthcare*, http:// truecostofhealthcare.net/the_pharmaceutical_industry/.

[9]V. Prasad and S. Mailankody, "Research and Development Spending to Bring a Single Cancer Drug to Market and Revenues after Approval," *JAMA Internal Medicine,* (September 11, 2017): doi:10.1001/jamainternmed.2017.3601.

[10]Herper, "The Cost of Creating a New Drug."

[11]Belk, "The Pharmaceutical Industry."

[12]Michael Kremer and Heidi Williams, "Incentivizing Innovation: Adding to the Tool Kit," *Innovation Policy and the Economy* 10, no. 1 (2010), http://www.jstor .org/stable/10.1086/605851.

[13]Priority Review Vouchers website, http://priorityreviewvoucher.org/.

[14]Amy Nordrum, "Drug Prices: World's Most Expensive Medicine Costs $440,000 a Year, but Is It Worth the Expense?," *International Business Times*, February 13, 2016, http://www.ibtimes.com/drug-prices-worlds-most-expensive-medicine-costs-440000-year-it-worth-expense-2302609.

[15]Ibid.

[16]Kelly Crowe, "How Pharmaceutical Company Alexion Set the Price of the World's Most Expensive Drug," *CBC News*, June 25, 2015, http://www.cbc .ca/news/health/how-pharmaceutical-company-alexion-set-the-price-of-the-world-s-most-expensive-drug-1.3125251.

[17]Ibid.

[18]David A. Hyman and William E. Kovacic, "Risky Business: Should the FDA Pay Attention to Drug Prices?," *Regulation* 40, no. 4 (2017): 22–26.

[19]Rachel Bluth, "Looking for Bargains, Many Americans Buy Medicines Abroad," *NPR*, December 17, 2016, http://www.npr.org/sections/ health-shots/2016/12/17/505690791/looking-for-bargains-many-americans-buy-medicines-abroad.

[20]Neil Osterweil, "The Letter (and Spirit) of Drug Import Laws," *WebMD*, (undated), https://www.webmd.com/healthy-aging/features/letter-and-spirit-of-drug-import-laws#1.

[21]*eDrugSearch.com*, "State-Sponsored Web Sites for Ordering Imported Drugs," https://edrugsearch.com/state-sponsored-web-sites-for-ordering-imported-drugs/. See also Phil Galewitz, "Cities, Counties and Schools Sidestep FDA

Canadian Drug Crackdown, Saving Millions," *Kaiser Health News*, December 8, 2017, https://khn.org/news/cities-counties-and-schools-sidestep-fda-canadian-drug-crackdown-saving-millions/.

[22]Phil Galewitz, "FDA Raids Florida Stores That Consumers Use to Buy Drugs from Canada," *Kaiser Health News*, November 20, 2017, https://khn.org/news/fda-raids-florida-stores-that-consumers-use-to-buy-drugs-from-canada/?utm_campaign=KHN%3A%20First%20Edition&utm_sour%E2%80%A6.

CHAPTER 20

[1]U.S. Department of Justice, Office of Public Affairs, "Former Wellcare Chief Executive Sentenced for Health Care Fraud," news release, http://www.justice.gov/opa/pr/former-wellcare-chief-executive-sentenced-health-care-fraud.

[2]Amy Sherman, "Rick Scott 'Oversaw the Largest Medicare Fraud in the Nation's History,' Florida Democratic Party Says," *PolitiFact Florida*, March 3, 2014, http://www.politifact.com/florida/statements/2014/mar/03/florida-democratic-party/rick-scott-rick-scott-oversaw-largest-medicare-fra/.

[3]Jeff Overley, "Ex-WellCare CEO Gets 3 Years for Medicaid Fraud," *Law360*, May 19, 2014, http://www.law360.com/articles/539387/ex-wellcare-ceo-gets-3-years-for-medicaid-fraud.

[4]Charles Babcock, "Fraud Trial for WellCare Ex-CEO Shows Medicaid Abuse," *Bloomberg.com*, November 19, 2012, http://www.bloomberg.com/news/articles/2012-11-20/fraud-trial-for-wellcare-ex-ceo-shows-medicaid-program-abuse.

[5]Ibid.

[6]Ibid.

[7]Kris Hundley, "WellCare Whistle-Blower Talks about His Corporate Double Life," *Tampa Bay Times*, July 3, 2010, http://www.tampabay.com/news/business/wellcare-whistle-blower-talks-about-his-corporate-double-life/1106867.

[8]Babcock, "Fraud Trial for WellCare Ex-CEO."

[9]Kris Hundley, "WellCare Whistle-Blower Talks about His Corporate Double Life," *Tampa Bay Times*, July 3, 2010, http://www.tampabay.com/news/business/wellcare-whistle-blower-talks-about-his-corporate-double-life/1106867.

[10]Ibid.

[11]Ibid.

[12]Ibid.

[13]Ibid.

[14]Jeff Harrington, "WellCare Health Plans Whistle-Blower to Receive about $21 Million," *Tampa Bay Times*, April 3, 2012, http://www.tampabay.com/news/business/wellcare-health-plans-whistle-blower-to-receive-about-21-million/1223263.

[15]Carol Gentry, "New Whistleblower Charges at WellCare," *Health News Florida*, November 4, 2014, http://health.wusf.usf.edu/post/new-whistleblower-charges-wellcare#stream/0.

[16]Anthony Brino, "Fraud Files: Trio of Managed Care Execs Head to the Slammer," *HeathcareITNews*, May 20, 2014, http://www.healthcareitnews.com/news/fraud-files-trio-managed-care-execs-head-slammer.

[17]Taxpayers Against Fraud Education Fund, "Whistleblower Stories," http://www.taf.org/whistleblower-stories#Thakur (visited November 23, 2016).

[18]U.S. Department of Justice, "Generic Drug Manufacturer Ranbaxy Pleads Guilty and Agrees to Pay $500 Million to Resolve False Claims Allegations, cGMP Violations and False Statements to the FDA," news release, May 13, 2013, https://www.justice.gov/opa/pr/generic-drug-manufacturer-ranbaxy-pleads-guilty-and-agrees-pay-500-million-resolve-false.

[19]Taxpayers Against Fraud Education Fund, "Whistleblower Stories."

[20]David Voreacos, "Florida Pharmacists Win $597 Million Blowing Whistle on Scheme," *Bloomberg Markets*, August 13, 2013, https://www.bloomberg.com/news/articles/2013-08-13/florida-pharmacists-win-597-million-blowing-whistle-on-scheme.

[21]Paul Heldman, "Firm to Pay $486m Fraud Settlement," *Sun Sentinel*, January 20, 2000, http://articles.sun-sentinel.com/2000-01-20/business/0001192012_1_fresenius-medical-care-health-care-fraud-nmc-medical-products.

[22]Ibid.

[23]Voreacos, "Florida Pharmacists Win $597 Million."

[24]Jessica Mason, "U.S. Chamber Works behind the Scenes to Gut Whistleblower Protections," *PRWatch*, April 29, 2016, http://www.prwatch.org/news/2016/04/13098/us-chamber-works-behind-scenes-gut-whistleblower-protections.

[25]Gregory Wallace, "$168 Million Payout to Johnson & Johnson Whistleblowers," *CNN Money*, November 4, 2013, http://money.cnn.com/2013/11/04/news/johnson-and-johnson-whistleblower-payout/index.html.

[26]Ed Cara, "How Did Dr. Farid Fata, America's Greater Cancer Fraudster, Get Away with It for So Long?," *Medical Daily*, July 7, 2015, http://www.medicaldaily.com/how-did-dr-farid-fata-americas-greatest-cancer-fraudster-get-away-it-so-long-341478.

[27]U.S. Department of Justice, "Fraud Statistics—Overview: October 1, 1987–September 30, 2015, 2015," https://www.justice.gov/opa/file/796866/download.

[28]David Freeman Engstrom, "Public Regulation of Private Enforcement: Empirical Analysis of DOJ Oversight of Qui Tam Litigation under the

False Claims Act," *Northwestern University Law Review* 107, no. 4 (2013): 1689, 1718–20.

[29]Voreacos, "Florida Pharmacists Win $597 Million."

[30]Ibid.

[31]Yuki Noguchi, "D.C. Law Firm's Big BlackBerry Payday: Case Fees of More Than $200 Million Are Said to Exceed Its 2004 Revenue," *Washington Post*, March 18, 2006, p. D03.

[32]*Whistleblowers, Qui Tam & False Claims Act Legal Blog*, "Immunity and Protection for Qui Tam Whistleblowers," Berger & Montague, P.C., http://www.bergermontague.com/practice-areas/whistleblowers,-qui-tam-false-claims-act/whistleblowers,-qui-tam-false-claims-act-legal-blog/immunity-and-protection-for-qui-tam-whistleblowers.

[33]Ibid.

[34]31 U.S.C. 3730(d)(3).

[35]Cong. Globe, 37th Cong., 3rd Sess. 955–56 (1863).

[36]Richard Kronick, "Projected Coding Intensity in Medicare Advantage," *Health Affairs*, 2017, http://content.healthaffairs.org/content/36/2/320.abstract; Fred Schulte, "Medicare Failed to Recover up to $125 Million in Overpayments from Private Insurers," *NPR.org*, http://www.npr.org/sections/health-shots/2017/01/06/508260306/medicare-failed-to-recover-up-to-125-million-in-overpayments-from-private-insure.

[37]Complaint, U.S. v. UnitedHealth Group, No. CV 16-08697 WMF (SSx) (C.D.Cal.May 16,2017),https://www.documentcloud.org/documents/3727655-Justice-Department-Complaint-Against.html. In October, 2017, the case was dismissed for failing to plead details of the alleged fraud with sufficient particularity. Erica Teichert, "UnitedHealth defeats Federal Medicare Advantage Suit," *Modern Healthcare*, October 6, 2017, http://www.modernhealthcare.com/article/20171006/NEWS/171009939. The DOJ dropped the lawsuit entirely in 2018.

[38]Better does not mean perfectly. Criminals sometimes fool private insurers too. For an example in which criminals are alleged to have billed private carriers for more than $100 million, see Jacob Batchelor,"Doctor Accused of Illegally Letting Assistants Do Surgeries," *Law360*, September 16, 2015, http://0-www.law360.com.tallons.law.utexas.edu/articles/703343/print?section=health. All payment systems experience some level of fraud, as we say in the text.

[39]Alex Wolf, "Fight for Conoco–Aetna Docs Erupts in $120M Kickbacks Suit," *Law360.com*, September 29, 2015, http://0-www.law360.com.tallons.law.utexas.edu/health/articles/708425/fight-for-conoco-aetna-docs-erupts-in-120m-kickbacks-suit.

CHAPTER 21

[1] *ValuePenguin*, "Average Cost of Homeowners Insurance (2017)," https://www.valuepenguin.com/average-cost-of-homeowners-insurance.

[2] Chris Conover, "Young People under Obamacare: Cash Cows for Older Workers," *Forbes*, November 27, 2012, https://www.forbes.com/sites/chrisconover/2012/11/27/young-people-under-obamacare-cash-cow-for-older-workers/#63f0498247fc.

[3] Ibid.

[4] Ibid.

[5] "Obamacare Architect: 'Lack of Transparency Is a Huge Political Advantage,'" *Real Clear Politics*, November 10, 2014, http://www.realclearpolitics.com/video/2014/11/10/obamacare_architect_lack_of_transparency_is_a_huge_political_advantage.html.

[6] David Grabowski, Jonathan Gruber, and Vincent Mor, "You're Probably Going to Need Medicaid," *New York Times*, June 13, 2017, https://nyti.ms/2tfTdFy.

[7] See, for example, Jay Bhattacharya and M. Kate Bundorf, "The Incidence of the Healthcare Costs of Obesity," NBER Working Paper no. 11303, National Bureau of Economic Research, May 2005, http://www.nber.org/papers/w11303.

[8] Tami Luhby, "Before Obamacare, Some Liked Their Health Care Plans Better," *CNN.com*, March 31, 2017, http://webcache.googleusercontent.com/search?q=cache:YteV7Tj1pMgJ:money.cnn.com/2017/03/31/news/economy/obamacare-health-care-plans/index.html=&cd=1&hl=en&ct=clnk&gl=us.

[9] Andrew McGill, "The Platinum Patients," *Atlantic*, June 2017, https://www.theatlantic.com/theplatinumpatients/.

[10] Carolyn Y. Johnson, "Half of Americans Are Responsible for Only 3 Percent of Health Care Costs," *Washington Post*, April 3, 2017, https://www.washingtonpost.com/news/wonk/wp/2017/04/03/most-americans-spend-little-on-health-care-and-that-hasnt-budged-in-37-years/?utm_term=.bf0b54e27098.

[11] Anita Soni, "Statistical Brief #470: Trends in the Five Most Costly Conditions among the U.S. Civilian Noninstitutionalized Population, 2002 and 2012," Agency for Healthcare Research and Quality, April 2015, https://meps.ahrq.gov/data_files/publications/st470/stat470.shtml.

[12] McGill, "The Platinum Patients."

[13] BlueCross BlueShield, "A Study of Cost Variations for Knee and Hip Replacement Surgeries in the U.S.," January 21, 2015, https://www.bcbs.com/about-us/capabilities-initiatives/health-america/health-of-america-report/study-cost-variations.

[14]James R. Healey, "Average New Car Price Zips 2.6% to $33,560," *USA Today*, May 4, 2015, https://www.usatoday.com/story/money/cars/2015/05/04/new-car-transaction-price-3-kbb-kelley-blue-book/26690191/.

[15]BlueCross BlueShield, "A Study of Cost Variations for Knee and Hip Replacement."

[16]Phil LeBeau, "New Car, New Reality: Auto Loan Borrowing Hits Fresh Highs," *CNBC.com*, June 2, 2016, http://www.cnbc.com/2016/06/02/us-borrowers-are-paying-more-and-for-longer-on-their-auto-loans.html.

[17]Linda Rath, "Knee Replacement and Revision Surgeries on the Rise," Arthritis Foundation, (undated), http://www.arthritis.org/living-with-arthritis/treatments/joint-surgery/types/knee/knee-replacement-younger-patients.php.

[18]Samuel Greengard, "Clinical Outcomes and Statistics of Knee Replacement," *Healthline.com*, February 18, 2015, http://www.healthline.com/health/total-knee-replacement-surgery/outcomes-statistics-success-rate.

[19]Christopher Kurz, Geng Li, and Daniel Vine, "The Young and the Carless? The Demographics of New Vehicle Purchases," *FEDS Notes*, Board of Governors of the Federal Reserve System, Washington, June 24, 2016, http://dx.doi.org/10.17016/2380-7172.1798.

[20]Examples include Carmen H. Rodriguez, "Without ACA Guarantees, 52 Million Adults Could Have Trouble Buying Individual Plans," *Kaiser Health News*, December 13, 2016, http://khn.org/news/without-aca-guarantees-52-million-adults-could-have-trouble-buying-individual-plans/; U.S. Department of Health and Human Services, Office of the Assistant Secretary for Planning and Evaluation, "At Risk: Pre-Existing Conditions Could Affect 1 in 2 Americans: 129 Million People Could Be Denied Affordable Coverage without Health Reform," (undated), https://aspe.hhs.gov/system/files/pdf/76376/index.pdf.

[21]Mark V. Pauly and Bradley Herring, *Pooling Health Insurance Risks*, (Washington: AEI Press), p. 18, https://www.aei.org/wp-content/uploads/2014/07/-pooling-health-insurance-risks_114406587191.pdf.

[22]Ibid.

[23]Greg Scandlen, *Myth Busters: Why Health Reform Always Goes Awry* (North Charleston, SC: CreateSpace Publishing, 2017).

[24]Letter from Douglas W. Elmendorf, Director of Congressional Budget Office, to Michael B. Enzi, Ranking Member, Committee on Health, Education, Labor, and Pensions, U.S. Senate, June 21, 2010, https://www.cbo.gov/sites/default/files/111th-congress-2009-2010/reports/06-21-high-risk_insurance_pools.pdf.

[25]U.S. Department of Health and Human Services, Office of Consumer Information and Insurance Oversight, "Pre-Existing Condition Insurance Plan Program; Interim Final Rule," 45 CFR Part 152, *Federal Register* 75 no. 146 (July 30, 2010):

45026, https://www.federalregister.gov/documents/2010/07/30/2010-18691/
pre-existing-condition-insurance-plan-program.

[26]Karen Pollitz, "High Risk Pools for Uninsurable Individuals," The Henry J.
Kaiser Family Foundation, February 2017, http://files.kff.org/attachment/Issue-
Brief-High-Risk-Pools-For-Uninsurable-Individuals.

[27]Wikipedia, "Michigan Stadium," https://en.wikipedia.org/wiki/Michigan_
Stadium.

[28]Farzon A. Nahvi, "Don't Leave Health Care to a Free Market," *New York
Times*, July 10, 2017, https://www.nytimes.com/2017/07/10/opinion/health-
insurance-free-market.html.

[29]John Cochrane, "After the ACA: Freeing the Market for Health Care" in
*The Future of Healthcare Reform in the United States*, ed. Anup Malani and Michael H.
Schill (Chicago: University of Chicago Press, 2015), pp. 161-201, https://faculty
.chicagobooth.edu/john.cochrane/research/papers/after_aca_published.pdf.

[30]Jonathan Gruber, "Health Care Reform Is a 'Three-Legged Stool': The
Costs of Partially Repealing the Affordable Care Act," Center for American
Progress, August 5, 2010, https://www.americanprogress.org/issues/healthcare/
reports/2010/08/05/8226/health-care-reform-is-a-three-legged-stool/.

## Chapter 22

[1]Gallup Editors, "Most Americans Practice Charitable Giving, Volunteerism,"
*Gallup*, December 13, 2013, http://www.gallup.com/poll/166250/americans-
practice-charitable-giving-volunteerism.aspx.

[2]This point has been made many times. Obamacare was subject to a similar moral critique. As John Goodman wrote, the insurance premium regulations
"[f]orce[d] young people to pay two or three times the real cost of their insurance
in order to subsidize older people who have more income and more assets." John
Goodman, "Is There a Moral Case for Obamacare?" National Center for Policy
Analysis, *Health Policy Blog*, July 6, 2011, http://healthblog.ncpa.org/is-there-a-
moral-case-for-obamacare/#sthash.7xxpksYB.dpuf.

[3]"Changes in U.S. Family Finances from 2010 to 2013: Evidence from the
Survey of Consumer Finances," *Federal Reserve Bulletin*, September 2014, https://
www.federalreserve.gov/pubs/bulletin/2014/pdf/scf14.pdf.

[4]Kaiser Family Foundation, "Poverty Rate by Age 2015," http://kff.org/
other/state-indicator/poverty-rate-by-age/?currentTimeframe=0.

[5]Elizabeth Arias, M. Heron, and J. Xu, "United States Life Tables," *National
Vital Statistics Reports* 66 no. 3 (April 11, 2017): Table 20, https://www.cdc.gov/
nchs/data/nvsr/nvsr66/nvsr66_03.pdf.

[6]Alyene Senger, "The Number of Workers per Medicare Beneficiary Is Fall-
ing," infographic in "Medicare at Risk: Visualizing the Need for Reform," *Heritage*

*Foundation*, May 22, 2012, http://dailysignal.com/2012/05/22/medicare-at-risk-visualizing-the-need-for-reform/.

[7]Centers for Medicare and Medicaid Services, "National Health Expenditures 2015 Highlights," https://www.cms.gov/Research-Statistics-Data-and-Systems/Statistics-Trends-and-Reports/NationalHealthExpendData/downloads/highlights.pdf.

[8]Phillip Longman, "Justice between Generations," *Atlantic Monthly*, 1985, https://www.theatlantic.com/past/docs/issues/96may/aging/longm.htm.

[9]Norman Daniels, *Am I My Parents' Keeper* (Oxford: Oxford University Press, 1988) p. 43.

[10]Ibid., 44–45.

[11]Singapore's mandatory savings program is described in William A. Haseltine, *Affordable Excellence: The Singapore Healthcare Story* (Washington: Brookings Institute, 2013). See also David Reisman, *Social Policy in an Ageing Society: Age and Health in Singapore* (Cheltenham: Edward Elgar, 2009). The program contains many elements that are not described here, some of which involve the state heavily in the regulation of the delivery of health care. See Ezra Klein, "Is Singapore's 'Miracle' Health Care System the Answer for America?," *Vox*, April 25, 2017, http://www.vox.com/policyandpolitics/2017/4/25/15356118/singaporehealthcaresystemexplained.

[12]Haseltine, *Affordable Excellence*.

[13]Reisman, *Social Policy*, pp. 37–38.

[14]Ibid.

[15]Drew Desilver, "5 Facts about Social Security," Pew Research Center, August 18, 2015, http://www.pewresearch.org/fact-tank/2015/08/18/5-facts-about-social-security/.

[16]Bob Sullivan, "The Future of U.S. Health Care? FSAs & HSAs," *Credit.com*, December 19, 2016, http://blog.credit.com/2016/12/the-future-of-u-s-health-care-account-based-health-plans-163671/.

[17]Kff.org, "Medicaid Spending per Full Benefit Enrollee. FY2011," http://kff.org/medicaid/state-indicator/medicaid-spending-per-full-benefit-enrollee/?currentTimeframe=0&selectedDistributions=total.

[18]Harold Pollack, Bill Gardner, and Timothy Jost, "Valuing Medicaid: Why We Need It, How We Should Improve It," *American Prospect*, July 26, 2015, http://prospect.org/article/valuing-medicaid.

[19]Matt Zwolinski, "The Pragmatic Libertarian Case for a Basic Income Guarantee," *Cato Unbound*, August 4, 2014, https://www.cato-unbound.org/2014/08/04/matt-zwolinski/pragmatic-libertarian-case-basic-income-guarantee.

[20]Pollack, Gardner, and Jost, "Valuing Medicaid," citing Benjamin D. Sommers, Katherine Baicker, and Arnold M. Epstein, "Mortality and Access to Care among

Adults after State Medicaid Expansions," *New England Journal of Medicine* 367 (2012): 1025–34, doi:10.1056/NEJMsa1202099.

[21]Thomas L. Hungerford and Rebecca Thiess, "Issue Brief #370: The Earned Income Tax Credit and the Child Tax Credit," *Economic Policy Institute*, September 25, 2013, http://www.epi.org/publication/ib370-earned-income-tax-credit-and-the-child-tax-credit-history-purpose-goals-and-effectiveness/.

[22]Ibid. On the health benefits of these cash transfers, see Hilary Hoynes, Doug Miller, and David Simon, "Income, the Earned Income Tax Credit, and Infant Health," *American Economic Journal: Economic Policy* 7, no. 1 (2015): 172–211, http://dx.doi.org/10.1257/pol.20120179; William N. Evans and Craig L. Garthwaite, "Giving Mom a Break: The Impact of Higher EITC Payments on Maternal Health," *American Economic Journal: Economic Policy* 6, no. 2 (2014): 258–90, http://dx.doi.org/10.1257/pol.6.2.258; Hilary Hoynes, Marianne Page, and Ann Stevens, "Can Targeted Transfers Improve Birth Outcomes? Evidence from the Introduction of the WIC Program," *Journal of Public Economics* 95, no. 7–8 (2011): 813–27; Hilary Hoynes, Diane Whitmore Schanzenbach, and Douglas Almond, "Long Run Impacts of Childhood Access to the Safety Net," NBER Working Paper no. 18535, National Bureau of Economic Research, 2013, https://gspp.berkeley.edu/assets/uploads/research/pdf/Hoynes-Schanzenbach-Almond-14.pdf. Even health care providers recognize the health-related benefits of nonmedical services. See Theresa Fraze, Valerie A. Lewis, Hector P. Rodriguez, and Elliott S. Fisher, "Housing, Transportation, and Food: How ACOs Seek to Improve Population Health by Addressing Nonmedical Needs of Patients," *Health Affairs* 35, no. 11 (2016): 2109–15.

[23]"Do EITC Recipients Use Their Tax Refunds to Get Ahead? Evidence from the Refund to Savings Initiative," Washington University in St. Louis, Center for Social Development, CSD Research Brief no. 15-38, July 2015. See also Andrew Goodman-Bacon and Leslie McGranahan, "How Do EITC Recipients Spend Their Refunds?" Federal Reserve Bank of Chicago, *Economic Perspectives* 38 (2008), https://www.chicagofed.org/publications/economic-perspectives/2008/2qtr2008-part2-goodman-etal.

[24]Amy Finkelstein, Nathaniel Hendren, and Erzo F. P. Luttmer, "The Value of Medicaid: Interpreting Results from the Oregon Health Insurance Experiment," NBER Working Paper no. 21308, National Bureau of Economic Research, June 2015, http://www.nber.org/papers/w21308.

[25]The Obamacare Medicaid expansion reduced the amount of uncompensated care provided by hospitals from $34.9 billion to $28.9 billion. Peter Cunningham, Robin Rudowitz, Katherine Young, et al., "Understanding Medicaid Hospital Payments and the Impact of Recent Policy Changes," Kaiser Family Foundation, June 9, 2016, http://kff.org/medicaid/issue-brief/understanding-medicaid-hospital-payments-and-the-impact-of-recent-policy-changes/.

These numbers must be taken with a grain of salt, because hospitals' reports of the cost of charity care are unreliable, but it is clear that the Medicaid expansion helped them financially.

[26]Ibid., citing Craig Garthwaite, Tal Gross, and Matthew J. Notowidigdo, "Hospitals as Insurers of Last Resort," NBER Working Paper No. 21290, National Bureau of Economic Research, June 2015, http://www.nber.org/papers/w21290.

[27]Pollack, Gardner, and Jost, "Valuing Medicaid."

[28]Kaiser Family Foundations, "Pulling It Together: A Public Opinion Surprise," April 4, 2011, http://kff.org/health-reform/perspective/pulling-it-together-a-public-opinion-surprise/.

[29]Mira Norton, Bianca DiJulio, and Mollyann Brodie, "Medicare And Medicaid At 50," Kaiser Family Foundation, July 17, 2015, http://kff.org/medicaid/poll-finding/medicare-and-medicaid-at-50/.

[30]U.S. Centers for Medicare and Medicaid Services, "NHE Fact Sheet," https://www.cms.gov/research-statistics-data-and-systems/statistics-trends-and-reports/nationalhealthexpenddata/nhe-fact-sheet.html. For a state-by-state breakdown, see MACPAC, "Medicaid Spending by State, Category, and Source of Funds," https://www.macpac.gov/publication/medicaid-spending-by-state-category-and-source-of-funds/.

[31]*Usgovernmentspending.com*, "Estimated vs. Actual Federal Spending for Fiscal Year 2017 from Federal Budgets," https://www.usgovernmentspending.com/federal_budget_estimate_vs_actual_2017.

[32]Erica L. Reaves and MaryBeth Musumeci, "Medicaid and Long-Term Services and Supports: A Primer," Kaiser Family Foundation, December 15, 2015, http://kff.org/medicaid/report/medicaid-and-long-term-services-and-supports-a-primer/. See also Kaiser Family Foundation, "Medicaid's Role in Meeting Seniors' Long-Term Services and Supports Needs," August 2, 2016, http://kff.org/medicaid/fact-sheet/medicaids-role-in-meeting-seniors-long-term-services-and-supports-needs/.

[33]Robert H. Brook, Emmett B. Keeler, Kathleen N. Lohr, et al., "Research Brief: The Health Insurance Experiment," RAND, 2006, https://www.r,and.org/pubs/research_briefs/RB9174.html.

[34]Allison K. Hoffman, "Three Models of Health Insurance: The Conceptual Pluralism of the Patient Protection and Affordable Care Act," *University of Pennsylvania Law Review* 159 (2011): 103–79; Allison K. Hoffman, "The Unhealthy Return to Individual Responsibility in Health Policy," *Regulatory Review*, January 16, 2017, https://www.theregreview.org/2017/01/16/hoffman-unhealthy-return-individual-responsibility-health-policy/.

[35]Ibid.

[36]Ibid.

[37]Brook et al., "Research Brief: The Health Insurance Experiment."

[38]Ibid.

[39]Ibid.

[40]U.S. Department of Veterans Affairs, "Budget in Brief 2017," 2016, https://www.va.gov/budget/docs/summary/Fy2017-BudgetInBrief.pdf; U.S. Department of Veterans Affairs, Veterans Health Administration, "Providing Health Care for Veterans," https://www.va.gov/health/.

[41]We have discussed quality problems at VHA hospitals in other writings. See, for example, David A. Hyman and Charles Silver, "The Poor State of Health Care Quality in the U.S.: Is Malpractice Liability Part of the Problem or Part of the Solution?," *Cornell Law Review* 90, no. 4 (2005): 893–994, http://scholarship.law.cornell.edu/cgi/viewcontent.cgi?article=2996&context=clr.

[42]Paul Giblin, "VA Patient Load Outpaced Budget, Led to Latest Scandal," *USA Today*, June 15, 2014, https://www.usatoday.com/story/news/nation/2014/06/15/va-patient-load-outpaced-budget/10553987/.

[43]Donovan Slack, "VA Failed to Report 90% of Potential Dangerous Medical Providers, GAO Confirms," *USA Today*, November 27, 2017, https://www.usatoday.com/story/news/politics/2017/11/27/va-failed-report-90-potentially-dangerous-medical-providers-gao-confirms/890582001/. See also U.S. Government Accountability Office, VA Health Care: Improved Policies and Oversight Needed for Reviewing and Reporting Providers for Quality and Safety Concerns, November 2017, https://www.gao.gov/assets/690/688378.pdf.

[44]Donovan Slack and Michael Sallah, "VA Conceals Shoddy Care and Health Workers' Mistakes," *USA Today*, October 11, 2017, https://www.usatoday.com/story/news/2017/10/11/va-conceals-shoddy-care-and-health-workers-mistakes/739852001/.

[45]Harlan Krumholz, "3 Things to Know Before You Judge VA Health System," *Forbes.com*, May 23, 2014, http://www.forbes.com/sites/harlankrumholz/2014/05/23/3-things-to-know-before-you-rush-to-judgment-about-va-health-system/#347d1f497660.

[46] Hyman and Silver, "The Poor State of Health Care Quality."

# INDEX

Note: Information in figures, notes, and tables is indicated by f, n, and t.

## ABOUT THE AUTHORS

David A. Hyman, MD, JD, is an adjunct scholar at the Cato Institute and a professor at Georgetown University Law Center. He teaches or has taught health care regulation, civil procedure, insurance, medical malpractice, law and economics, professional responsibility, consumer protection, and tax policy. While serving as special counsel to the Federal Trade Commission, Professor Hyman was principal author and project leader for the first joint report ever issued by the Federal Trade Commission and Department of Justice, "Improving Health Care: A Dose of Competition" (2004). He is also the author of *Medicare Meets Mephistopheles*, which was selected by the U.S. Chamber of Commerce/National Chamber Foundation as one of the top 10 books of 2007.

Charles Silver, MA, JD, is an adjunct scholar at the Cato Institute and holds the Roy W. and Eugenia C. McDonald Endowed Chair in Civil Procedure at the University of Texas School of Law, where he teaches about civil litigation, health care policy, legal ethics, and insurance. His writings on class actions and other aggregate proceedings, litigation finance, medical malpractice, and legal and medical ethics have appeared in leading peer-reviewed journals and law reviews. In 2009, the Tort Trial & Insurance Practice Section of the American Bar Association awarded him the Robert B. McKay Law Professor Award for outstanding scholarship on tort and insurance law.

# Cato Institute

Founded in 1977, the Cato Institute is a public policy research foundation dedicated to broadening the parameters of policy debate to allow consideration of more options that are consistent with the principles of limited government, individual liberty, and peace. To that end, the Institute strives to achieve greater involvement of the intelligent, concerned lay public in questions of policy and the proper role of government.

The Institute is named for *Cato's Letters*, libertarian pamphlets that were widely read in the American Colonies in the early 18th century and played a major role in laying the philosophical foundation for the American Revolution.

Despite the achievement of the nation's Founders, today virtually no aspect of life is free from government encroachment. A pervasive intolerance for individual rights is shown by government's arbitrary intrusions into private economic transactions and its disregard for civil liberties. And while freedom around the globe has notably increased in the past several decades, many countries have moved in the opposite direction, and most governments still do not respect or safeguard the wide range of civil and economic liberties.

To address those issues, the Cato Institute undertakes an extensive publications program on the complete spectrum of policy issues. Books, monographs, and shorter studies are commissioned to examine the federal budget, Social Security, regulation, military spending, international trade, and myriad other issues. Major policy conferences are held throughout the year, from which papers are published thrice yearly in the *Cato Journal*. The Institute also publishes the quarterly magazine *Regulation*.

In order to maintain its independence, the Cato Institute accepts no government funding. Contributions are received from foundations, corporations, and individuals, and other revenue is generated from the sale of publications. The Institute is a nonprofit, tax-exempt, educational foundation under Section 501(c)3 of the Internal Revenue Code.

CATO INSTITUTE
1000 Massachusetts Ave., N.W.
Washington, D.C. 20001
www.cato.org